SAMUEL J. FOMON, M.D.

Professor of Pediatrics, The University
of Iowa College of Medicine, Iowa City

INFANT NUTRITION

W. B. SAUNDERS COMPANY

Philadelphia and London, 1967

W. B. Saunders Company: West Washington Square
                         Philadelphia, Pa. 19105

                         12 Dyott Street
                         London W.C.1

Infant Nutrition

© 1967 by W. B. Saunders Company. Copyright under the International Copyright
Union. All rights reserved. This book is protected by copyright. No part of it may
be duplicated or reproduced in any manner without written permission from the pub-
lisher. Made in the United States of America. Press of W. B. Saunders Company.
Library of Congress catalog card number 67–14822.

To Betty

PREFACE

In much of North America, the United Kingdom, the Scandinavian countries, western Europe and several other parts of the world, vitamin A intoxication is more common than vitamin A deficiency and overnutrition is likely to be encountered more frequently than undernutrition. In these countries, where major nutritional deficiency diseases in infancy are no longer prevalent, relatively little effort needs to be expended in nutritional measures aimed at preservation of life and immediate health. Physicians and nutritionists may therefore find time and energy to pursue important questions that have long been ignored: Do the type of fat and amount of cholesterol fed during early life contribute to the incidence of atherosclerosis among adults? Is the salt content of the infant's diet of significance in relation to subsequent development of hypertension? Are eating habits developed during infancy and childhood important determinants of later obesity? Our inability to provide satisfactory answers to these questions at present indicates the scope of work remaining to be done in the field of infant nutrition.

Meanwhile, it is possible to provide at least a partial answer to many of the questions that trouble the thoughtful physician, nutritionist and dietitian. A working definition of failure to thrive can be offered so that one may distinguish between slow rates of growth that may yet be considered normal and those slightly slower rates that are to be considered abnormal. A tentative definition of obesity in infancy can be presented.

Requirements and advisable intakes of individual nutrients can be tentatively specified and those circumstances delineated in which

v

vitamin or mineral supplementation is desirable. Measures for elimination of iron deficiency anemia and for assuring an adequate intake of fluoride can be summarized. Differences between the many commercially available formulas can be critically assessed and situations identified in which a specified formula is likely to be preferable to other formulas. Nutritional considerations relating to time of introduction into the diet of cereal and strained foods and choices among the many available strained foods can be examined.

It is for persons troubled by these questions that an attempt has been made to assemble current information relating to infant nutrition in technologically advanced nations. Perhaps a greater understanding of infant nutrition by physicians, nutritionists and dietitians will constitute an early step toward the goal of achieving optimal nutrition in infancy.

S. J. F.

ACKNOWLEDGMENTS

It is not really possible to separate completely the material of this book from the research effort of the Infant Metabolism Unit, Department of Pediatrics, University of Iowa. The reporting is that of a single individual but the thoughts are those of many, tempered and modified by endless discussions.

Dr. Charles D. May originally interested me in the field of infant nutrition and provided the needed support and guidance during the early years of our studies. Dr. George M. Owen, first a postdoctoral research fellow and later a coinvestigator in the program, was a constant source of inspiration and stimulation during his years with us. During the past few years I have had the great pleasure of sharing direction of the program with Dr. L. J. Filer, Jr. His influence in expanding the scope of our research is readily apparent to all who are familiar with our program.

The almost unique capabilities of Mrs. Lora N. Thomas and her nursing staff in the Metabolic Unit have made possible a continuing series of studies of normal full-size infants. Mr. Robert L. Jensen's supervision of our laboratory has assured a high degree of quality control in the face of an immense volume of work and considerable diversity of methodology. During the past few years Mr. Dean W. Andersen has been responsible for an increasing share of the laboratory supervision, thereby contributing greatly to recent expansion in laboratory aspects of the program. The assistance of Mr. Ronald R. Rogers during the past two years has been a particular asset.

Many contributions have been made by our research assistants, our several postdoctoral research fellows, technicians and secretaries.

In the preparation of the book itself enormous help has been given by Dr. Filer, who has read each chapter, detected errors, called my attention to additional pertinent references and served as chief critic. Miss Beverly Collins has painstakingly proofread the entire manuscript.

Finally, two individuals have made the book possible by seeing that I had the time to write it: Dr. Donal Dunphy, who is chairman of the Department of Pediatrics, University of Iowa, and Mrs. Betty Fomon, who is co-chairman of my family.

S. J. F.

CONTENTS

Chapter One

Recent History
and Current Trends

Until the latter half of the nineteenth century breast feeding was essential to infant survival, and when the mother was unable to breast feed, the only satisfactory alternative was employment of a wet nurse. However, since the nutritional status of wet nurses was often poor (some suffered from tuberculosis or other chronic disease) and many were unreliable, this solution to the problem was far from ideal. Attempts at feeding an infant by bottle almost uniformly led to death. Nursing from the udders of goats, cows or asses was attempted but only rarely was successful.

Wide-scale success with bottle feeding became possible through application of newer knowledge in four separate areas: (1) development of sanitary standards for handling of milk; (2) development of easily cleansed and sterilized bottles and nipples; (3) alteration of curd tension of milk; and (4) adequate vitamin supplementation. Major advances in each of these areas occurred late in the nineteenth century and during the first two decades of the twentieth century with the result that formula feeding has been extensively and successfully practiced during the past 40 or 50 years (Fig. 1–1). During the last 15 or 20 years, rapid advances in technology and packaging have resulted in major changes in infant feeding practices.

Sanitation

Controlled heating of a liquid to eliminate pathogenic bacteria

1

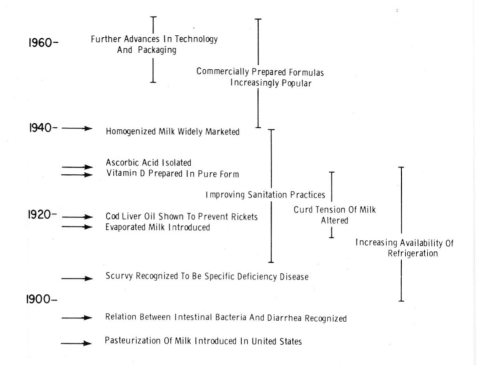

1960–   Further Advances In Technology
        And Packaging

        Commercially Prepared Formulas
        Increasingly Popular

1940– → Homogenized Milk Widely Marketed

        Ascorbic Acid Isolated
        Vitamin D Prepared In Pure Form

        Improving Sanitation Practices

1920– → Cod Liver Oil Shown To Prevent Rickets
         Evaporated Milk Introduced

        Curd Tension Of Milk
        Altered

        Increasing Availability Of
        Refrigeration

        Scurvy Recognized To Be Specific Deficiency Disease

1900–

        Relation Between Intestinal Bacteria And Diarrhea Recognized

        Pasteurization Of Milk Introduced In United States

1880–

Figure 1–1. Some advances and trends in infant feeding from the late 1800's to the present.

was introduced in Germany in 1882 and in the United States in 1891, although widespread use of pasteurization* was not practiced until considerably later. Poorly designed, narrow-mouth feeding bottles and such sucking devices as rubber tubing attached to the bottle were used during the latter part of the nineteenth century and the first decade of the twentieth and contributed to bacterial contamination. Because purchase of milk on a daily basis was usually not feasible and refrigeration was often inadequate, it is not surprising that problems in bacterial contamination of milk were frequent even when milk had been pasteurized (Davison, 1935). Identification of the colon bacillus and related organisms toward the end of the nineteenth century and the demonstration that bloody diarrhea in infants was often caused by organisms of the dysentery group gave impetus to public health measures that gradually resulted, during the early part of the twentieth century, in better control of water supplies and more efficient disposal of sewage.

_____

*Now defined as heating to 61° C for 30 minutes.

In the 1920's the combination of progress in sanitary control of milk production, water supplies, and sewage disposal, increasing availability of refrigeration, better design of feeding bottles and introduction of a variety of methods for modifying curd tension resulted in generally successful bottle feeding. With the introduction of evaporated milk in 1920 there became available a source of milk with relatively low curd tension that was bacteriologically safe, at least until the time the can was opened.

Curd Tension

When milk is coagulated, as occurs when it comes into contact with the hydrochloric acid of the stomach, the precipitate (curd) contains most of the casein and calcium of the milk, while the watery portion contains whey proteins and most of the milk sugar. When fresh, unprocessed cow milk is coagulated, the curd is tough and rubbery and can be demonstrated by standard testing procedures to have high resistance to stirring (i.e., high curd tension). Fresh human milk, on the other hand, contains a relatively small amount of casein and forms a soft, flocculent curd. Processing of cow milk— acidification, dilution, boiling, modification of mineral composition, treatment with enzymes, homogenization—results in a softer curd that is more easily digested by the small infant.

Acidification of milk became popular about 1920 and was believed to exert its beneficial action through reduction of the buffering capacity. The high buffering capacity of unacidified cow milk had long been blamed for promotion of bacterial growth, diminution in flow of pancreatic juice and bile and inhibition of gastric digestion (Marriott, 1927). However, reduction of curd tension was almost certainly the major beneficial effect of acidification of milk, whereas inhibition of growth of pathogenic bacteria was a secondary advantage, and diminution of buffering capacity was probably of little consequence.

Although a method for homogenization of milk was demonstrated at the World's Fair in Paris in 1900, practical application of the method on a wide scale was not feasible until about 1921, when adequate means were found for sterilizing the equipment (Trout, 1950). Widespread marketing of homogenized milk began about 1940.

The impact on infant feeding of the introduction of evaporated milk in the late 1920's can be appreciated from published comments of some of the leading pediatricians of the time. Marriott and Schoenthal (1929) observed that

> ...evaporated milk mixtures were uniformly well digested....There were no cases in which it was found necessary to substitute some other form of milk for the evaporated milk because of untoward

symptoms or failure to do well. The results of evaporated milk feeding of newly born infants appear to us to indicate that this form of milk is readily digestible and well utilized by very young infants.

Brennemann (1929) described his observations as

... the most startling I have ever encountered in more than twenty-five years of hospital experience in feeding ward babies. The interns had often asked me to show them a normal stool such as I had told them all babies had in private practice and I had had great difficulty in meeting their request. At one swoop I was able to show them normal, yellow, smooth, well formed or thick pasty stools with a perfect putrefactive bouquet in practically every one of these babies.

The low incidence of gastrointestinal disturbances was commented upon by many observers.

Vitamin Deficiencies

Only two vitamin deficiency diseases are likely to have contributed significantly to lack of success in early attempts at bottle feeding. These are scurvy and rickets.

Scurvy was described in the Ebers Papyrus written about 1500 B.C. (Major, 1945), and the protective role of lemon juice was recognized at least by 1600 A.D. during the first expedition of the East India Company (Vogel, 1933). Bachstrom in 1734 stated that "... this evil is solely owing to a total abstinence from fresh vegetable food, and greens; which is alone the true primary cause of the disease" (Stewart and Guthrie, 1953). However, it was not until 1906 that Hopkins postulated that infantile scurvy was a deficiency disease due to lack of some essential food substance, the exact nature of which was not known. Ascorbic acid was isolated in 1928 by Szent-Györgyi although it was not identified as ascorbic acid until 1930. Its structural formula was established in 1933 by Herbert.

In a series of reports published between 1908 and 1912, the Russian pediatrician, Schabad, demonstrated that cod liver oil was effective in curing and preventing rickets (Holt, 1963). Mellanby (1920) demonstrated that the active substance was a fat-soluble vitamin. Vitamin D was prepared in pure form in 1931.

Although deficiencies of vitamins other than C and D were probably not of major significance in the lack of success of bottle feeding before the twentieth century, the discovery of vitamins and description of their role exerted a major influence on the history of modern infant nutrition. Before the importance of various vitamins was recognized, attention was centered on the harmfulness of having too much of certain foods. In the 1920's the emphasis shifted to the harmfulness of having too little. Today, the philosophy of avoiding nutritional deficiency is so firmly established that it undoubtedly contributes to our national problem of overnutrition and, once again, it seems necessary to emphasize the possibility that one may ingest too much as well as too little.

Trends in Feeding by Breast and Bottle

With the increasing safety and convenience of formula feeding during the past 30 years and the failure of various investigators to provide evidence of definite superiority of breast feeding over formula feeding, most physicians have been unenthusiastic in promotion of breast feeding. Decision to feed by breast or bottle has been left largely to the mother. Information regarding trends in breast feeding in the United States is available from several sources (Bain, 1948; Jackson et al., 1956; Meyer, 1958b; Salber et al., 1958; Robertson, 1961; Salber and Feinleib, 1966; Cox, 1966). In Britain, as in the United States, breast feeding is less common in the lower socioeconomic classes (Newson and Newson, 1962).

Frequency of breast feeding during the newborn period decreased from approximately 65 per cent in the 1940's (Bain, 1948) to 30 per cent in 1958 and 26 per cent in 1965 (Fig. 1–2). Since 1958 the frequency of breast feeding at age one month has remained constant at about 20 per cent of the infant population and a further decrease to 8 or 10 per cent of the infant population has occurred by age four months (Fig. 1–3). Data in Figure 1–3 indicating that at age six months only about 5 per cent of infants are breast fed are in agreement with a recently published report by Salber and Feinleib (1966).

Social class is an important variable influencing the incidence of breast feeding. From 1930 until about the middle of the 1940's, incidence of breast feeding was greatest in the lower social classes but, at present, women of upper social classes and especially wives of students exhibit the highest incidence of breast feeding (Salber and Feinleib, 1966).

Trends in types of formulas fed to newborn infants have been reported (Meyer, 1958a, 1960, 1965a, 1965b; Robertson, 1961; Cox, 1966); data for the years 1958 through 1965 are shown in Figure 1–3. Commercially prepared formulas are fed to about 50 per cent of infants during the first two months of life and to smaller percentages of infants as age increases. Evaporated milk is fed to slightly more than 25 per cent of the infants during the first few months of life and to smaller percentages of older infants. As a consequence of the decreased proportion of infants fed at the breast or fed commercially prepared formulas after three months of age, the percentage of in-

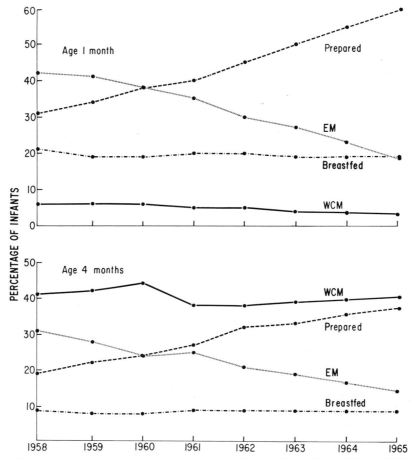

Figure 1-2. Percentages of infants in the United States from 1958 to 1965 receiving various milks or formulas. WCM indicates whole cow milk with or without added carbohydrate; EM indicates evaporated milk and water with or without added carbohydrate, and Prepared indicates commercially prepared formulas in ready-to-use form or requiring only the addition of water before they are ready to feed. Data of Cox, 1966.

fants receiving homogenized whole cow milk increases steeply, reaching nearly 40 per cent by four months of age, and nearly 70 per cent by six months of age.

With the relatively recent introduction of iron-fortified commercially prepared formulas, it seems likely that this convenient method of administration of iron will be responsible for some prolongation of formula feeding, with the result that an increasing number of infants will continue to receive a formula until four or five months of age and there will not be a discontinuation of formula feeding in favor of whole milk at age two to three months as commonly occurs at present.

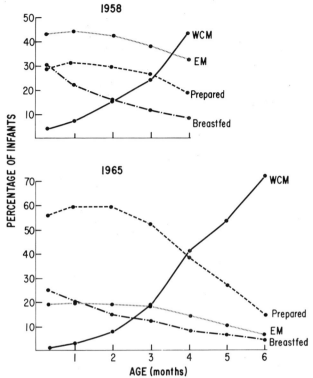

Figure 1-3. Trends in infant feeding between 1958 and 1965. Types of feeding are the same as in Figure 1-2. Data of Cox, 1966.

Trends in Feeding of Foods Other Than Milk or Formula

Until about 1920 solid foods were seldom offered to infants before one year of age (Committee on Nutrition, 1958). In 1935 Marriott suggested that six months was the proper age for introduction of solid foods and in 1937 the A.M.A. Council on Foods stated that pediatricians favored feeding of strained fruits and vegetables at about four to six months of age. Beal (1957) demonstrated in an upper socioeconomic group in Denver that strained foods were offered to the infant at increasingly early ages during the years 1946 through 1955. Among pediatricians responding to a survey in 1954, feeding of solids was recommended before three months of age by 88 per cent and before eight weeks of age by 66 per cent (Butler and Wolman, 1954). More recently, Epps and Jolley (1963) have reported that approximately 83 per cent of infants between one and two months of age when seen for a first visit in the Child Health

Clinics of the District of Columbia Department of Public Health had already begun to receive solid foods (Table 1–1). In the United States at the present time, the six-month-old infant probably receives approximately one-third of this caloric intake from non-milk sources (Filer and Martinez, 1964).

*Table 1–1. Incidence of Solid Feeding of Infants at Time of First Clinic Visit**

Age (months)	Number of Infants	Percentage Receiving Solids
< 1	12	66.7
1–2	226	82.7
2–3	152	96.1
3–4	65	100.0
4–5	27	96.3
5–6	18	100.0

*Data of Epps and Jolley (1963).

That extremely early introduction of cereal and strained foods is possible has been demonstrated by Sackett (1956), who routinely begins feeding cereal on the second or third day of life, and introduces vegetables at age 10 days, strained meat at age 14 days, and fruit at age 17 days. There can no longer be doubt that infants tolerate strained foods early in life. Advantages or disadvantages of such early introduction of foods other than milk or formula remain to be determined.

Recent Trends

Feeding of infants in hospitals has undergone major changes in the past 15 years. Commercial formula services (private enterprises now operating in a number of metropolitan centers)* are equipped to provide a variety of formulas to hospitals so that many hospitals in such areas have discontinued their own activities in formula preparation (Committee on Nutrition, 1965). By purchasing formulas rather than preparing these intramurally, the hospital is able to use for other purposes the space previously allocated to hospital formula preparation. In some instances it has proved economically bene-

*At the time of publication of the report by the Committee on Nutrition (1965), such services were available in the following metropolitan areas: Phoenix, Arizona; the Los Angeles, San Diego, and San Francisco areas in California; Miami, Florida; Chicago and Peoria, Illinois; Baltimore, Maryland; Brockton, Massachusetts; Kansas City, Missouri; New York City; Cincinnati, Ohio; Allentown, Lancaster, and Philadelphia, Pennsylvania; and Seattle, Washington.

ficial to purchase formulas rather than to maintain and staff a unit for this purpose (Schenkweiler et al., 1960; Howley and Lewis, 1965).

It is evident that a commercial formula service is able to influence to some extent the choice of formula utilized by a hospital. Thus, if an evaporated milk formula is offered at 9 cents per bottle while a commercially marketed prepared formula is offered at 12 cents per bottle, the less expensive formula is likely to be chosen. Manufacturers of specific prepared formulas have, therefore, intoduced competing feeding systems.

In 1961 the Mead Johnson Company introduced the Beneflex system of feeding in which bulk quantities of any infant formula manufactured by that company could be transferred aseptically to feeders suitable to the needs of individual infants. More recently, sterile ready-to-feed formulas have been supplied to hospitals by a number of manufacturers in disposable bottles with disposable or reusable nipples. Early in 1965 ready-to-feed formulas supplied by manufacturers were utilized by about the same number of hospitals as were supplied by commercial formula services. Developments in this area have progressed so rapidly in the past two years that it is difficult to predict the future of feeding of infants in hospitals.

Commercial formula services have for several years supplied formulas to limited numbers of infants living at home. In the past few years makers of some ready-to-feed formulas have begun to market their products in disposable bottles through drug stores, grocery stores and supermarkets. At present, cost of these items is sufficiently high to limit widespread acceptance, but there is a strong suggestion that such innovations in packaging are likely to exert major influences on practices of infant feeding in the future.

REFERENCES

A.M.A. Council on Foods: Strained fruits and vegetables in the feeding of infants. J.A.M.A. *108*:1259, 1937.

Bain, K.: The incidence of breast feeding in hospitals in the United States. Pediatrics 2:313, 1948.

Beal, V. A.: On the acceptance of solid foods, and other food patterns, of infants and children. Pediatrics *20*:448, 1957.

Brennemann, J.: The curd and the buffer in infant feeding. J.A.M.A. 92:364, 1929.

Butler, A. M., and Wolman, I. J.: Trends in the early feeding of supplementary foods to infants; and analysis and discussion based on a nationwide survey. Quart. Rev. Pediat. 9:63, 1954.

Committee on Nutrition, American Academy of Pediatrics: On the feeding of solid foods to infants. Pediatrics *21*:685, 1958.

Committee on Nutrition, American Academy of Pediatrics: Prepared infant formulas and commercial formula services. Pediatrics *36*:282, 1965.

Cox, David O., Ross Laboratories, Columbus, Ohio. Report of market research data. Personal communication, 1966.

Davison, W.: Elimination of milk-borne disease. Amer. J. Dis. Child. 49:72, 1935.

Epps, R. P., and Jolley, M. P.: Unsupervised early feeding of solids to infants. Med. Ann. District Columbia 32:493, 1963.

Filer, L. J., Jr., and Martinez, G.: Intake of selected nutrients by infants in the United States. Clin. Pediat. 3:633, 1964.

Herbert, R. W., Hirst, E. L., Percival, E. G. V., Reynolds, R. J. W., and Smith, F.: Constitution of ascorbic acid. J. Soc. Chem. Ind. 52:221, 1933.

Holt, L. E., Jr.: Letter to Editor: Let us give the Russians their due. Pediatrics 32:462, 1963.

Hopkins, F. G.: The analyst and the medical man. Analyst 31:385, 1906.

Howley, M. P. F., and Lewis, M. N.: Comparison of hospital-prepared formulas with prebottled infant formulas. Hosp. 39:97, 1965.

Jackson, E. B., Wilkin, L. C., and Auerbach, H.: Statistical report on incidence and duration of breast feeding in relation to personal-social and hospital maternity factors. Pediatrics 17:700, 1956.

Major, R. H.: Classic Descriptions of Disease, with Biographical Sketches of the Authors. Springfield, Illinois, Charles C Thomas, 1945.

Marriott, W. M.: Preparation of lactic acid mixtures for infant feeding. J.A.M.A. 89:862, 1927.

Marriott, W. M.: Infant Nutrition. A Textbook of Infant Feeding for Students and Practitioners of Medicine. 2nd ed. St. Louis, The C. V. Mosby Co., 1935.

Marriott, W. M., and Schoenthal, L.: An experimental study of use of unsweetened evaporated milk for the preparation of infant feeding formulas. Arch. Pediat. 46:135, 1929.

Mellanby, E.: Accessory food factors (vitamines) in the feeding of infants. Lancet 1: 856, 1920.

Meyer, H. F.: Infant feeding practices in hospital maternity nurseries. A survey of 1,904 hospitals involving 2,225,000 newborn infants. Pediatrics 21:288, 1958a.

Meyer, H. F.: Breast feeding in the United States: extent and possible trend. A survey of 1,904 hospitals with two and a quarter million births in 1956. Pediatrics 22:116, 1958b.

Meyer, H. F.: Infant Foods and Feeding Practice. Springfield, Ill., Charles C Thomas, 1960.

Meyer, H. F.: The new ready-to-feed formulas. Some pertinent considerations. Clin. Pediat. 4:376, 1965a.

Meyer, H. F.: Survey of hospital nursery ready-to-feed milk mixtures. Hosp. 39:60, 1965b.

Newson, L. J., and Newson, E.: Breast-feeding in decline. Brit. M. J. 2:1744, 1962.

Robertson, W. O.: Breast feeding practices: some implications of regional variations. Am. J. Public Health 51:1035, 1961.

Sackett, W. W., Jr.: Use of solid foods early in infancy. G.P. 14:98, 1956.

Salber, E. J., Stitt, P. G., and Babbott, J. G.: Patterns of breast feeding. I. Factors affecting the frequency of breast feeding in the newborn period. New England J. Med. 259:707, 1958.

Salber, E. J., and Feinleib, M.: Breast-feeding in Boston. Pediatrics 37:299, 1966.

Schenkweiler, L., Hixson, H. H., Paxon, H. H., Clark, J. R., Berke, M., and Hosford, R. F.: Six administrators look at infant formula costs. Hosp. 34:46, 1960.

Stewart, C. P., and Guthrie, P. (eds.): Lind's Treatise on Scurvy. A Reprint of the First Edition of a Treatise of the Scurvy. Edinburgh, University Press, 1953.

Szent-Györgyi, A.: Observations on the function of peroxidase systems and the chemistry of adrenal cortex: Description of new carbohydrate derivative. Biochem. J. 22:1387, 1928.

Trout, G. M.: Homogenized Milk. A Review and Guide. East Lansing, Michigan State College Press, 1950.

Vogel, K.: Scurvy—"The plague of the sea and the spoyle of mariners." Bull. New York Acad. Med. 9:459, 1933.

Chapter Two

Normal Growth
and Failure to Thrive

When an infant who was full size at birth reaches three months of age and weighs only 4 kg, the conclusion that he has failed to thrive is justified even if measurement of length has been so inaccurate as to be useless. Thus, in technically underdeveloped countries in which a relatively high percentage of one-year-old infants weigh between 6 and 7 kg, it has proved simple and practical to describe failure to thrive in terms of the number of infants whose weights were 30 or 40 per cent or more below the average expected weight for age.

Such crude methods of evaluation are of relatively little value to the practitioner in technically highly developed countries in which the more frequent problem is one of distinguishing between slow rates of growth that may yet be considered within the normal range and those slightly slower rates of growth that are to be considered abnormal. An attempt will be made in this chapter to define normal rates of growth and failure to thrive.

Growth in Weight and Length

In an extensive and scholarly analysis of published reports, Meredith (1965) has shown that size at a specified age during infancy is not highly correlated with size at some subsequent age or with rate of gain between the time of the first measurement and a subsequent age. Thus, the assumption that a particular infant may be expected to progress along a specified growth channel is erroneous. If weight is recorded at the thirtieth percentile at age one month and at the tenth percentile at age four months, the physician is likely to experience difficulty in deciding whether growth has been within normal limits. The material that will be presented on incremental growth has been assembled in an effort to aid the practitioner in making such decisions.

Since growth retardation is among the earliest evidences of nutritional deficiency — whether such deficiency relates to total caloric intake or to intake of a specific essential nutrient — evaluation of dietary adequacy must include analysis of growth. Animal studies are of great value, but final appraisal must include observations with normal infants. Therefore, data on normal *rates* of growth (not merely ranges of normal body size at specified ages) are essential both for the investigator in infant nutrition and for the practitioner.

Incremental Growth in Weight

Although there are obvious practical problems and inconveniences involved in the use of incremental growth data rather than in merely plotting size on a growth chart, use of incremental data is strongly recommended because of its much greater sensitivity as an index of failure to thrive. As will be discussed, Tables 2–1 and 2–2 are considered helpful in arriving at a diagnosis of failure to thrive in infancy. Proper use of these tables requires the following steps:

1. *Age is recorded in days.*
2. *Weight is recorded in grams.*
3. *Gain in weight between two ages is divided by the number of days elapsed to obtain a result expressed as grams per day.*

If weight of a male infant was 4000 gm at 30 days of age and 5610 gm at 91 days of age, average daily gain in weight during this interval of 61 days will have been 1600 gm divided by 61 days, or 26 gm/day. By consulting Table 2–1, A, it will be found that the 10th percentile value for gain in weight during the age interval 28 to 84 days is 24.7 gm/day. Therefore, the rate of gain of the infant being considered was well within the range encountered in normal infants.

As may be seen from Table 2–1 and Figure 2–1, rates of gain in weight during successive 28-day intervals demonstrate progressive decrease with increasing age. Between 28 and 56 days of age 90 per cent of male infants demonstrated gains in weight greater than 26 gm/day, but only 10 per cent demonstrated similar rates of gain between 140 and 168 days of age.

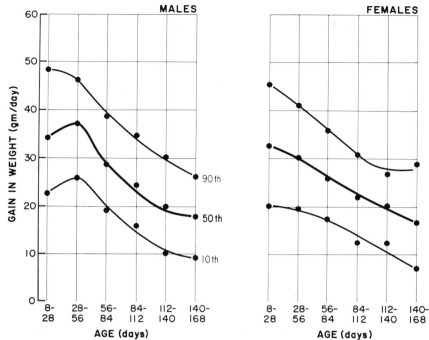

Figure 2–1. Rates of gain in weight of normal infants during successive 28-day intervals. The 10th, 50th and 90th percentile values for each sex are based on 100 to 120 infants in the first four age intervals and on 85 to 100 infants in the last two age intervals.

Incremental Gain in Length

Incremental data on length during infancy will be of little value if length cannot be measured regularly with an error no greater than 0.5 cm. Therefore, unless it is practical to employ a sound procedure for measurement, it is probably preferable to rely on incremental weight data and to ignore length.

Satisfactory measurement requires two individuals and a measuring device such as that depicted in Figure 2–2, with a fixed headpiece and movable footpiece. One examiner holds the infant's head firmly against the headpiece of the measuring device while the other grasps the ankles of the infant with one hand and the movable footpiece with the other. The infant's lower extremities are stretched and the footpiece pressed firmly against the soles of the feet. A reading of length is then made. The examiners next exchange positions and repeat the procedure. With practice, two examiners can regularly record measurements that agree within 0.5 cm (Meredith and Goodman, 1941).

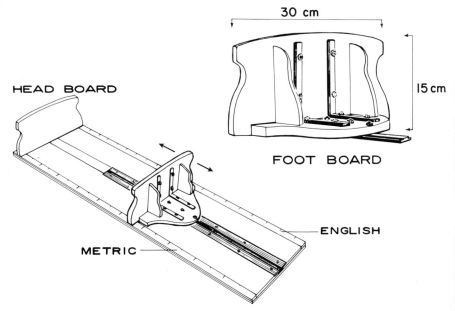

Figure 2-2.   Apparatus used for measurement of length.

Data on rates of change in length at various ages are presented in Tables 2–1 and 2–2. Because changes in length in 28 days are relatively small even during the early months of life and because well trained individuals may occasionally disagree in measurement of the same infant by as much as 0.5 cm, conclusions regarding change in length should ordinarily be based on observations over a period of at least 56 days during the first three months of life and on observations over approximately 90 days later in the first year.

Rate of Gain in Weight in Relation to Choice of Feeding

Although other investigators have reported greater gains in weight by infants fed evaporated milk formulas than by infants who are breast fed (Mellander et al., 1959), the author and his associates have been unable to confirm this observation. As may be seen from Figure 2–3, rates of gain in weight for breast-fed infants were similar to those for infants receiving several different formulas in the age intervals of 8 to 112 and 28 to 112 days.

(*Text continued on page 22.*)

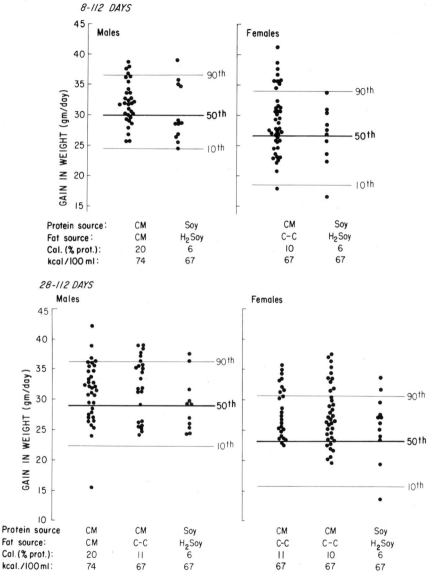

Figure 2–3. Rates of gain in weight of normal infants receiving various diets during the age periods 8 to 112 days (upper) and 28 to 112 days (lower). The 10th, 50th and 90th percentile values from the study of 40 breast-fed males and 29 breast-fed females are indicated. CM indicates cow milk, H₂Soy indicates partially hydrogenated soy oil, and C-C indicates corn and coconut oils.

Table 2–1.   *Average Daily Change in Weight (gm/day) and Length (mm/day) Between Selected Ages During Early Infancy* †*

		WEIGHT: Males					
		28 days	56 days	84 days	112 days	140 days	168 days
Birth	−2 S.D.	6.1	17.4	19.4	20.5	19.7	18.9
	10th	12.7	22.6	24.5	24.1	23.2	21.4
	25th	19.8	26.7	26.6	26.0	24.8	23.5
	50th	25.2	30.9	30.3	29.6	28.3	26.4
	75th	32.5	36.2	34.4	32.6	30.8	28.8
	90th	37.0	40.6	38.5	35.2	33.4	31.7
	+2 S.D.	45.1	45.9	42.3	38.6	36.4	34.3
8 days	−2 S.D.	15.4	21.7	21.9	22.6	21.1	19.8
	10th	22.7	27.1	26.8	25.8	24.1	22.1
	25th	27.2	31.0	29.4	28.1	25.9	24.1
	50th	34.1	35.7	32.9	31.3	29.4	27.2
	75th	43.3	40.4	37.6	34.1	31.8	29.8
	90th	48.6	46.0	41.5	37.8	33.9	32.2
	+2 S.D.	54.8	50.5	45.0	40.2	37.4	35.1
28 days	−2 S.D.	—	20.2	20.1	20.7	18.7	17.5
	10th	—	26.6	24.7	24.0	22.0	20.4
	25th	—	31.8	28.1	26.5	24.0	23.4
	50th	—	37.5	33.8	30.4	28.0	25.7
	75th	—	42.7	37.0	34.8	32.0	29.5
	90th	—	46.6	40.6	36.9	34.8	32.8
	+2 S.D.	—	54.0	45.8	40.5	37.8	35.3
56 days	−2 S.D.	—	—	13.4	15.5	14.3	13.4
	10th	—	—	19.3	19.0	18.7	17.4
	25th	—	—	23.9	22.8	21.1	19.8
	50th	—	—	28.9	27.1	24.0	22.7
	75th	—	—	33.9	31.2	29.1	27.0
	90th	—	—	38.7	35.0	33.0	31.3
	+2 S.D.	—	—	44.3	38.9	36.0	33.9
84 days	−2 S.D.	—	—	—	10.1	10.4	10.0
	10th	—	—	—	16.1	15.6	14.0
	25th	—	—	—	20.9	18.6	17.6
	50th	—	—	—	24.4	22.2	21.2
	75th	—	—	—	28.9	26.5	24.2
	90th	—	—	—	34.1	30.2	29.1
	+2 S.D.	—	—	—	39.5	35.2	32.7
112 days	−2 S.D.	—	—	—	—	4.6	7.6
	10th	—	—	—	—	10.2	10.8
	25th	—	—	—	—	14.3	15.7
	50th	—	—	—	—	20.0	19.7
	75th	—	—	—	—	26.8	22.8
	90th	—	—	—	—	30.5	27.6
	+2 S.D.	—	—	—	—	37.0	31.6
140 days	−2 S.D.	—	—	—	—	—	2.7
	10th	—	—	—	—	—	9.1
	25th	—	—	—	—	—	14.3
	50th	—	—	—	—	—	18.6
	75th	—	—	—	—	—	24.2
	90th	—	—	—	—	—	26.8
	+2 S.D.	—	—	—	—	—	34.0

Table 2–1. *Average Daily Change in Weight (gm/day) and Length (mm/day) Between Selected Ages During Early Infancy*† (cont.)*

		WEIGHT: Females					
		28 days	56 days	84 days	112 days	140 days	168 days
Birth	−2 S.D.	6.4	13.0	15.5	15.7	15.4	15.7
	10th	14.1	18.8	20.0	19.1	19.8	19.3
	25th	18.6	22.6	23.9	22.9	21.9	20.5
	50th	23.8	26.8	26.8	25.8	24.5	22.8
	75th	28.0	31.9	30.4	29.0	28.6	26.7
	90th	36.3	36.7	35.7	33.4	32.3	30.1
	+2 S.D.	41.9	41.3	38.9	36.4	35.0	32.0
8 days	−2 S.D.	12.0	16.6	17.6	18.0	17.2	17.3
	10th	20.2	23.3	22.7	22.0	21.4	20.5
	25th	27.6	27.0	26.0	25.1	23.3	22.2
	50th	32.9	32.2	30.0	27.5	25.8	23.9
	75th	39.1	36.9	34.3	31.3	30.1	28.6
	90th	45.5	42.3	37.8	35.2	33.7	30.8
	+2 S.D.	55.1	47.4	42.5	38.7	36.7	33.3
28 days	−2 S.D.	—	13.1	16.2	16.1	15.4	15.5
	10th	—	19.8	20.5	19.7	19.1	18.4
	25th	—	25.2	24.9	23.5	21.7	20.6
	50th	—	30.2	28.6	26.9	24.5	22.7
	75th	—	35.5	33.2	29.8	27.8	26.2
	90th	—	41.1	36.4	33.6	32.0	29.4
	+2 S.D.	—	47.2	41.0	37.2	35.0	31.7
56 days	−2 S.D.	—	—	12.4	13.5	13.3	13.4
	10th	—	—	17.7	17.5	17.0	16.8
	25th	—	—	23.0	20.8	19.7	18.7
	50th	—	—	26.3	24.4	23.2	21.2
	75th	—	—	30.5	28.6	26.5	25.3
	90th	—	—	36.0	31.6	29.6	27.5
	+2 S.D.	—	—	41.5	35.9	33.6	30.6
84 days	−2 S.D.	—	—	—	8.8	10.8	11.1
	10th	—	—	—	12.7	15.0	14.5
	25th	—	—	—	18.2	17.9	17.0
	50th	—	—	—	22.9	21.1	19.6
	75th	—	—	—	28.0	25.5	23.5
	90th	—	—	—	31.1	28.8	26.5
	+2 S.D.	—	—	—	36.2	32.5	29.4
112 days	−2 S.D.	—	—	—	—	8.7	9.5
	10th	—	—	—	—	12.9	12.9
	25th	—	—	—	—	16.1	15.0
	50th	—	—	—	—	20.2	18.7
	75th	—	—	—	—	23.7	22.0
	90th	—	—	—	—	27.1	24.9
	+2 S.D.	—	—	—	—	31.5	28.0
140 days	−2 S.D.	—	—	—	—	—	2.1
	10th	—	—	—	—	—	7.5
	25th	—	—	—	—	—	12.5
	50th	—	—	—	—	—	16.4
	75th	—	—	—	—	—	21.4
	90th	—	—	—	—	—	28.7
	+2 S.D.	—	—	—	—	—	33.3

Table 2–1. *Average Daily Change in Weight (gm/day) and Length (mm/day) Between Selected Ages During Early Infancy*† (cont.)*

		LENGTH: Males				
		56 days	84 days	112 days	140 days	168 days
Birth	−2 S.D.	0.8	1.0	0.9	0.8	0.8
	10th	1.0	1.0	0.9	0.9	0.8
	25th	1.1	1.1	1.0	1.0	0.9
	50th	1.3	1.2	1.1	1.0	1.0
	75th	1.4	1.2	1.2	1.1	1.0
	90th	1.4	1.3	1.2	1.1	1.1
	+2 S.D.	1.6	1.4	1.3	1.2	1.2
28 days	−2 S.D.	—	0.7	0.8	0.8	0.7
	10th	—	0.9	0.9	0.8	0.8
	25th	—	1.0	1.0	0.9	0.9
	50th	—	1.1	1.0	1.0	0.9
	75th	—	1.2	1.1	1.1	1.0
	90th	—	1.3	1.2	1.1	1.0
	+2 S.D.	—	1.5	1.2	1.2	1.1
56 days	−2 S.D.	—	—	0.8	0.7	0.6
	10th	—	—	0.8	0.7	0.7
	25th	—	—	0.9	0.8	0.8
	50th	—	—	1.0	0.9	0.8
	75th	—	—	1.1	1.0	0.9
	90th	—	—	1.1	1.0	1.0
	+2 S.D.	—	—	1.2	1.1	1.0
84 days	−2 S.D.	—	—	—	0.6	0.6
	10th	—	—	—	0.6	0.6
	25th	—	—	—	0.8	0.7
	50th	—	—	—	0.8	0.8
	75th	—	—	—	0.9	0.9
	90th	—	—	—	1.0	0.9
	+2 S.D.	—	—	—	1.0	1.0
112 days	−2 S.D.	—	—	—	—	0.5
	10th	—	—	—	—	0.5
	25th	—	—	—	—	0.6
	50th	—	—	—	—	0.7
	75th	—	—	—	—	0.8
	90th	—	—	—	—	0.9
	+2 S.D.	—	—	—	—	0.9

Table 2-1. *Average Daily Change in Weight (gm/day) and Length (mm/day) Between Selected Ages During Early Infancy*† (cont.)*

LENGTH: Females

		56 days	84 days	112 days	140 days	168 days
Birth	−2 S.D.	0.8	0.9	0.8	0.8	0.7
	10th	0.9	0.9	0.9	0.9	0.8
	25th	1.1	1.0	1.0	0.9	0.9
	50th	1.2	1.1	1.0	1.0	0.9
	75th	1.3	1.2	1.1	1.1	1.0
	90th	1.4	1.2	1.2	1.1	1.1
	+2 S.D.	1.6	1.3	1.2	1.2	1.1
28 days	−2 S.D.	−	0.8	0.7	0.7	0.6
	10th	−	0.8	0.8	0.8	0.7
	25th	−	0.9	0.9	0.8	0.8
	50th	−	1.0	0.9	0.9	0.8
	75th	−	1.1	1.0	1.0	0.9
	90th	−	1.2	1.1	1.0	1.0
	+2 S.D.	−	1.2	1.1	1.1	1.0
56 days	−2 S.D.	−	−	0.7	0.7	0.6
	10th	−	−	0.7	0.7	0.7
	25th	−	−	0.8	0.8	0.7
	50th	−	−	0.9	0.8	0.8
	75th	−	−	1.0	0.9	0.9
	90th	−	−	1.1	1.0	0.9
	+2 S.D.	−	−	1.1	1.1	1.0
84 days	−2 S.D.	−	−	−	0.6	0.5
	10th	−	−	−	0.6	0.6
	25th	−	−	−	0.7	0.7
	50th	−	−	−	0.8	0.7
	75th	−	−	−	0.9	0.8
	90th	−	−	−	1.0	0.9
	+2 S.D.	−	−	−	1.0	0.9
112 Days	−2 S.D.	−	−	−	−	0.3
	10th	−	−	−	−	0.5
	25th	−	−	−	−	0.6
	50th	−	−	−	−	0.7
	75th	−	−	−	−	0.8
	90th	−	−	−	−	0.9
	+2 S.D.	−	−	−	−	1.1

*Values are based on observations of approximately 100 infants in each age group. Values given are the mean minus two standard deviations, the 10th, 25th, 50th, 75th and 90th percentiles, and the mean plus two standard deviations.
†Unpublished data of Fomon et al., 1966.

Table 2–2. Rate of Gain in Length and Weight at Three-month and Six-month Intervals During the First Year of Life

Age (months)	Number of Infants		−2 Standard Deviations		Percentiles					+2 Standard Deviations	
	Milbank*	Fels*	Milbank	Fels	10th	25th	50th	75th	90th	Milbank	Fels
White Males											
Change in Length (mm/day)											
0–3	243		0.7							1.1	
0–6	217		0.8							1.2	
3–6	209	126		0.3†	0.56	0.60	0.70	0.79	0.87		0.8†
3–9		118		0.4	0.51	0.55	0.60	0.65	0.74		0.8
6–9		128		0.2	0.38	0.44	0.51	0.59	0.66		0.5
6–12	127	121		0.3†	0.36	0.41	0.47	0.50	0.56		0.6†
9–12		119		0.1	0.24	0.33	0.40	0.48	0.57		0.5
Change in Weight (gm/day)											
0–3	264		13.2							31.8	
0–6	238		17.6							35.1	
3–6	212	126		8.3†	15.0	16.7	20.3	24.2	28.8		24.6†
3–9		118		10.3	13.1	15.3	18.0	20.5	23.0		25.8
6–9		128		3.3	8.3	12.0	15.3	18.4	22.7		19.5
6–12	132	121		5.5†	7.7	9.8	12.5	15.2	17.2		20.5†
9–12		119		0.5	5.5	7.2	9.9	12.3	15.4		14.7

Table 2–2. *Rate of Gain in Length and Weight at Three-month and Six-month Intervals During the First Year of Life (continued)*

White Females

Age (months)	Number of Infants		−2 Standard Deviations		Percentiles					+2 Standard Deviations	
	Milbank*	Fels*	Milbank	Fels	10th	25th	50th	75th	90th	Milbank	Fels
Change in Length (mm/day)											
0–3	207		0.6							1.1	
0–6	173		0.7							1.1	
3–6	203	112		0.3†	0.52	0.60	0.69	0.78	0.89		0.7†
3–9		109		0.4	0.47	0.53	0.58	0.64	0.66		0.7
6–9		108		0.2	0.34	0.41	0.48	0.58	0.67		0.6
6–12	122	101		0.3†	0.37	0.42	0.47	0.51	0.55		0.6†
9–12		102		0.2	0.28	0.39	0.46	0.52	0.60		0.5
Change in Weight (gm/day)											
0–3	248		11.2							27.8	
0–6	212		14.7							32.0	
3–6	204	112		7.1†	13.8	16.1	19.7	24.0	27.9		24.1†
3–9		109		9.1	12.5	14.0	17.3	19.8	22.7		25.2
6–9		108		4.0	9.3	11.8	14.4	17.4	20.4		17.9
6–12	120	101		5.6†	8.1	10.0	11.8	14.6	17.2		19.6†
9–12		102		0.8	4.2	7.6	11.0	14.0	16.3		15.4

*Milbank data from Kasius et al. (1957); Fels data from Garn & Rohmann (1966b); percentiles are from Fels study.
†Based on data of Milbank and Fels studies combined.

FAILURE TO THRIVE

Definition of Failure to Thrive

The term "failure to thrive" has frequently been used loosely to indicate growth failure, with no delineation of the boundary between normal and abnormal rates of growth. It is proposed, tentatively, that failure to thrive be defined as a rate of gain in length and/or weight less than the value corresponding to two standard deviations below the mean during an interval of at least 56 days for infants less than three months of age and during an interval of at least three months for older infants. Values two standard deviations below the mean in length and weight for various age intervals are presented in Tables 2–1 and 2–2. The longer the interval of observation, the more conclusive the diagnosis. It is suggested that infants gaining in length or weight at rates less than the 10th percentile values be regarded as suspect. Such infants deserve more careful and more frequent medical evaluation than do other infants.

Definition of Obesity

A satisfactory definition of obesity must almost certainly be expressed in terms of percentage of body weight accounted for by fat. Because the fat content of the body of living subjects is difficult to estimate, it is suggested that, tentatively, obesity be defined as a gross discrepancy between length and weight (Table 2–3). The extent of discrepancy in percentile values for length and weight listed in the table is sufficiently great that nearly all infants classified on this basis will be likely to have excessive body content of fat. However, many obese infants may not be so classified with these criteria. For example, the infant with length less than the 10th percentile value and weight just below the 50th percentile might be quite obese. Neither does the table permit a diagnosis of obesity to be made in an infant whose length exceeds the 75th percentile value. Development of a more satisfactory definition of obesity in infancy must be considered an important area for further study.

Genetic Influences

As may be seen from Table 2–4, Garn and Rohmann (1966a) have demonstrated that body lengths of siblings during infancy are similar. For boys the slope of infant length on midparental height is 0.196 at birth (r = 0.56) and 0.305 at age one year (r = 0.61). Although of value in assessing size of groups of infants, these correlations have relatively slight predictive value when applied to individuals. Parent-specific data for *rate of gain* in length and weight of infants are not yet available.

Table 2-3. *Tentative Definition of Obesity*[*]

Age (months)	Males Length (cm) less than	Males Weight (kg) more than	Females Length (cm) less than	Females Weight (kg) more than
Birth	48.1	3.4	47.8	3.4
	48.9	3.8	48.4	3.6
	50.3	4.1	50.2	3.9
	51.7	4.3	50.9	4.1
1	52.0	4.3	50.4	4.0
	53.4	4.6	52.3	4.3
	54.6	4.9	54.0	4.5
	55.9	5.4	55.1	5.0
3	58.4	6.1	56.4	5.6
	59.6	6.6	58.2	6.0
	60.9	7.1	59.7	6.3
	62.7	7.5	61.3	6.8
6	64.8	8.1	63.3	7.5
	66.2	8.7	64.5	8.0
	67.6	9.1	66.0	8.3
	69.4	9.9	67.6	9.1
9	69.2	9.3	67.5	8.7
	70.8	10.0	68.4	9.2
	72.3	10.7	70.0	9.6
	73.4	11.3	71.9	10.5
12	72.8	10.5	71.2	9.7
	74.7	11.3	72.8	10.4
	76.3	11.5	74.4	10.7
	77.8	12.8	76.1	11.9

[*]The table is based on combined data for white infants from the studies of Kasius et al., (1957) and Garn and Rohmann (1966b). At each age, the values for length for each sex are the 10th, 25th, 50th and 75th percentiles while the values for weight are the 50th, 75th and 90th percentiles and the mean plus two standard deviations.

Classification of Failure to Thrive

Causes for the failure of infants to thrive may be listed in four categories:

1. Amounts of ingested food are too small to support normal rates of growth even in infants whose requirements are average.
2. Vomiting reduces the net intake of food and reduces intake of nutrients below the requirements of the average infant.
3. Fecal losses of energy are sufficiently great to reduce the net intake to a level insufficient to promote normal growth of the average infant.
4. Energy requirements are unusually high.

A combination of two or more of these factors may also occur.

Table 2–4. *Relation of Infant's Length to Length of Sibling and Height of Parents*

Correlations	Age Birth n	Age Birth r	Age 6 months n	Age 6 months r	Age 12 months n	Age 12 months r
Sibling						
sister-sister	45	0.52	75	0.52	74	0.54
brother-brother	59	0.52	73	0.44	74	0.35
sister-brother	113	0.54	156	0.49	154	0.39
Parent-child						
father-son		0.14		0.33		0.36
mother-son		0.15		0.26		0.28
father-daughter		0.14		0.29		0.34
mother-daughter		−0.06		0.14		0.23
midparent*-son		0.18		0.38		0.42
midparent*-daughter		0.05		0.28		0.34

*"Midparent" height refers to mean height of parents.
Data of Garn and Rohmann, 1966a.

By far, the majority of infants who fail to thrive do so because food intake is low. Obviously, the conclusion that failure to thrive may be attributed to low dietary intake is only the first step in arriving at a satisfactory diagnosis. The problem can, however, be restated from the more general, "Why has the infant failed to achieve a normal rate of growth?" to the somewhat more specific, "Why has the infant failed to obtain an adequate caloric intake?" Stated in this manner, the answer may become obvious: the diet is poorly devised; feeding technique is poor; the infant is neglected; the infant has a congenital malformation or an acute or chronic disease.

In addition to a careful history and physical examination in which particular attention is given to the central nervous system, the following diagnostic studies have been found useful for diagnosis in infants who fail to thrive because of low caloric intake: concentration of hemoglobin, total and differential leukocyte count, stained smear of blood, erythrocyte sedimentation rate, urinalysis, roentgenogram of chest, serum concentration of urea nitrogen, skin tests for tuberculosis and histoplasmosis. When these diagnostic measures fail to provide a clue to the nature of the problem, roentgenographic study of the gastrointestinal tract after administration of barium may be useful.

When vomiting occurs with sufficient frequency and in sufficient quantity to reduce the net intake of calories below the amounts usually accepted by normal infants, further study may be directed toward causes of vomiting rather than toward the more general area of failure to thrive.

When net caloric intake is adequate (amount of food accepted is within normal limits and vomiting does not account for an important loss of energy), metabolic balance studies are desirable to determine fecal loss of fat and nitrogen. Fortunately, except in those patients with cystic fibrosis of the pancreas (which is readily diagnosed without the aid of metabolic balance studies), excessive fecal losses comprise a relatively small percentage of cases of failure to thrive in infancy.

Little information is available concerning failure to thrive because of unusually high energy requirements. It seems reasonable to assume that infants with muscular hypertonia or spastic cerebral palsy may have high energy requirements because of constant muscular contractions. Similarly, infants with congenital heart disease and tachypnea may, in fact, be constantly exercising and may demonstrate markedly elevated energy requirements. Rates of oxygen consumption per unit of body weight have been shown to be high in malnourished infants (Montgomery, 1962), in those with severe congenital heart disease (Pittman and Cohen, 1964; Lees et al., 1965) and in those whose birth weights are low in relation to gestational age (Sinclair and Silverman, 1966). Management of such infants often requires use of calorically concentrated formulas.

Growth of Body Components

Methods now available for determining chemical composition of the living subject are not generally suitable for wide scale clinical application. Therefore, clinical appraisal of growth is at present largely limited to evaluation of size and of rate of change in length and weight. As methods for assessing body composition become standardized and simplified, a broader concept of normal growth may be expected to develop. Even now, research in this area is progressing actively and a chapter dealing with normal growth would seem incomplete without at least a brief review of information on body composition of the normal infant at various ages. Of the several approaches possible for determining body composition of the living infant, a few will be discussed in the section that immediately follows and others will be mentioned in relation to consideration of the male reference infant and of sex-related differences that occur in infancy.

Urinary Excretion of Hydroxyproline

In the past few years much interest has been expressed in urinary excretion of hydroxyproline as a chemical index of growth.

Collagen accounts for about 25 per cent of total body proteins of adult men (Widdowson and Dickerson, 1960), but may be as much as 44 per cent of total body proteins of the infant with severe malnutrition (Picou et al., 1965). It is found primarily in skin, tendons, cartilage, blood vessels, connective tissue, organ capsules and bone matrix. Nearly all the hydroxyproline in vertebrates is found in collagen (Prockop, 1964), and endogenous hydroxyproline excreted in urine almost certainly represents products of collagen degradation or, possibly, precursors of collagen. Newly formed collagen is soluble in neutral salt solutions and is metabolically quite active; mature collagen is insoluble and metabolically inert. Urinary excretion of endogenous hydroxyproline reflects predominantly the rate at which soluble collagen is being formed and degraded.

Hydroxyproline is excreted in the urine primarily in the form of peptides. Increased rates of excretion are observed during periods of rapid synthesis of collagen, as occurs during normal growth and during periods of rapid degradation of collagen, as in severe burns (Smiley and Ziff, 1964). Decreased rates of excretion are characteristic of growth failure resulting from nutritional deficiency (Whitehead, 1965; Picou et al., 1965) or from pituitary dwarfism.

When growing subjects receive a collagen-free diet and are not affected by those few specific abnormalities that result in excessive rates of degradation of collagen, rates of urinary excretion probably reflect rates of collagen synthesis in the body. Serial studies of urinary excretion of endogenous hydroxyproline in normal infants may, therefore, aid in defining the pattern of growth of this body component during early life. In addition, establishment of a range of values for urinary excretion of endogenous hydroxyproline by normal infants of various ages may be useful in interpreting results obtained with infants who fail to thrive or are suspected of various disorders of collagen metabolism.

A summary of data from serial study of 29 normal male infants is presented in Table 2–5. Each of nine male infants was studied on five to seven occasions between the ages of 20 and 120 days, a period during which rates of excretion are influenced relatively little by age. When the mean urinary excretion of hydroxyproline for each infant was plotted against the rate of gain in body length of that infant, a high degree of correlation was demonstrated (r = 0.78) (Fig. 2–4). Correlation between mean rate of urinary excretion of hydroxyproline and gain in weight was much less (r= 0.26). Since much of the growth of collagen during early life is accounted for by growth of long bones, it is not surprising that rate of urinary excretion of hydroxyproline and rate of growth in length should be related.

Table 2–5. *Summary of Data on Urinary Excretion of Hydroxyproline by Normal Male Infants**

Age (days)	Number of Subjects	Number of Studies	Excretion of Hydroxyproline† (mg/day)	
			Mean	Standard deviation
4–8	22	22	32.1	5.9
10–19	9	11	42.1	8.0
22–60	9	22	49.3	10.9
63–120	9	31	46.7	8.6
121–180	7	25	43.0	10.0

*Data of Younoszai et al., 1967.
†Average daily excretion during three days of observation.

Urinary Excretion of Endogenous Creatinine

Approximately 98 per cent of creatine in the body exists in muscle and about 2 per cent of total body creatine is converted to creatinine each day and excreted in the urine (Borsook and Dubnoff, 1947). A high correlation between urinary excretion of endogenous creatinine and fat-free body mass has been demonstrated by Kumar et al. (1959) in the rat and by Van Niekerk et al. (1963) in sheep carcasses. These studies have been performed with animals receiving diets free of creatine and creatinine. The influence of dietary creatine and creatinine in increasing urinary excretion of creatinine has been demonstrated by Bleiler and Schedl (1962).

Figure 2–5 presents data on urinary excretion of endogenous creatinine by normal infants studied during the first 18 months of life. To the extent that such urinary excretion reflects muscle mass, it would appear that muscle mass, as a percentage of body weight, de-

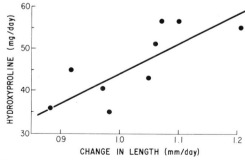

Figure 2–4. Relation between urinary excretion of endogenous hydroxyproline and rate of gain in length of normal male infants between 20 and 120 days of age. Each point represents the mean urinary excretion of hydroxyproline during five, six or seven 72-hour periods of urine collection. Data of Younoszai et al., 1967.

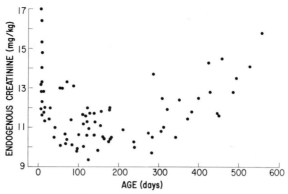

Figure 2–5.   Urinary excretion of endogenous creatinine by normal male infants.

creases until nearly one year of age and then rather rapidly increases. Data at present apply to relatively few infants, but studies of this type may in the future help to provide additional insight into composition of weight gained during infancy.

Oxygen Consumption

Rate of consumption of oxygen by infants in the resting thermoneutral state probably reflects body mass of actively metabolizing tissue and is, therefore, of interest in relation to body composition, even though "actively metabolizing tissue" cannot be anatomically defined. Severely malnourished infants (Montgomery, 1962), those of low birth weight in relation to gestational age (Sinclair and Silverman, 1966) and those with severe congenital heart disease (Pittman and Cohen, 1964; Lees et al., 1965) have been shown to have relatively high rates of oxygen consumption per unit of body weight.

Total Body Potassium

In normal individuals of a specified age, potassium concentration of fat-free body mass is remarkably constant. Therefore, if body content of potassium can be determined and if a reasonable estimate of potassium concentration of fat-free body mass can be made for the age in question, calculation of fat-free body mass is possible. By subtracting fat-free body mass from whole body weight, the fat content of the body can be determined.

Because the naturally occurring radioisotope ^{40}K occurs in the body in fixed proportion to total potassium, whole body counting for ^{40}K has been useful in study of body composition of adults and older children (Forbes, 1962) and, more recently, in study of severely malnourished infants (Garrow, 1965). Further refinements of the difficult techniques involved in such investigations may be anticipated and will undoubtedly contribute greatly to knowledge of body composition of the living subject.

Cell Number and Cell Size

Because deoxyribonucleic acid (DNA) is located almost entirely within the nucleus of the cell, because the amount of DNA per nucleus of a species is constant (except for germ cells), and because most tissues and organs have one nucleus per cell, the number of nuclei and, hence, the number of cells in an organ may be estimated. Thus, the content of DNA per gram of the organ in question is divided by the DNA content per nucleus of that species (6.2 $\mu\mu$g for the rat) to give the number of nuclei per gram of organ weight. Cell size as well as cell number can, of course, be calculated.

Patterns of increase in cell number and cell size in various organs during normal growth of the rat have been described by Enesco and Leblond (1962) and by Winick and Noble (1965, 1966a, 1967). During prenatal and early postnatal development all organs appear to grow by cell division alone. Gradually a shift occurs to a pattern of increasing cell size as the major component of growth. This shift occurs first in brain and lung and last in skeletal muscle. A similar sequential pattern of hyperplasia, hyperplasia plus hypertrophy and, finally, hypertrophy alone has been described for rat placenta (Winick and Noble, 1966b) and human placenta (Winick et al., 1967).

Caloric restriction during the period of cellular hyperplasia in rats results in decreased ultimate body size, decreased size of individual organs and reduction in cell number in these organs without major change in cell size (Winick and Noble, 1966a). Conversely, overfeeding during the period of cellular hyperplasia results in greater ultimate stature with larger numbers of cells in the various organs (Winick and Noble, 1967).

Pituitary insufficiency imposed on mice at birth results in gross reduction in muscle cell size for age, but if imposed at weaning exerts only slight influence on muscle cell size (Cheek et al., 1965a and b). When growth failure results from malnutrition imposed on the individual after the neonatal period, cell size rather than cell number is reduced (Waterlow and Weisz, 1956; Mendes and Waterlow, 1958).

It seems possible that knowledge of cell number and cell size in one or more organs or tissues of infants who are small for age may provide considerable insight into the nature of growth failure (Cheek and Cooke, 1964) and might be of predictive value in relation to results of therapeutic measures. For example, muscle cells of certain children who have congenital heart disease and failure to thrive have been shown to be decreased in number but normal or somewhat increased in size (Cheek et al., 1966). One may speculate that such children are unlikely to attain normal ultimate stature even if the congenital heart disease is corrected.

Male Reference Infant

An estimate (Fomon, 1967) of body composition of the male reference infant between birth and one year of age is presented in Table 2–6 and Figure 2–6. Since body water increases less rapidly than body weight, body water, expressed as a percentage of body weight, decreases. While the percentage of body weight accounted for by body water is decreasing, fat and protein are accumulating rapidly so that percentage composition of the body at age two months is quite different from that at birth. After two months of age, percentage of body weight accounted for by fat continues to increase until six months of age, then decreases slightly, while percentage of protein increases most rapidly between six and 12 months of age. From Figure 2–7 it may be seen that the body weight of the male reference infant at age one year is considered to be the sum of three equal increments of 3.5 kg. The first 3.5 kg, synthesized between conception and birth, is high in water, relatively low in lipid and protein. The second 3.5 kg, synthesized between birth and age four months, is relatively low in water and protein, exceptionally high in lipid. The third 3.5 kg, synthesized between four and 12 months of age, is intermediate in content of water and lipid and quite high in content of protein. Fat-free body mass accounts for 89.0 per cent, 59.2 per cent

*Table 2–6. Body Composition of Male Reference Infant**

Age (months)	Body Weight (kg)	Composition of Body (gm/100 gm)			
		Water	Fat	Protein	Other
birth	3.50	75.1	11.0	11.4	2.5
2	5.45	63.7	22.4	11.4	2.5
4	7.10	60.2	25.9	11.4	2.5
6	8.28	59.9	25.3	12.3	2.5
8	9.08	59.6	24.8	13.1	2.5
10	9.82	59.3	24.5	13.7	2.5
12	10.50	59.0	23.9	14.6	2.5

*From Fomon, S. J.: Pediatrics, 1967, to be published.

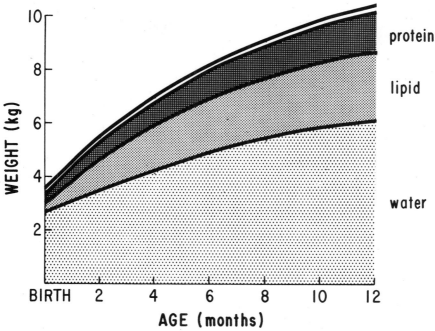

Figure 2–6. Total body weight and estimated amounts of water, fat and protein from birth to one year of age (see Table 2–6). (From Fomon, S. J.: Pediatrics, 1967, to be published.)

and 80.1 per cent, respectively, of weight gain in the three age intervals.

Although fat-free body mass accounts for a greater percentage of weight gain between four and 12 months of age than between birth and four months of age, daily rate of gain in fat-free body mass is greater during the first four months of life. Thus, assuming that a few days will elapse after birth before weight gain begins and that weight gain may not occur during a day or two of minor illness during the first four months of life, perhaps 115 days are available for tissue synthesis in this interval. If synthesis of fat-free body mass is 2072 gm (3.5 kg × 59.2 per cent FFBM) in four months, the rate of synthesis will be approximately 18 gm of fat-free body tissue daily. Assuming 235 days available for tissue synthesis between four and 12 months of age, the rate of synthesis will be approximately 12 gm daily (3.5 kg × 80.1 per cent ÷ 235 days). Similarly, rate of gain in protein may be calculated to be approximately 3.5 gm/day during the first four months of life and 3.1 gm/day between four and 12 months of age.

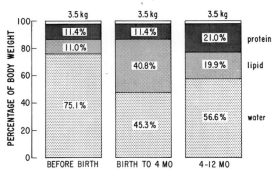

Figure 2-7. Composition of weight gain of the "male reference infant." (From Fomon, S. J.: Pediatrics, 1967, to be published.)

Significance of Adipose Tissue

Information is not available on the extent of variation in body composition of presumably normal infants. However, one may speculate that if the average infant, represented by the reference infant, is approximately 26 per cent fat at age four months, apparently normal infants at this age may vary from perhaps 18 to 34 per cent fat. Since fat makes up about 47 per cent of adipose tissue at six months of age (Dju, 1953; Dju et al., 1958), adipose tissue might account for 37 per cent of body weight in one infant and nearly 70 per cent in another. The consequences of such differences are unknown. The thick layer of subcutaneous adipose tissue of the relatively fat infant may be beneficial in some circumstances by contributing to efficient conservation of body heat, but it may make him particularly vulnerable to hyperpyrexia when ill or exposed to elevated environmental temperature.

Diet and Body Composition

The literature provides many examples of the influence of seemingly minor variations in composition of the diet on the rate of growth and the body composition of animals. Among the most dramatic and puzzling examples are the findings of Dymsza et al. (1964) with respect to studies of artificial feeding of rats from birth until 22 days of age—the usual time of weaning. Weight gain with the basal diet was considerably less than that of control rats nursed by their mothers (Fig. 2-8). Supplementation of the basal diet with 5 per cent by weight of rat milk (but not by 1 per cent or by 10 per cent) was found to eliminate this difference in weight gain.

That weight gain is only one aspect of growth is well illustrated by body composition studies of these infant rats. Although the arti-

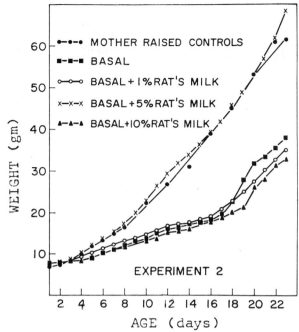

Figure 2–8. Comparative growth curves of infant rats fed various diets. (From Dymsza, H. A., Czajka, D. M., and Miller, S. A.: J. Nutrition 84:100, 1964.)

ficially fed rats whose diets were supplemented with 5 per cent rat milk were most similar in rate of gain in weight to breast-fed control rats, they resembled the breast-fed controls least in percentage composition of the carcass. Fat comprised 8 to 9 per cent of carcass weight of the breast-fed controls and of the slowly growing rats fed the basal diet either unsupplemented or supplemented with 1 per cent or 10 per cent rat milk. Quite in contrast, fat comprised 14 per cent of carcass weight of rats fed the basal diet supplemented with 5 per cent rat milk.

Whether such differences in rates of growth and body composition during infancy have fundamental physiologic significance in terms of subsequent incidence of disease and longevity is unknown. However, the possibility that important later consequences may result from early diet must be taken into consideration in seeking a definition of optimal nutrition in infancy.

Sex-related Differences

Commonly employed charts for plotting length and weight indicate that infant boys are inclined to be somewhat larger than infant girls. Factors responsible for these differences are probably gonadal in origin but the mechanism is unknown. It has been demonstrated that in the case of lambs (Donald and Purser, 1956) and of human infants (Karn, 1952, 1953), prenatal growth of a twin is influenced not only by its own sex, but by the sex of its co-twin. Thus, in the case of twin lambs, birth weight superiority of males over females is twice as great in mixed-sex twins as in like-sex twins. In human twins, birth weights of males have been reported to be significantly greater when the co-twin is a female than when the co-twin is another male (Karn, 1952, 1953). However, sex of the co-twin did not appear to exert a significant influence on weight of a female twin. Not only are boys slightly larger than girls at birth, but rates of gain in length and weight are greater during the early months of life. The extent of the difference in rates of gain in weight may be seen from Tables 2–1 and 2–2 and from Figure 2–1. Between 28 and 56 days of age, the median rate of gain in weight is 38 gm/day for boys and 31 gm/day for girls. Between 140 and 168 days of age, corresponding rates of gain are 20 and 16 gm/day.

Although it is frequently assumed that important sex-related differences in body composition are not present during infancy or early childhood, available data provide convincing evidence that a sex-related difference in body composition is, in fact, present during early infancy (Owen et al., 1966). Possibly the factors responsible for this difference in body composition are similar to those responsible for the larger mean weight and length of male than of female infants at birth and the more rapid rates of gain in weight of male than of female infants during early life. In any case, the existence of a sex-related difference in body composition during infancy strongly suggests that fundamental physiologic processes differ between infant boys and girls.

Data demonstrating sex-related differences in body composition during infancy are derived both from whole body chemical analyses and from various indirect measurements that can be carried out during life. Indirect measurements include studies of total body water; measurement of urinary excretion of endogenous creatinine as an index of muscle mass and of urinary excretion of endogenous hydroxyproline as an index of rate of synthesis of collagen; skinfold thickness determined with calipers; and widths of skin-plus-adipose tissue, muscle and bone from roentgenograms. Activity of serum alkaline phosphatase and pseudocholinesterase among normal breast-fed infants is greater for males than for females (Garry et al., 1966).

Existence of sex-related differences in body composition during infancy indicates a need for investigation of fundamental physiologic processes responsible for the observed differences. Sex-related differences in physiologic functions during infancy may have implications of far greater importance than differences in body composition. Definite sex-related differences in susceptibility to certain infectious diseases (Thompson et al., 1963; Washburn et al., 1965*) and the well-recognized sex-related differences in incidence of such disorders as hypertrophic pyloric stenosis suggest the need for intensified investigation of other sex-related differences during infancy.

As we increase our knowledge of normal growth and physiology during infancy, it may prove that management (including feeding) optimal for one sex is not optimal for the other. Certainly the demonstration of sex-related differences in body composition during infancy, together with well-recognized sex-related differences in neonatal mortality and in the incidence of certain diseases, strongly suggests that fundamental physiologic processes differ between infant boys and girls.

REFERENCES

Bleiler, R. E., and Schedl, H. P.: Creatinine excretion: Variability and relationships to diet and body size. J. Lab. & Clin. Med. 59:945, 1962.

Borsook, H., and Dubnoff, J. W.: The hydrolysis of phosphocreatine and the origin of urinary creatinine. J. Biol. Chem. 168:493, 1947.

Cheek, D. B., and Cooke, R. E.: Growth and growth retardation. Ann. Rev. Med. 15: 357, 1964.

Cheek, D. B., Graystone, J., and Mehrizi, A.: The importance of muscle cell number in children with congenital heart disease. Bull. Johns Hopkins Hosp. 118:140, 1966.

Cheek, D. B., Powell, G. K., and Scott, R. E.: Growth of muscle mass and skeletal collagen in the rat. I. Normal growth. II. The effect of ablation of the pituitary, thyroid or testes. Bull. Johns Hopkins Hosp. 116:378, 1965a.

Cheek, D. B., Powell, G. K., and Scott, R. E.: Growth of muscle cells (size and number) and liver DNA in rats and Snell Smith mice with insufficient pituitary thyroid or testicular function. Bull. Johns Hopkins Hosp. 117:306, 1965b.

Dju, M. Y.: Tocopherol content of human tissues from conception to old age. Doctoral thesis. University of Rochester, 1953.

Dju, M. Y., Mason, K. E., and Filer, L. J., Jr.: Vitamin E (Tocopherol) in human tissues from birth to old age. Amer. J. Clin. Nutr. 6:50, 1958.

Donald, H. P., and Purser, A. F.: Competition in utero between twin lambs. J. Agric. Sci. 48:245, 1956.

Dymsza, H. A., Czajka, D. M., and Miller, S. A.: Influence of artificial diet on weight gain and body composition of the neonatal rat. J. Nutrition 84:100, 1964.

Enesco, M., and Leblond, C. P.: Increase in cell number as a factor in the growth of the organs and tissues of the young male rat. J. Embryol. Exp. Morph. 10:530, 1962.

Fomon, S. J.: Body composition of the infant. Part I: The male "reference infant." In Falkner, F. (ed.): Human Development, Philadelphia, W. B. Saunders Co., 1966.

Fomon, S. J.: Body composition of the male reference infant. Borden Award Address. To be published. Pediatrics, 1967.

---

*Although the original publication includes only seven references, reprints of the paper list 430.

Fomon, S. J., Thomas, L. N., and Filer, L. J., Jr.: Growth of normal infants during the first five months of life. Unpublished, 1966.

Forbes, G. B.: Methods for determining composition of the human body. With a note on the effect of diet on body composition. Pediatrics 29:477, 1962.

Garn, S. M., and Rohmann, C. G.: Interaction of nutrition and genetics in the timing of growth and development. Pediat. Clin. North America 13:353, 1966a.

Garn, S. M., and Rohmann, C. G.: Personal communication concerning infant growth data of the Fels Institute, 1966b.

Garrow, J. S.: Total body-potassium in kwashiorkor and marasmus. Lancet 2:455, 1965.

Garry, P. J., Routh, J. I., and Fomon, S. J.: Influence of age and sex on activity of alkaline phosphatase and pseudocholinesterase of normal breastfed infants. Unpublished, 1966.

Karn, M. N.: Birth weight and length of gestation of twins, together with maternal age, parity and survival rate. Ann. Eugenics. 16:365, 1952.

Karn, M. N.: Twin data: a further study of birth weight, gestation time, maternal age, order of birth, and survival. Ann. Eugenics. 17:233, 1953.

Kasius, R. V., Randall, A., IV, Tompkins, W. T., Wiehl, D. G.: Maternal and infant nutrition studies at Philadelphia Lying-In Hospital. Newborn studies. V. Size and growth of babies during the first year of life. Milbank Mem. Fund Quart. 35:323, 1957.

Kumar, I., Land, D. G., and Boyne, A. W.: The determination of body composition of living animals. The daily endogenous creatinine excretion as a measure of body composition in rats. Brit. J. Nutr. 13:320, 1959.

Lees, M. H., Bristow, J. D., Griswold, H. E., and Olmsted, R. W.: Relative hypermetabolism in infants with congenital heart disease and undernutrition. Pediatrics 36:183, 1965.

Mellander, O., Vahlquist, B., and Mellbin, T. and collaborators: Breast feeding and artificial feeding: a clinical, serological, and biochemical study of 402 infants, with a survey of the literature. The Norbotten study. Acta Paediatrica. Suppl. 116, 1959.

Mendes, C. B., and Waterlow, J. C.: The effect of a low protein diet, and of refeeding on the composition of liver and muscle in the weanling rat. Brit. J. Nutr. 12:74, 1958.

Meredith, H. V.: Selected anatomic variables analyzed for interage relationships of the size-size, size-gain, and gain-gain varieties, in Advances in Child Development and Behavior, Lipsitt, L. P. and Spiker, C. C., (eds.), New York, Academic Press Inc., 2:221, 1965.

Meredith, H. V., and Goodman, J. L.: A comparison of routine hospital records of birth stature with measurements of birth stature obtained for longitudinal research. Child. Develop. 12:175, 1941.

Montgomery, R. D.: Changes in the basal metabolic rate of the malnourished infant and their relation to body composition. J. Clin. Invest. 41:1653, 1962.

Owen, G. M., Filer, L. J., Jr., Maresh, M., and Fomon, S. J.: Body composition of the infant. Part II: Sex-related difference in body composition in infancy. In Falkner, F., (ed.): Human Development, Philadelphia, W. B. Saunders Company, 1966.

Picou, D., Alleyne, G. A. O., and Seakins, A.: Hydroxyproline and creatine excretion in infantile protein malnutrition. Clin. Sci. 29:517, 1965.

Pittman, G. J., and Cohen, P.: The pathogenesis of cardiac cachexia. New England J. Med. 271:403, 453, 1964.

Prockop, D. J.: Isotopic studies on collagen degradation and the urine excretion of hydroxyproline. J. Clin. Invest. 43:453, 1964.

Sinclair, J. C., and Silverman, W. A.: Intrauterine growth in active tissue mass of the human fetus, with particular reference to the undergrown baby. Pediatrics 38:48, 1966.

Smiley, J. D., and Ziff, M.: Urinary hydroxyproline excretion and growth. Physiol. Rev. 44:31, 1964.

Thompson, D. J., Gezon, H. M., Hatch, T. F., Rycheck, R. R., Rogers, K. D.: Sex distribution of staphylococcus aureus colonization and disease in newborn infants. New England J. Med. 269:337, 1963.

Van Niekerk, B. D. H., Reid, J. T., Bensadoun, A., and Paladines, O. L.: Urinary creatinine as an index of body composition. J. Nutr. 79:463, 1963.

Washburn, T. C., Medearis, D. N., Jr., Childs, B.: Sex differences in susceptibility to infections. Pediatrics 35:57, 1965.

Waterlow, J. C., and Weisz, T.: The fat, protein and nucleic acid content of the liver in malnourished human infants. J. Clin. Invest. 35:346, 1956.

Whitehead, R. G.: Hydroxyproline creatinine ratio as an index of nutritional status and rate of growth. Lancet 2:567, 1965.

Widdowson, E. M., and Dickerson, J. W. T.: The effect of growth and function on the chemical composition of soft tissues. Biochem. J. 77:30, 1960.

Winick, M., and Noble, A.: Quantitative changes in DNA, RNA and protein during prenatal and postnatal growth in the rat. Developmental Biol. 12:451, 1965.

Winick, M., and Noble, A.: Quantitative changes in DNA, RNA and protein during normal growth of rat placenta. Nature (in press) 1966b.

Winick, M., and Noble, A.: Cellular response in rats during malnutrition at various ages. J. Nutrition 89:300, 1966a.

Winick, M., Coscia, A., and Noble, A.: Cellular growth in human placenta. I. Normal placental growth. Pediatrics 39:248, 1967.

Winick, M., and Noble, A.: Cellular response with increased feeding in neonatal rats. J. Nutrition 91:179, 1967.

Younoszai, M. K., Andersen, D. W., Filer, L. J., Jr., and Fomon, S. J.: Urinary excretion of hydroxyproline by normal infants during the first six months of life. To be published, 1967.

Chapter Three

Requirements, Recommended Dietary Allowances, and Advisable Intakes

The *requirement* of an individual for a specific nutrient may be defined as the least amount of that nutrient that will promote an optimal state of health. *"Recommended Dietary Allowances"* apply to a table of values periodically published by the Food and Nutrition Board, National Academy of Sciences—National Research Council. These recommendations, drawn up for the guidance of those charged with food procurement for groups of persons, do not necessarily apply to individuals. The designation *"advisable intakes"* is utilized in this book to indicate the amounts of various nutrients recommended for the individual. While both the Recommended Dietary Allowance and the advisable intake will be greater than the requirement, the Recommended Dietary Allowance usually will exceed the advisable intake because of the necessity for using broader age classifications and because of a natural tendency to overestimation of desirable intakes in food procurement. Unless clear distinction is made between these terms, confusion will result.

Meaning of "Requirements"

The requirement of an individual for a specific nutrient has already been defined. The meanings of the terms "requirement" and "minimal requirement" for an individual are identical.

As knowledge of nutrition increases, we may expect to achieve a more enlightened definition of the optimal state of health with respect to individual nutrients. At present, the requirement is necessarily determined primarily on the basis of freedom from all evidences of undernutrition attributable to deficiency of that particular nutrient. For some nutrients, these evidences of undernutrition are clinically detectable; but for others, biochemical evaluation is considerably more sensitive.

The requirement for a specified nutrient is clearly not an absolute value independent of other variables. In fact, the requirement actually has direct application only to those exact circumstances under which it was determined and, parenthetically, it is for this reason that tables of values for guidance of food procurers (Recommended Dietary Allowances) and tables of advisable intakes for infants such as those included in this book are of more practical value than requirement figures.

Not only does requirement frequently vary with age, size, rate of growth and level of activity, but relationships between various nutrients are of major importance. Requirements for various vitamins depend on intake of total calories, protein, fat, carbohydrate, specific amino acids and other vitamins (Gershoff, 1964). For example, because thiamine functions as an essential coenzyme in decarboxylation reactions, its requirement is related to the carbohydrate content of the diet; tryptophan, a niacin precursor, can substitute for part or all of the requirement for niacin. Requirements for individual amino acids increase when total protein content of the diet increases and requirement for one essential amino acid is related to intakes of others. Deficiency symptoms arising from inadequate intake of two essential amino acids may be aggravated by supplementing the diet with only one of these essential amino acids. In addition, the non-essential sulfur-containing amino acid, cystine, can substitute for a major portion of the requirement for the essential sulfur-containing amino acid, methionine.

Mineral imbalances may be far more common and important than we now recognize (Hoekstra, 1964). The tendency to think of calcium and phosphorus as a closely related pair of nutrients has been gradually superseded by an awareness of the close relationship of a tetrad of nutrients: calcium, phosphorus, magnesium and zinc. We do not know how many other major minerals and trace minerals must be considered before full understanding of these relationships is possible.

When discussing a nutrient requirement for a particular age group rather than for an individual, knowledge of the fiftieth percentile requirement of those in that age group (one half of normal individuals of the age will have greater requirements and one half will have lesser requirements) may be of particular value in certain instances, whereas knowledge of an intake that will fulfill the needs of nearly all normal individuals may be more significant in other circumstances.

Unfortunately, the designation, "daily requirement," may imply that deficiency will develop rather rapidly if this intake is not regularly achieved each day. Actually, for most vitamins and for certain other nutrients, an intake twice the daily requirement on one day will obviate the need for any intake of that nutrient on the next day. For example, sufficient amounts of most of the fat-soluble vitamins can be stored in the body to protect the individual for months against evidences of deficiency.

Although knowledge of requirements for specific nutrients may be of less immediate practical value than knowledge of the recommendations for intakes of these nutrients by some committee of experts, any such recommendations must ultimately be based on data concerning requirements. Without appreciation of the degree of confidence one may have in the stated value for requirement and without some knowledge of the philosophy which the committee or individual has employed in converting data on requirements into recommendations, any table of values will be of little use.

Meaning of "Recommended Dietary Allowances"

The Food and Nutrition Board of the National Academy of Sciences — National Research Council revises at regular intervals the publication, "Recommended Dietary Allowances." Since the text of the document reviews the deliberations of its various subcommittees, this publication has contributed greatly to knowledge of requirements for various nutrients (Food and Nutrition Board, 1964). The summary table presenting the recommended dietary allowances has, unfortunately, often been misused. The introduction to the booklet clearly specifies the intended use:

> The allowances are intended to serve as goals toward which to aim in planning food supplies and as guides for the interpretation of food consumption records of groups of people. Actual nutritional status of groups of people or individuals must be judged on the basis of physical, biochemical, and clinical observations combined with observations on food or nutrient intakes. If the recommended allowances are used as reference standards for interpreting records of food consumption, it should not be assumed that food practices are necessarily poor or that malnutrition exists because the recommendations are not completely met.

In guidance of those responsible for purchase of food for groups of individuals, simplicity must be a primary goal, and it is neither practical nor necessary to distinguish between the two-month-old and the four-month-old infant. If the four-month-old is adequately provided for, the purchase of a moderate excess for the two-month-old is of little concern.

Definition of "Advisable Intake"

If the requirement for a particular nutrient were the same under all conditions of diet, activity, environmental temperature and rates of growth; if all individuals in an age group had exactly the same requirement; and if optimal health with respect to that nutrient could be accurately defined, the advisable intake of a nutrient would be identical to the daily requirement. None of these suppositions is true.

The author has therefore arbitrarily selected as the advisable intake for most nutrients a value approximately twice the estimated requirement. Ideally, this estimated requirement would be the average requirement (i.e., 50 per cent of normal individuals of the specified age will have a greater requirement) determined under normal conditions of living and while receiving a diet providing adequate but not lavish amounts of all essential nutrients. It is presumed that requirements of nearly all normal individuals of the stated age under nearly all variations of living conditions will be satisfied by intakes twice the average requirement.

That such knowledge of average requirements in infancy is not available with respect to most nutrients is an indication of the need for much additional investigation. Meanwhile, it is necessary to utilize the best information available with the anticipation that revision of the values will be necessary at frequent intervals.

Two classes of exceptions must be mentioned with respect to the general concept that advisable intakes are to be considered approximately twice the average requirement. First, for some nutrients the margin between the requirement and the amount producing adverse effects is too narrow to warrant a twofold factor. Examples are total caloric intake, of which twice the average requirement is too great to represent an advisable intake, and fluoride, of which twice the requirement (for caries inhibition) may be responsible for a greater than desirable degree of mottling of the dental enamel. Second, it is apparent that the breast-fed infant consumes completely adequate amounts of certain nutrients during the early months of life even though such intakes may be less than twice the estimated requirement. In these instances, the intake of the breast-fed infant will be assumed to be the advisable intake unless other known differences between human milk and other infant diets suggest the need for greater intakes by the infant who is not breast fed.

When a young infant is breast-fed by a healthy, well-nourished mother and receives an adequate caloric intake from this source, requirements for most specific nutrients appear to be fulfilled. With the exceptions of iron, fluoride and vitamin D, there would seem to be no justification for supplementation of the diet of the breast-fed infant. Stated in another way, advisable intakes for all specific essential nutrients (with the exceptions noted) are provided during at least the first four or five months of life by breast feeding in adequate amounts.

As will be discussed in Chapter Eleven, considerable variability in composition of human milk supplied by different women causes some difficulty in establishing the intakes of various nutrients from an "adequate quantity" of human milk. With respect to some nutrients (e.g., vitamin A), it is apparent that an adequate caloric intake from human milk provides several times the required amounts. The advisable intake will then be set as twice the best available estimate of requirement.

Finally, in consideration of most nutrients it must be emphasized that an intake somewhat in excess of the requirement presents no known hazard and is to be preferred to long-continued ingestion of a diet providing a slight deficiency of the nutrient.

MEANS OF ACHIEVING ADVISABLE INTAKES. If readily available basic foods cannot be easily combined to provide all the essential nutrients, supplements of the lacking substances must be added in some manner. When a specific deficiency is identified as causing widespread ill health and is attributed to a general insufficiency, the inclination is to correct the deficiency by some sort of public health measure, such as enrichment of basic foods. This approach is considered preferable if enrichment is technically feasible and if individual prescription of a required dietary supplement proves undependable because of complexities in educating physicians regarding the need or because their instructions are not followed.

In the case of rickets, the prevalence of the disorder and the uncertainty that adequate prevention could be achieved by individual prescription of a dietary supplement made it seem reasonable to fortify virtually the entire milk supply with vitamin D. Similarly, addition of fluoride to drinking water has contributed to decreased incidence of dental caries.

The public health approach is not without problems. When many foods and separate supplements provide the full requirement of an essential nutrient and these foods are pushed with vigor for a place in the market, corresponding effort is required to prevent excessive intake. Many older infants and preschool children now receive several times the advisable intake of vitamin D (Committee on Nutrition, 1963). The essential role of the physician in educating parents in this respect is apparent.

REFERENCES

Committee on Nutrition, American Academy of Pediatrics: The prophylactic requirement and the toxicity of vitamin D. Pediatrics 31:512, 1963.

Food and Nutrition Board: Recommended Dietary Allowances. 6th ed. Washington, D.C., National Academy of Sciences—National Research Council, Publication 1146, 1964.

Gershoff, S. N.: Effects of dietary levels of macronutrients on vitamin requirements. Fed. Proc. 23:1077, 1964.

Hoekstra, W. G.: Recent observations on mineral interrelationships. Fed. Proc. 23: 1068, 1964.

Chapter Four

Voluntary Food Intake and Its Regulation

The quantity of food willingly accepted by an infant is determined to a large extent by basal caloric needs plus requirements for growth and muscular activity. Such factors as caloric concentration of the feeding, acceptability of a food (determined by taste, consistency and nutritional adequacy), and emotional factors also influence the quantity of food consumed and the total caloric intake.

In contrast to the situation with most individual nutrients, mild excess of *caloric* intake is likely to be just as undesirable as mild deficiency. A reasonable recommendation for caloric intake should, therefore, provide for the needs of as many infants as possible while risking overnutrition in as few as possible. A recommendation that is sufficient for nearly all normal individuals of a particular age group will almost certainly be excessive for many. Since it is not yet possible to make a recommendation for intake of calories on the basis of probable later consequences of mild overnutrition or mild undernutrition during infancy, the question of advisable intakes is approached on the basis of intakes observed in normal thriving infants fed ad libitum. These intakes are almost certainly adequate for the great majority of infants; whether they are excessive cannot yet be stated.

Formula Intake During Early Infancy

Amounts of formula consumed by normal infants will be influenced by age of introduction of cereal and strained foods and enthusiasm for these foods demonstrated by the parent or other individual responsible for feeding the infant. Table 4–1 and Figure 4–1 indicate volumes of intake and Figure 4–2 caloric intakes of normal full-size infants whose sole source of calories was milk or formula fed ad libitum at concentration of 67 kcal/100 ml (Fomon et al., 1964). Attention is called to the extent of individual variability in intake. For example, Table 4–1 indicates that 10 per cent of the infants accepted no more than 164 ml/kg/day (equal to 110 kcal/kg/day) between one and two months of age while 10 per cent of infants of the same age accepted at least 220 ml/kg/day (147 kcal/kg/day).

Differences in per kilogram intake are even more impressively related to age than to individual variability. From Figure 4–2 it may be seen that the great majority of infants ingested more than 120 kcal/kg/day during the first 60 days of life, but that relatively few accepted this level of caloric intake after 100 days of age.

As will be discussed in Chapter Six, fecal loss of fat may be considerable with some feedings, especially during the first month of life. When fecal fat loss is high, intake may be expected to be somewhat increased.

Since the quantity of food an infant will consume voluntarily is determined by bulk as well as by energy needs, caloric intakes depend to some extent on caloric concentrations of foods in the diet. Table 4–1 and Figures 4–1 and 4–2, therefore, are not predictive of intakes by infants fed formulas other than those providing 67 kcal/

Table 4–1. *Volume of Intake by Normal Infants Fed Ad Libitum* *

| Age | *Percentile Values for Volume of Intake (ml/kg/day)* | | | | |
	10th	25th	50th	75th	90th
5–12 days†	105	120	145	180	195
1 wk–1 mo	172	184	199	220	224
1 mo–2 mo	164	174	189	205	220
2 mo–3 mo	145	155	174	190	199
3 mo–4 mo	134	148	158	170	180
4 mo–5 mo	132	138	149	158	172

*Milk or formula at 67 kcal/100 ml provided sole source of calories.

†Data of Faber (1922) from study of 85 normal infants: other data are those of Fomon, Owen and Thomas (1964) from serial study of 82 infants.

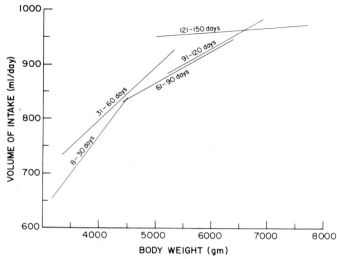

Figure 4–1. Volume of intake by normal infants receiving milk or formula as sole source of calories. The calculated regressions of volume of intake on body weight at various ages are shown. (From Fomon, S. J., et al.: Am. J. Dis. Child. *108*:601, 1964.)

100 ml nor are they predictive of caloric intakes by infants receiving appreciable amounts of cereal or strained foods.

Caloric Concentration of Formula

Total caloric intakes of full-size infants and of infants of low birth weight fed ad libitum have been shown to be influenced to a major extent by the caloric concentration of the formula. When a relatively dilute formula is offered, infants seem unwilling or unable to ingest the amounts of formula required to achieve caloric intakes

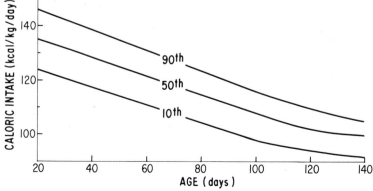

Figure 4–2. Caloric intake in relation to age of normal infants receiving milk or formula as sole source of calories. The 10th, 50th and 90th percentiles are indicated.

equal to those accepted by infants receiving the more commonly utilized formulas that provide 67 kcal/100 ml. Conversely, when calorically more concentrated formulas are offered, infants do not greatly decrease their volumes of intake. Caloric intakes are, therefore, considerably larger when feedings high in calories are offered.

Full-size infants receiving a relatively dilute formula (50 kcal/100 ml) were found by Doxiadis and Paschos (1962) to accept larger volumes than did those receiving a more concentrated formula (73 kcal/100 ml). However, the increased volume of intake by those receiving the dilute feeding was insufficient to compensate for the difference in caloric density so that total caloric intake was significantly less than that of infants receiving the more concentrated feed-

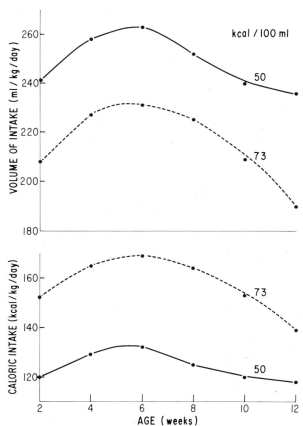

Figure 4–3. Influence of two levels of caloric concentration of feeding on volume of intake and intake of calories by full-term infants fed ad libitum (Data of Doxiadis and Paschos, 1962).

ing (Figure 4–3).* Mean rate of gain in weight by infants receiving the dilute feeding was approximately 72 per cent as great as that by the infants fed 73 kcal/100 ml.

Reports of most investigators suggest that when concentrated formulas (133 kcal/100 ml) are fed ad libitum to infants of low birth weight, rates of gain in weight are more rapid than those of infants of similar weight fed less concentrated formulas (67 kcal/100 ml). Results of observations by several investigators are presented in Table 4–2. Infants fed formulas supplying 67 kcal/100 ml had lesser caloric intakes than those fed more concentrated formulas. Weight gains were consistently more rapid in infants receiving the greater caloric intakes provided by more concentrated formulas.

Strained Foods

It seems probable that caloric density of foods offered to the infant modify total caloric intake to an important extent whether these foods happen to be liquid (that is, milk or formula) or solids (cereal or strained foods). Choice of solids and time of introduction of such foods in the diet, therefore, exert important influences on caloric intakes. The belief that young infants are unable to utilize tongue action to transfer foods from the front to the back of the mouth (Committee on Nutrition, 1958) no longer seems tenable. Time of introduction of solid foods must therefore be based on other considerations.

Physicians have ordinarily failed to appreciate the great variation in caloric concentrations of strained foods. As may be seen from Table 4–3 and Appendix I (p. 280), several strained foods, especially vegetables and some of the strained "breakfasts" and "dinners," offer fewer calories per unit of volume than does milk. However, greater caloric intakes per unit of volume are afforded by cereal as ordinarily fed and by most strained foods. Caloric concentrations are greatest in the case of egg yolk, meats (but not all "meat dinners"), cereals and "desserts." With these foods, caloric intakes per unit of volume range from one and one-half to three times that provided by milk.

The extent to which choice of strained foods can modify caloric intake may be illustrated by considering a hypothetic infant who receives 700 ml of milk (67 kcal/100 ml) and 300 gm of other foods. If his mother selects egg yolk, meats, cereal, desserts, "meat dinners,"

---

*No explanation can be given for the high volumes of intake observed in infants fed the formula providing 73 kcal/100 ml. Despite the high caloric intakes, mean rates of gain in weight (28.1 gm/day during the first three months of life) were less than those observed by the author and his associates in a larger group of normal full-size infants (Table 2–1, Chapter Two).

Table 4-2. *Influence of Two Levels of Caloric Concentration of Formula on Rate of Gain in Weight of Premature Infants*

Number of Infants	Initial Weight (gm)	Formula Concentration (kcal/100 ml)	Caloric Intake (kcal/kg/day)	Weight Gains (gm/day)	Comment	Investigators
10	1120–2040	133	155–180*	44	Growth rates of long bones not significantly different in two groups	Snyderman & Holt (1961)
11	1360–1930	67	120–130*	27		
115	1360–1770	138†	281	42	Values for weight gain calculated from assumed mean birth weight of 1565 gm and mean number of days to reach weight of 2500 gm	Falkner et al. (1962)
90	1360–1770	86‡	231	29		
11	1301–1700	133		42	Caloric intakes by infants receiving 133 kcal/100 ml twice as great as those by infants receiving 67 kcal/100 ml; growth rates of long bones not significantly different in two groups.	Combes & Pratt (1961)
13	1301–1700	67		32		

*After 10 days of age
†Mean value (range: 100–158).
‡Mean value (range: 67–100).

Table 4–3.   *Caloric Value of Strained Foods*
*Commercially Prepared for Infants**

Food	Caloric Concentration (kcal/100 gm)	Comments and Caloric Concentrations of Exceptions
Egg yolk	194–213	With or without bacon
Meats	90–138	Chicken, 121–138; beef heart and veal as low as 70
Cereals	108–112	1 part dry cereal, 6 parts milk Gerber high protein, 95; wet-packed cereals (including cereals with fruit or egg yolk and bacon), 72–96
Desserts (puddings, custards, etc)	82–113	Gerber fruit custard, 68; pineapple custard, 70
"Meat Dinners" or "High Meat Dinners"	63–85	Heinz and Beech-Nut products containing chicken, turkey or ham, 93–119
Fruit	65–86	Prunes, plums and fruit with cereal, 89–115
"Breakfasts" and "Dinners"	29–73	Label on jar distinguishes these from "Meat Dinners" or "High Meat Dinners" Heinz peas, vegetables and bacon, 93 Beech-Nut creamed cottage cheese food with pineapple juice, 90
Vegetables	24–53	Beech-Nut creamed corn, 85; Heinz creamed peas, 79; all brands potatoes, sweet potatoes, peas, 50–71
Juices Heinz Gerber Beech-Nut	23–55 34–47 51–67	Grape, 72; prune, 76 Orange with apricot, banana, pineapple, or prune, 80–87

*Data from Beech-Nut Professional and Consumer Services (1964), Gerber Professional Relations Department (1965) and Heinz International Research Center (1960).

and "high meat dinners" as the major items in his diet, total caloric intake will almost certainly average more than 800 kcal/day. However, if she selects predominantly vegetables, "breakfasts," "dinners" and fruit, it is unlikely that he will receive more than 700 kcal/day.

Data of Epps and Jolley (1963) concerning types of foods being fed to infants at the time of their first visit to a clinic in Washington,

D. C., are of interest. As may be seen from Table 4–4, the majority received cereal or other strained foods during the early months of life; between one and two months of age all but 39 of 226 infants were receiving foods other than milk or formula. Of infants receiving solid foods, nearly all of those between one and four months of age received cereal. Percentages of infants fed fruit, vegetables and meat increased with increasing age.

An indication of the approximate costs of foods fed to infants has been included in a publication of the Maternal and Child Health and Food and Nutrition Sections of the American Public Health Association (1966). From the data presented in this publication it may be seen that cereals commercially prepared for infants are inexpensive, strained meats and egg yolks are expensive, and other foods are intermediate in cost.

Caloric Intakes by Infants Receiving Mixed Diets

As might be anticipated on the basis of the previous discussion, normal full-size infants fed cereal and strained foods in appreciable quantities in addition to milk or formula generally accept greater caloric intakes than those whose only or principal food is milk or formula. Figure 4–4 summarizes data on intake of calories reported by several groups of investigators.

The greater caloric intakes by some infants (Beal, 1953; Rueda-Williamson and Rose, 1962) than by others (Fomon et al., 1964) are probably due, at least in part, to augmentation of caloric intake in the former group by feeding of cereal and strained foods. Data accumulated by Filer and Martinez (1964) from a study of 4146 "representative" infants between five and eight months of age (mean age

Table 4–4. Types of Foods in Diets of Normal Infants at Time of First Visit to Clinic*

Age (months)	Total	No Solids	Cereal	Fruit	Vegetables	Meat
			Number of Infants†			
1–2	226	39	186	94	26	3
2–3	152	6	144	116	60	17
3–4	65	0	64	61	39	18

*Data of Epps and Jolley, 1963.
†A few infants received meat or table foods.

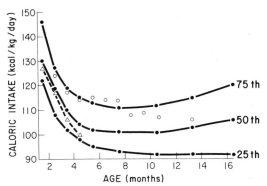

Figure 4–4. Caloric intakes by normal full-term infants studied by several investigators. Solid lines indicate 25th, 50th and 75th percentiles reported by Beal (1953) from serial study of 46 infants; open circles indicate 50th percentile values reported by Rueda-Williamson and Rose (1962) from study of 67 infants. The interrupted line indicates 50th percentile values reported by Fomon et al. (1964) from study of infants receiving milk or formula as sole source of calories (see Table 4–1 and Figure 4–1).

6.8 months) suggest that the values reported by Beal may, in fact, be reasonably characteristic of the general population. In Beal's sample of 18 boys and 28 girls, median intake was 750 kcal/day for infants five to six months of age and 825 kcal/day for infants six to nine months of age. Filer and Martinez reported mean values of 846 kcal/day for boys and 798 kcal/day for girls at a mean age of 6.8 months. The data of Guthrie (1963) are generally similar.

Skim Milk versus Whole Milk

A question not infrequently asked by parents concerns the substitution of skim milk for whole milk in the feeding of infants. Presumably, parents (and some physicians) decide that skim milk is preferable to whole milk as a basic component of the infant's diet either because they wish to prevent excessive weight gain through reduction in caloric intake or because they wish to decrease the quantity of saturated fatty acids in the diet. Consideration of the consequences of such substitution on caloric intake of the infant clearly indicates the need for attention to the choice of solid foods for the infant.

If one assumes that a four-month-old infant weighing 7 kg ingests the amounts and types of food indicated in Table 4–5, he would receive 147 gm of food and 107 kcal/kg. These intakes fall at about the 50th percentile values for normal infants. Protein, carbohydrate and fat contribute 18, 42, and 40 per cent, respectively, of the calories. If this hypothetic infant were given exactly the same food except

Table 4–5. *Caloric Intake of Hypothetic Four-month-old Infant Weighing Seven Kilograms*

Food	Amount (gm)	Energy (kcal)	Protein (gm)	Carbo-hydrate (gm)	Fat (gm)
Whole milk	780	523	25.7	37.4	28.9
Rice cereal	50				
cereal, 7 gm		26	0.8	5.5	0.3
whole milk, 43 gm		29	1.4	2.1	1.6
Applesauce	134	117	0.3	28.4	0.3
Strained beef with vegetables	64	52	4.2	3.5	2.4
	1028	747	32.4	76.9	33.5
			(18% of calories)	(42% of calories)	(40% of calories)

that whole milk was replaced by an equal volume of skim milk (33 kcal/100 ml), he would receive only 67 kcal/kg.

If skim milk replaced whole milk in the diet indicated in Table 4–5 and intakes of other foods were doubled, an adequate caloric intake would be achieved (101 kcal/kg) but food intake would increase to 180 gm/kg, probably greater than a substantial percentage of infants can tolerate. In addition, the diet would be deficient in essential fatty acids (Chapter Six) and relatively high in protein and renal solute load (Chapter Nine).

Employment of half-skim (50 kcal/100 ml) rather than skim milk in the diet and inclusion of foods exceptionally high in caloric density (Table 4–3) would reduce the necessity for ingestion of large quantities of food, but the diet would probably remain deficient in essential fatty acids. Addition of a small amount of corn oil could correct the latter deficiency.

It is therefore *possible* to devise a satisfactory diet based on skim milk or half-skim milk, but considerable care will be required. The infant must not be permitted to drink so much skim milk or half-skim milk (with their low caloric densities) that he will be unable to consume an adequate quantity of foods of higher caloric density. Selection of certain strained foods and avoidance of others is more important than with diets based on whole milk. Altogether, it seems that management becomes quite complicated when whole milk is eliminated from the diet. Even if the goals of weight control and reduction in dietary intake of saturated fatty acids could be shown to be desirable during infancy, the adverse effects of a poorly devised diet would almost certainly overshadow any benefit.

Attitude of Individual Caring for Infant

The attitude of the individual who feeds the infant is undoubtedly reflected to some extent in the volume of formula consumed. Infants studied by Fomon et al. (1964) were fed the largest volume of milk or formula they would accept consistently rather than the least amount that would seem to relieve hunger. According to another philosophy of feeding, 56 infants between 29 and 56 days of age studied by Brown et al. (1960) were offered approximately 165 ml/kg/day of formula, and this volume was not increased unless excessive crying between feedings suggested that the infants were dissatisfied.* Under these circumstances, the median intake was 168 ml/kg/day, a value considerably less than the median intake of 189 ml/kg/day reported by Fomon et al. (1964) (Table 4–1).

Similarly, the question of whether infants are reluctant to accept food from the spoon until 2 1/2 to 3 1/2 months of age (Beal, 1957) or accept it readily at two to three days of age (Sackett, 1962) probably depends largely on the attitude of the individual feeding the infant.

Although physical characteristics of the food, such as consistency and lumpiness, are clearly important in feeding of small infants, acceptance of various food items by infants may depend more on maternal attitudes than on the infant himself. Manufacturers of strained foods for infants have long recognized that taste and odor of the products must be acceptable to mothers as well as to infants. If a product seems particularly unattractive to a mother, she is likely to interpret the infant's response to it as unfavorable.

In considering foods of equal caloric concentration per unit of volume, data are not available to indicate relative satiety values. We do not know, for example, whether feeding 100 gm of strained fruit providing 67 kcal/100 gm contributes more to satiety than does feeding an equal quantity of milk.

Studies of experimental animals as well as clinical observations of human subjects of various ages suggest that deficiency of any essential nutrient in the diet may be associated with decreased food intake (Committee on Nutrition, 1964). Much further study is needed in relation to this and other factors determining food intake by infants.

Recommendations

Since the infant's caloric intake may be greatly modified by such factors as the age at which cereal or strained foods are introduced, the choice of such foods and the extent of substitution of

---

*Personal communication from Dr. G. W. Brown.

other foods for milk, the physician should be prepared to offer some direction to parents in relation to these aspects of infant feeding. As indicated at the beginning of the chapter, no firm basis yet exists for making a recommendation concerning desirable caloric intakes for infants. Only tentative recommendations can be offered. For full-term infants the data of Fomon et al. (Fig. 4–1) and of Beal (Fig. 4–4) may serve as general guides indicating suitable caloric intakes by infants believed to be thriving. When intakes are greatly in excess of the 75th or considerably less than the 25th percentile values, some adjustment of caloric intake may be desirable because of the possible danger of permanent nutritional imprinting (Chapter Fourteen). Rates of gain in weight and the relation between rates of gain in length and in weight should probably be taken into consideration before adjusting the diet. It seems doubtful that caloric intake should be limited when an infant is growing extremely rapidly in both length and weight. On the other hand, the combination of large caloric intake and rapid gain in weight in the absence of rapid change in length suggests overfeeding and may warrant some reduction in caloric intake.

Practical measures for increasing caloric intake include early introduction of cereal and strained foods, use of a formula more concentrated than 67 kcal/100 ml, and choice of strained foods rich in calories rather than those relatively poor in calories (Table 4–3 and Appendix I). Caloric intakes may be decreased by substitution of strained foods of low caloric value for a portion of the milk intake and for high-caloric strained foods.

Special considerations pertaining to infants of low birth weight are given in Chapter Thirteen.

REFERENCES

Committee on Nutrition, American Academy of Pediatrics: Factors affecting food intake. Pediatrics 33:135, 1964.

Committee on Nutrition, American Academy of Pediatrics: On the feeding of solid foods to infants. Pediatrics 21:685, 1958.

Beal, V. A.: Nutritional intake of children. J. Nutr. 50:223, 1953.

Beal, V. A.: On the acceptance of solid foods, and other food patterns, of infants and children. Pediatrics 20:448, 1957.

Beech-Nut Professional and Consumer Services: Nutritive Values and Ingredients of Beech-Nut Baby Foods. New York, Beech-Nut Baby Foods, 1964.

Brown, G. W., Tuholski, J. M., Sauer, L. W., Minsk, L. D., and Rosenstern, I.: Evaluation of prepared milks for infant nutrition; use of the Latin square technique. J. Pediat. 56:391, 1960.

Combes, M. A., and Pratt, E. L.: Premature infants and concentrated feeding. Am. J. Dis. Child. 102:610, (Abstract.) 1961.

Doxiadis, S. A., and Paschos, A.: Feeding behavior and growth in the first three months of life. *In* Merminod, A. (ed.): Modern Problems in Pediatrics. New York, Karger, Vol. 7, 1962, p. 202.

Epps, R. P., and Jolley, M. P.: Unsupervised early feeding of solids to infants. Med. Ann. District Columbia 32:493, 1963.

Faber, H. K.: Food requirements in new-born infants. Am. J. Dis. Child. 24:56, 1922.

Falkner, F., Steigman, A. J., and Cruse, M. O.: The physical development of the premature infant. I. Some standards and certain relationships to caloric intake. J. Pediat. 60:895, 1962.

Filer, L. J., Jr., and Martinez, G.: Intake of selected nutrients by infants in the United States. Clin. Pediat. 3:633, 1964.

Fomon, S. J., Owen, G. M., and Thomas, L. N.: Milk or formula volume ingested by infants fed ad libitum. Am. J. Dis. Child. 108:601, 1964.

Gerber Professional Relations Department: Nutritive Values of Gerber Baby Foods. Fremont, Michigan, Gerber Products Co., 1965.

Guthrie, H. A.: Nutritional intake of infants. J. Am. Dietet. A. 43:120, 1963.

Heinz International Research Center and Heinz Research Fellowship of Mellon Institute: Nutritional Data. 4th ed. Pittsburgh, H. J. Heinz Co., 1960.

Maternal and Child Health and Food and Nutrition Sections, American Public Health Association: Economy and nutrition in feeding of infants. Am. J. Public Health 56:1756, 1966.

Rueda-Williamson, R., and Rose, H. E.: Growth and nutrition of infants. The influence of diet and other factors of growth. Pediatrics 30:639, 1962.

Sackett, W. W.: Bringing Up Babies: A Family Doctor's Practical Approach to Child Care. New York, Harper & Row, 1962, p. 55.

Snyderman, S. E., and Holt, L. E., Jr.: The effect of high caloric feeding on the growth of premature infants. J. Pediat. 58:237, 1961.

Chapter Five

Protein

Since most infants in technically advanced countries receive diets that provide abundant amounts of high quality protein, problems of gross protein deficiency and amino acid deficiency are infrequently met. Nevertheless, an understanding of protein needs, both quantitatively and qualitatively, is essential in evaluation of new infant formulas that continue to appear on the market, in management of infants who are unwilling or unable to accept usual diets and in management of those with exceptional requirements, as in phenylketonuria and other disorders characterized by specific defects in amino acid metabolism.

For a complete presentation of current concepts in protein metabolism the reader is referred to the excellent publication of Munro and Allison (1964). The present chapter emphasizes some of the aspects believed of most value in relation to infant nutrition. These include methods commonly used for estimating protein quality, nature of essential amino acids, meaning of amino acid imbalance and factors modifying requirements for amino acids and protein. In the light of these considerations, tentative statements will be made about requirements and advisable daily intakes of protein and amino acids.

Calculated Protein Intake

The protein content of a food is generally estimated on the basis of analysis of the food for nitrogen, together with a calculation based on the assumption that nitrogen accounts for approximately 16 per cent by weight of protein. A factor of 6.25 (100 ÷ 16 = 6.25) is therefore commonly used for conversion of nitrogen to protein in infants' diets; use of this factor will rarely result in important error when dietary protein is of high quality. In the case of proteins of lesser quality, the factor 6.25 may not be appropriate since the assortment of amino acids varies from protein to protein and each amino acid has its own ratio of nitrogen to total weight. McCance and Widdowson (1960) have suggested a factor of 5.5 for gelatin and 5.7 for cereals. Although certain foods contain significant amounts of non-protein nitrogen (e.g., 20 per cent of the nitrogen in human milk), a portion of the non-protein nitrogen may consist of free amino acids that are utilized by the body in nearly the same manner as protein; some of the remainder can probably also be utilized for tissue synthesis (Snyderman et al., 1962).

Essential Amino Acids

Essential amino acids are those that "cannot be synthesized by the animal body from materials readily available at a speed commensurate with the demands for normal growth" (Rose, 1938). For the human infant these amino acids are arginine, isoleucine, leucine, lysine, methionine, phenylalanine, threonine, tryptophan, valine and histidine. Omission of any essential amino acid has been found to result in immediate and complete cessation of growth (or, in the case of arginine, reduced rate of growth). Histidine is essential for the human infant but apparently can be synthesized adequately by the adult.

Since two of the nonessential amino acids, tyrosine and cystine, can be formed by the human body only from phenylalanine and methionine, respectively, the requirements for phenylalanine and methionine are modified by the amounts of tyrosine and cystine in the diet. In addition, since tryptophan functions as a precursor of niacin, dietary intake of niacin is important in establishing the requirement for tryptophan.

As defined by Harper (1964a), amino acid toxicity (or antagonism) applies to adverse effects resulting from administration of excessive amounts of an amino acid; amino acid imbalance applies to conditions of amino acid deficiency in which the evidences of deficiency are exaggerated by administration of one or more amino acids. An example of amino acid imbalance is presented in Table 5–1. Rats in group 1 received a diet deficient in threonine while those in group 2 received a diet equally deficient in threonine but supplemented

Table 5–1. Effects of Amino Acid Imbalance on Weight Gain of Rats*

Group	Diet	Weight Gain in 2 Weeks (gm)
1	6% casein	18
2	6% casein, amino acid mixture	10
3	6% casein, amino acid mixture, threonine	21

*Data of Harper et al. (1964b).

with other indispensable amino acids. This amino acid supplementation resulted in further depression of growth rate, which was overcome (group 3) by administering a supplement of threonine.

In technically advanced countries where infants receive proteins of high quality, amino acid deficiency or imbalance is extremely rare. However, with the ever-increasing list of congenital metabolic disorders of amino acid metabolism, an understanding of deficiency and imbalance seems essential if we are to design and evaluate special diets for individuals with these disorders.

Protein Quality

Tests with Animals

The quality of a protein depends on its ability to supply essential amino acids in sufficient amounts to fulfill all the requirements for maintenance and growth. Terms most widely employed in discussions of protein quality are protein efficiency ratio (PER), biologic value (BV), true digestibility (D), net protein utilization (NPU), chemical score and nitrogen balance. These are defined in the chapter appendix (page 76).

Ideally, proteins to be used for feeding human infants should be evaluated in the normal human infant. However, the difficulty in devising sound experiments is exceptionally great, and practical considerations make it essential that all initial studies be done with experimental animals. Since, with few exceptions, the growing human subject closely resembles the growing rat in metabolic utilization of food proteins, a number of tests of protein quality have been developed with the weanling rat as the assay animal.

The method most widely used for determining quality of protein is the PER, which relates rate of gain in weight of weanling rats to amount of protein consumed under standardized conditions (see chapter appendix). Concentration of protein in the diet is less than that required for maximal growth rates of the animals.

Although a number of criticisms have been raised concerning the method (Mitchell, 1944; Bender and Doell, 1957), only three seem to be of major significance with respect to evaluation of protein quality for the human infant or child. First, since PER varies with dietary level of protein, results of the standardized assay with rats may not be predictive of the relative values of these proteins under the conditions obtaining when they are fed to the human infant. Second, the weanling rat probably requires proportionately more of its protein intake for maintenance and less for growth than is true of the human infant. Quality of a protein for growth may not be identical to quality for maintenance. Third, requirements of growing rats for certain essential amino acids are different from those of the human infant; for example, the growing rat probably requires more of the sulfur-containing amino acids than does the human infant.

In spite of these limitations, the PER may be assumed to provide a generally useful index of the amount of the limiting essential amino acid in the diet. Among its major advantages are simplicity, convenience and the widespread use of standardized methods.

Chemical Score

Since a protein of high quality is one that supplies all essential amino acids in relation to their need for maintenance and growth, the relative amounts of various amino acids in the protein has been employed as the basis for several scoring systems. Such systems have compared the concentration of a limiting essential amino acid in a test protein with its concentration in a reference protein. The reference protein has generally been whole egg or a hypothetic protein in which ratios between concentrations of amino acids are identical to the supposed requirement ratios. In general, the higher the protein score, the higher the biologic value, although proteins such as zein and maize, each devoid of one essential amino acid, have some biologic value in spite of a protein score of zero.

Three major limitations of chemical scoring should be noted: (1) Protein quality may be altered without change in content of specific amino acids. For example, the influence of moist heat in the processing of soy protein is beneficial since it inactivates a trypsin inhibitor that otherwise interferes with protein quality. Thus, protein quality is improved without change in protein score. Conversely, various amino acids may become unavailable to the organism because of the Maillard reaction in which amino acids combine with sugars in the presence of heat. This reaction is particularly likely to affect the availability of lysine, methionine and cystine. Thus, even a protein supplying generous amounts of all essential amino acids might prove inadequate because of unavailability of one or more essential amino acids. Carpenter (1958, 1960) has reported a method that may be suitable for estimating the proportion of lysine molecules damaged by heat, but convenient methods for estimating availability of other amino acids have not been developed. (2) Requirement for nitrogen may in some circumstances be limiting even though requirements for all essential amino acids are met (Snyderman et al., 1962). Such nitrogen could be supplied as essential or nonessential amino acids and, apparently, to some extent as forms other than amino acids (for example, urea, ammonia). (3) The chosen reference protein may not, in fact, reflect the amino acid requirements of the individual for the purpose intended. Requirements probably differ for growth and for maintenance; therefore, a reference protein reflecting requirements of the human adult may not be completely satisfactory as an indication of the needs of the rapidly growing human infant.

Adequacy of Protein Intake Studied With Human Infants

Growth of Human Infants

When a diet is grossly deficient in protein or in one of the essential amino acids, growth will fail to progress normally. However, in the presence of mild protein deficiency, it is possible that growth in length and weight will proceed normally. Quite possibly the composition of such weight gain will be abnormal, but such abnormality is unlikely to be detected by clinical appraisal. Under certain circumstances (to be discussed) serum concentrations of albumin may prove to be more sensitive than growth rate as an index of protein nutritional status and as a means of comparing the nutritional adequacy of two diets.

Development of various techniques for determining body composition of the normal infant will in the future permit estimation of changes in certain body components as well as in body weight. As discussed in Chapter Two, serial studies of total body water have already provided useful data. Rates of urinary excretion of endogenous creatinine and hydroxyproline by infants of the same age and sex may reflect, respectively, relative amounts of muscle and rates of synthesis of collagen. When reliable estimates of total body potassium of infants can be made by whole body counting for ^{40}K, an estimate of fat-free body mass will also be possible. Thus, in the future it seems probable that the quality of protein may be assessed in normal infants on the basis of gain in fat-free dry tissue rather than on the basis of gain in total weight.

Nitrogen Balance Studies With Human Infants

Nitrogen balance is affected by many factors, including age, state of health, nitrogen content of diet, amino acid deficiency or imbalance, deficiency of other essential dietary factors, and caloric intake. Failure to control these variables has often led to misinterpretation of data from nitrogen balance studies. In addition, rate of synthesis of body protein may be overestimated if based on calculations involving nitrogen balance studies (Wallace, 1959; Fomon and Owen, 1962a).

Requirements for satisfactory studies with infants are as follows: (1) Groups of infants should be matched with respect to age, size and state of health. Lack of general availability of normal full-size infants for such studies means that infants of low birth weight or infants recovering from disease are generally utilized, and the difficulty in matching groups of such subjects is great. The practice of studying two diets alternately with the same subject, although possibly desirable in studies of infants older than six months of age, is of little value with small infants. Differences in nitrogen balance among carefully matched infants of the same age are likely to be less than differences in nitrogen balance recorded with the same infant at different ages. (2) Diets should be identical in protein concentration and, as nearly as possible, in other constituents. Comparisons of protein quality are more sensitive when performed at an intake of protein approximating the requirement than when intake is considerably in excess of the requirement. Ad libitum feeding is more practical than pair feeding. (3) In analyzing the data, both age and nitrogen intake must be considered. With identical intakes per kilogram of body weight, retention of nitrogen per kilogram will be greater for younger than for older infants.

The relation between retention of nitrogen and intake of nitrogen by normal infants receiving protein from various sources is illustrated in Figure 5–1.

In prolonged feeding studies of normal full-size infants, nitrogen balance appears to be less sensitive than serum concentration of albumin as an index of nutritional adequacy of the diet. (See page 65.) However, in studies of infants recovering from protein-calorie malnutrition, nitrogen balance studies may be of considerable value in comparison of nutritional quality of feedings (Scrimshaw et al., 1958; Bressani, 1960; Hansen and Freesemann, 1960; Rice and Flodin, 1960; Waterlow and Wills, 1960).

Serum Concentrations of Protein

Although normal concentration of albumin in serum does not guarantee normal nutritional status with respect to protein, abnormally low concentrations strongly imply inadequate nutritional status. Values characteristic of normal infants as presented in Tables 5–2 to 5–6 are therefore of interest.

Concentrations of total protein and albumin in the serum of normal full-size infants decrease rather abruptly after birth and then

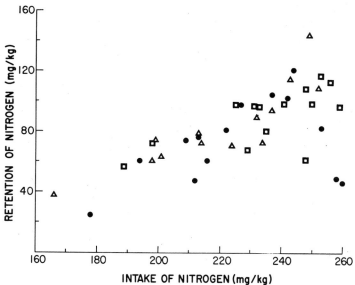

Figure 5–1. Relation of retention of nitrogen to intake of nitrogen by infants 29 to 84 days of age. Each point indicates results of one three-day nitrogen balance study with an infant fed pooled human milk (dots) (Fomon and May, 1958), a formula with protein from cow milk (squares) (Fomon, 1960; Fomon and Owen, 1962b) or a formula with protein from soy (triangles) (Fomon, 1959; Fomon et al., 1964; Fomon and Filer, unpublished).

Table 5–2. *Concentrations of Total Protein and Albumin in Relation to Age of Normal Full-Size Infants**

Age	Number of Subjects†	Total Protein (gm/100 ml)		Albumin (gm/100 ml)	
		Mean	Standard deviation	Mean	Standard deviation
<36 hr	142 & 113	6.47	0.52	4.33	0.38
8 days	161 & 130	6.02	0.43	4.00	0.36
1 mo‡	124	5.81	0.36	4.17	0.34
2 mo	91 & 87	6.07	0.39	4.45	0.39
3 mo	78 & 74	6.19	0.35	4.59	0.44
4 mo	75 & 59	6.32	0.43	4.73	0.50
5 mo	60 & 49	6.55	0.44	4.81	0.55
6 mo	49 & 45	6.56	0.48	4.81	0.47
7 mo	39 & 30	6.75	0.47	4.93	0.55
8 mo	34 & 31	6.73	0.40	5.08	0.36
9 mo	23 & 22	6.75	0.44	4.96	0.39
10 mo	18 & 11	7.09	0.42	5.16	0.15
11 mo	11 & 9	6.80	0.42	5.20	0.47
12–18 mo	18	7.05	0.41	5.16	0.22
adult	31	7.21	0.39	4.87	0.25

*Data of Levin et al., 1959.

†When two numbers are given, the first applies to total protein, the second to albumin.

‡The designation 1 month indicates that infant is at least one month of age, but has not yet reached two months of age.

gradually increase (Table 5–2 and Fig. 5–2). Concentrations of albumin equal to those of the adult are achieved by about five months of age. During the first few months of life, concentrations of both total protein and albumin are less for infants of low birth weight than for full-size infants (Table 5–3). Sex-related differences in concentration of serum proteins have not been demonstrated (Levin et al., 1959; Rogers et al., 1967).

Serum concentrations of globulins as reported by various investigators from studies with free or paper electrophoresis are indicated in relation to age in Tables 5–4 and 5–5. Particularly noteworthy is the initial rapid and later more gradual decrease in concentration of gamma globulin during the first six months of life.

Table 5–6 and Figure 5–3 present observations on the relation between diet during the early months of life and concentrations of proteins in serum of 112-day-old infants as determined by serum electrophoresis on cellulose acetate. Mean concentration of albumin in serum of the breast-fed infants was significantly greater than that of infants fed evaporated milk (t = 2.84; p < 0.01), Similac PM 60/40

Table 5–3. *Concentrations of Total Protein and Albumin in Relation to Age of Infants With Birth Weight Less Than 2500 Grams**

Age	Number of Subjects[†]	Total Protein (gm/100 ml)		Albumin (gm/100 ml)	
		Mean	Standard deviation	Mean	Standard deviation
<36 hr	24 & 15	6.05	0.77	3.93	0.60
8 days	61 & 45	5.44	0.55	3.63	0.40
1 mo[‡]	90 & 87	5.33	0.53	3.96	0.46
2 mo	69 & 67	5.71	0.41	4.30	0.36
3 mo	49 & 44	5.96	0.45	4.61	0.45
4 mo	52 & 44	6.19	0.43	4.60	0.43
5 mo	36 & 33	6.35	0.52	4.68	0.49
6 mo	28 & 22	6.51	0.38	4.84	0.37
7 mo	24 & 24	6.62	0.43	4.99	0.42
8 mo	29 & 26	6.62	0.36	5.02	0.36
9 mo	20 & 17	6.64	0.39	5.02	0.41
10 mo	11 & 11	6.86	0.52	5.04	0.14
11 mo	10 & 7	6.93	0.46	5.08	0.24
12–17 mo	16 & 14	7.00	0.38	5.21	0.23

*Data of Levin et al., 1959.

†The first number applies to determinations of total protein, the second to determinations of albumin.

‡The designation 1 month indicates that infant is at least one month of age, but has not yet reached two months of age.

(t = 2.22; p < 0.05) an experimental formula (CP 29A) providing 11 per cent of calories from soy isolate (t = 2.39; p < 0.02), or an experimental formula providing 6 per cent of calories from soy isolate (t = 5.55; p < 0.001).

The nutritional implications of the higher serum concentrations of albumin in breast-fed infants than in those receiving the other feedings cannot be stated at present. With respect to the soy isolate formula providing 6 per cent of calories from protein, concentrations of albumin appear to be consistently low: all values were below the median for breast-fed infants and nine of 23 values were below the range encountered with breast-fed infants. It seems probable that these low concentrations of albumin in the serum reflect nutritional inadequacy of the feeding. If so, serum concentration of albumin in this instance proved to be a more sensitive index of nutritional adequacy of the diet than were rates of gain in length and weight (Fig. 2–3) or nitrogen balance studies (Fig. 5–1).

Table 5-4. *Total Protein and Protein Fractions in Serum in Relation to Age as Determined by Various Investigators Using Free Electrophoresis**

Author	Serum or Plasma	No. of Cases	Age	Protein (g./100 ml.)					
				Total	Albumin	α_1-globulin	α_2-globulin	β-globulin	γ-globulin
Longsworth et al. (1945)	Serum	11	Cord blood	6.17	3.82	0.29	0.49	0.60	0.97
Knapp and Routh (1949)	Plasma	11	6–46 weeks	6.36	3.92	0.43	0.82	0.74	0.21
	,,	10	1–4 years	7.20	4.37	0.46	0.77	0.80	0.52
Levin et al. (1950)	Serum	Pool of 50	0–36 hours	6.52	3.71		0.76	0.91	1.14
	,,	Pool of 50	7–9 days	6.11	3.25		0.84	1.07	0.95
	,,	Pool of 33	28–59 days	6.01	3.86		0.94	0.73	0.48
Ewerbeck and Levens (1950)	Serum	7	Cord blood	5.8	3.70		0.50	0.38	1.21
Imperato (1951)	Serum	17	Cord blood	5.27	3.36		0.32	0.42	1.18
	,,	2	2–4 days	5.41	3.45		0.52	0.31	1.14
	,,	6	9–23 days	4.99	3.14		0.62	0.44	0.79
	,,	7	27 days–2 months	5.01	3.41		0.58	0.45	0.57
	,,	6	2–6 months	5.42	3.66		0.75	0.57	0.44
	,,	7	6–10 months	5.85	3.68		0.76	0.57	0.84
	,,	9	1–2 years	6.02	3.78		0.74	0.65	0.84
Norton et al.† (1952)	Serum	3	1–3 days	6.20	3.59	0.36	0.54	0.79	0.87
	,,	11	5–12 days	5.69	3.60	0.30	0.51	0.60	0.66
	,,	16	15–30 days	5.12	3.18	0.33	0.61	0.60	0.42
	,,	7	31–65 days	4.54	2.82	0.40	0.54	0.56	0.23
Caspani et al.‡ (1953)	Serum	8	Cord blood	6.43	3.82	0.40	0.52	0.59	1.09
	,,	6	1 month–1 year	6.67	4.0	0.49	0.80	0.69	0.70
	,,	5	1½–5 years	7.39	4.42	0.41	1.07	0.85	0.75
	,,	3	9–13 years	7.12	3.86	0.57	0.91	0.84	0.93

*From Levin et al., 1959. (Courtesy of Privy Council – Medical Research Council Special Report Series, No. 296. Her Majesty's Stationery Office.)
†Premature infants.
‡Calculated from authors' data.

Table 5-5. *Total Protein and Protein Fractions in Serum of Full-Size Infants in Relation to Age**

Age	No. of Observations	Protein (g./100 ml.)					
		Total Protein	Albumin	α_1-globulin	α_2-globulin	β-globulin	γ-globulin
		Paper electrophoresis					
Cord blood	21	6·25	3·77	0·20	0·58	0·50	1·20
0–36 hours	8	6·10	3·61	0·23	0·52	0·62	1·12
7–9 days	5	5·65	3·15	0·21	0·60	0·67	1·02
28 days–under 2 months .	7	5·75	3·86	0·12	0·62	0·62	0·53
Calendar months { 2–under 3 .	13	5·84	3·67	0·19	0·75	0·71	0·52
3–under 4 .	5	6·04	3·70	0·20	0·91	0·76	0·47
4–under 6 .	8	6·25	4·08	0·18	0·78	0·78	0·43
6–under 8 .	10	6·56	4·13	0·17	0·80	0·87	0·59
8–under 10 .	8	6·56	4·02	0·20	0·87	0·83	0·64
10–under 13 .	6	6·48	4·15	0·18	0·72	0·80	0·63
13–under 24 .	5	6·93	4·27	0·24	0·73	0·97	0·72
Adults	6	7·32	4·57	0·23	0·57	0·88	1·07
		Free electrophoresis on pooled sera					
0–36 hours	50	6·52	3·71		0·76	0·91	1·14
7–9 days	50	6·11	3·25		0·84	1·07	0·95
28 days–under 2 months .	33	6·01	3·86		0·94	0·73	0·48

*From Levin et al., 1959. (Courtesy of Privy Council–Medical Research Council Special Report Series, No 296, Her Majesty's Stationery Office.)

Table 5–6. *Concentrations of Proteins in Sera of Normal
112-Day-Old Infants in Relation to Feeding**

Feeding†	Number of Subjects	Total Protein (gm/100 ml)	Albumin (gm/100 ml)	Globulins (gm/100 ml)			
				α_1	α_2	β	γ
Breast fed	64	6.37 (0.54)‡	4.36 (0.39)	0.17 (0.03)	0.91 (0.16)	0.63 (0.15)	0.31 (0.10)
EM	26	6.10 (0.56)	4.01 (0.36)	0.13 (0.06)	0.88 (0.17)	0.72 (0.13)	0.37 (0.12)
PM 60/40	24	6.03 (0.66)	4.04 (0.46)	0.17 (0.06)	0.85 (0.19)	0.59 (0.11)	0.34 (0.09)
CP 29-A	10	5.92 (0.31)	4.02 (0.15)	0.18 (0.05)	0.74 (0.10)	0.67 (0.06)	0.30 (0.09)
3207 H	23	5.50 (0.39)	3.72 (0.27)	0.19 (0.02)	0.77 (0.14)	0.53 (0.14)	0.28 (0.07)

*Data of Rogers et al., 1967
†Formulas provided approximately 67 kcal/100 ml., CP 29-A and 3207 H are experimental formulas made from soy isolate fortified with methionine. 3207 H provided 6 per cent of calories from protein and CP 29-A provided 11 per cent of calories from this source. EM refers to equal parts of evaporated milk and water without added carbohydrate. PM 60/40 is Similac PM 60/40 (Table 11–8).
‡Values in parentheses are standard deviations.

Concentration of Urea Nitrogen in Serum

Concentration of urea nitrogen in serum reflects recent dietary intake of protein (or nitrogen) rather than nutritional status with respect to protein. Without knowledge of the intake of protein, it is quite impossible to interpret the concentration of urea nitrogen in serum. As may be seen from Table 5–7 and Figure 5–4, among healthy breast-fed infants (6 to 7 per cent of calories from protein) only about 2.5 per cent were found to have serum concentrations greater than 12 mg/100 ml (mean plus two standard deviations). When 20 per cent of calories were derived from protein, all but 2.5 per cent had concentrations greater than 12 mg/100 ml. Thus, in the breast-fed infant, a concentration of urea nitrogen of 14 mg/100 ml is suggestive of renal disease or abnormally low fluid intake. This same concentration of urea nitrogen would fall at about the *lower* limit of the normal range for infants fed evaporated milk and water without added carbohydrate, i.e., 20 per cent of calories from protein.

Several investigators (Omans et al., 1961; Williams, 1963) have demonstrated that quite high concentrations of urea nitrogen may be found in sera of infants of low birth weight when feedings provide 20 per cent or more of the calories from protein.

(*Text continued on page 72.*)

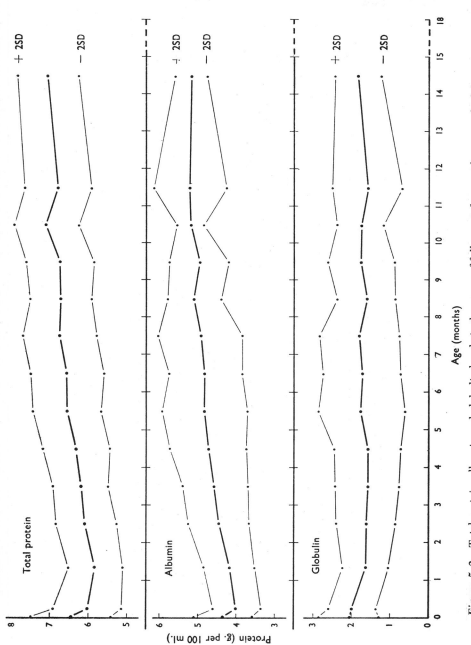

Figure 5–2. Total protein, albumin and globulin levels in the serum of full term infants, with two standard deviations on either side: birth to 18 months of age. (Courtesy of Privy Council – Medical Research Council Special Report Series, No. 296, Her Majesty's Stationery Office, 1959.

Table 5-7. *Concentration of Urea Nitrogen in Serum in Relation to Intake of Protein*

Diet	Concentration of Urea Nitrogen (mg/100 ml)								
	Age 8–60 days			Age 61–120 days			Age 121–182 days		
(% of calories) from protein	Number	Mean	Standard Deviation	Number	Mean	Standard Deviation	Number	Mean	Standard Deviation
20	95	24.3	5.4	102	19.6	3.7	100	17.4	3.7
9–11	133	10.4	2.9	173	10.1	3.0	154	9.8	2.8
6–7	276	7.0	2.5	257	6.6	2.6	169	7.3	3.7
1–2*	–	–	–	13	2.8	1.6	–	–	–

Data of Fomon (1961) and unpublished data of Nelsen and Owen and of Fomon and Filer (Pediatric Metabolic Unit, University of Iowa). All infants fed ad libitum, 67 cal/100 ml.

*Infants received this diet for only 4–6 days. All other diets had been fed for weeks or months.

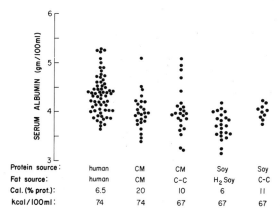

Figure 5–3. Concentrations of albumin in sera of 112-day-old infants in relation to feeding. CM refers to cow milk, C-C refers to corn and coconut oils and H₂Soy refers to partially hydrogenated soy oil.

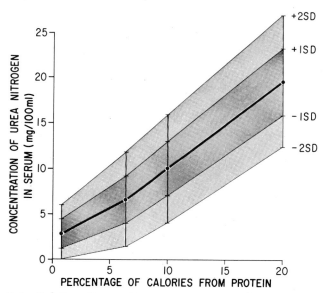

Figure 5–4. Relation of urea nitrogen concentration of serum to protein content of the diet during ad libitum feeding. Values pertain to infants 61 to 120 days of age (Table 5–4).

Comparison of Protein Quality in Human Milk, Cow Milk and Soy

Whey Protein Versus Casein

Proteins of human milk and cow milk are classified into two major categories: casein (the protein in the curd) and whey. Since whey is the predominant protein of human milk while casein is the predominant protein of cow milk, a comparison of nutritive value of these proteins for the human infant is of some importance. Lactalbumin, a major constituent of whey, was once considered nutritionally superior to casein for feeding of infants. However, when combined with a liberal intake of protein, casein and lactalbumin were shown to be equally effective in maintaining nitrogen balance in man (Mueller and Cox, 1947a and b). Furthermore, addition of small amounts of cystine or methionine, although improving the nutritive value of casein for the rat and dog to a value equivalent to that of lactalbumin, did not alter the nutritive value of casein for man (Cox et al., 1947). The greater requirement of fur-bearing animals than of man for sulfur-containing amino acids is presumably related to the relatively high concentration of cystine in hair.

Earlier work by Gordon et al. (1937) demonstrated that the protein of cow milk was as effective as that of human milk in promoting nitrogen retention by infants of low birth weight. This work has been confirmed more recently in studies with full-size infants (Barness et al., 1957; Fomon, 1960; Fomon and Owen, 1962b). Rates of gain in length and weight by full-size infants receiving 6 to 7 per cent of calories from cow milk protein or soy protein have been found to be similar to those by breast-fed infants (Fig. 2–3). The relation between retention of nitrogen and intake of nitrogen is also the same (Fig. 5–1). As will be discussed in Chapter Eleven, formulas are now commercially available in which the ratio of whey protein to casein is similar to that of human milk. A study in which one group of premature infants was fed such a formula and another group was fed a formula containing cow milk protein failed to demonstrate a difference between the two groups in rate of growth, nitrogen balance or food efficiency (Barness et al., 1963).

Data discussed previously in this chapter demonstrate that concentrations of albumin are significantly less than in sera of infants fed human milk. The conclusion that these proteins are of similar nutritional quality for the human infant therefore does not seem justified.

Requirements and Advisable Intakes of Protein

Requirements

The practical value of estimating requirements for protein by infants of various ages is obvious for countries in which protein is in short supply. However, even in countries with abundant food supplies, in certain instances optimal management requires that only the minimal safe intake (i.e., the requirement) of protein be fed. This may be true, for example, in phenylketonuria, leucine-sensitive hypoglycemia and various other disorders of amino acid metabolism. In addition, knowledge of the requirement is essential if a reasonable statement is to be made about advisable dietary intake.

As discussed in Chapter Two, rate of increase in protein of the male reference infant averages about 3.5 gm/day during the first four months of life. The data of Droese and Stolley (1966) suggest that nitrogen loss from the skin may average approximately 0.5 gm/day during this interval. Total needs, excluding losses in urine and feces, therefore average 4.0 gm/day.

When infants are fed human milk or formulas with similar concentrations of protein, retention of nitrogen averages about 45 per cent of intake during the first four months of life (Fomon and May, 1958; Fomon, 1959, 1960; Fomon and Owen, 1962b). Therefore, dietary intake of protein of 8.9 gm/day will be necessary to achieve a retention of 4.0 gm/day (i.e., the amount required for growth and losses from skin). Although, as previously discussed, metabolic balance studies are likely to overestimate the amount of nitrogen actually retained, urinary and fecal losses of nitrogen by breast-fed infants (and those receiving formulas providing similar intakes of protein) are undoubtedly greater than endogenous amounts. It is therefore unlikely that average requirements are greater than 8.9 gm/day.

Since median caloric intakes of normal infants during the first four months of life average about 540 kcal/day (Chapter Four), it is apparent that protein must account for approximately 6.5 per cent of caloric intake. Thus, with median caloric intakes of 132, 122 and 103 kcal/kg/day at ages one, two and four months (Fig. 4–2), requirements for protein will be 2.2, 2.0 and 1.7 gm/kg/day, respectively (Table 5–8).

Although the infant is larger at six to 12 months than at age four to five months of age and therefore requires greater amounts of protein for maintenance, rate of growth is much less and protein requirement for synthesis of new tissue is undoubtedly less. As indicated in Chapter Two, average rate of protein synthesis of the male

*Table 5–8. Estimated Requirements and
Advisable Intakes of Protein*

Age (months)	Estimated Requirement (gm/day)	(gm/kg/day)	Advisable Intakes° (gm/day)	(gm/kg/day)
1	10	2.2	14	3.0
2	11	2.0	15	2.7
4	12	1.7	16	2.3
6	12	1.6	16	2.2
8	12	1.3	16	1.8
10	12	1.2	16	1.6
12	12	1.2	16	1.6

°For infants not breastfed but receiving protein of high nutritional quality.

reference infant has been estimated to be 3.5 gm/day between birth and four months of age, and 3.1 gm/day between four and 12 months of age. Considering these decreased needs for synthesis of new tissue, total intakes of protein adequate for the four-month-old infant will probably be adequate for the six-, eight- and 10-month-old infant. On this basis, the *average* requirements for protein by the solely breast-fed infant throughout the first year of life is estimated to be *no more than* that indicated in Table 5–8.

Although the protein of cow milk has not been demonstrated to be nutritionally equivalent to the protein of human milk for the human infant, it is unlikely that the requirement is much greater when cow milk or other proteins of high quality, as determined in animal studies, are employed. Therefore, when management of infants with particular metabolic or other abnormalities is facilitated by use of a diet relatively low in protein, amounts of protein corresponding to the estimated requirement given in Table 5–8 are probably reasonable. For normal infants and others for whom there is no need to restrict intake of protein, higher intakes are to be preferred.

Advisable Intakes of Protein

Considerable clinical experience with formulas in which 9 per cent of calories are provided by protein from cow milk suggests that such feedings are completely adequate. Advisable intakes for the first five months of life have therefore been calculated from data on volumes of milk or formula ingested by infants fed ad libitum (Chapter Four) and on the assumption that 9 per cent of caloric intake is supplied from protein. For the reasons previously discussed, total daily requirement for protein is assumed to remain constant after five months of age, and advisable intakes for protein, expressed as grams per day, are also assumed to remain constant through the second half of the first year of life. Advisable intakes of protein at various ages are listed in Table 5–8.

Requirements and Advisable Intakes of Amino Acids

As is true for requirements of most nutrients, amino acid requirements are modified substantially by existing conditions. Requirements of infants cannot be estimated from results of studies with adults; results of studies with high intakes of amino acids or calories are not predictive of results with low intakes of amino acids or calories, and results with mixtures of amino acids are not predictive of results with whole proteins. Unfortunately, most studies of amino acid requirements have been carried out with mixtures of essential amino acids supplied in relatively generous amounts. Such studies (Holt and Snyderman, 1961; Snyderman et al., 1961a and b, 1963, 1964a and b) may have limited relevance to requirements for amino acids when infants receive restricted amounts of high quality proteins in an otherwise adequate diet.

An alternate approach to estimation of requirements for essential amino acids is provided by feeding human milk or other proteins at approximately the protein concentration of human milk. If infants fed in this manner maintain normal protein nutritional status, it can be concluded that requirements for essential amino acids are no greater under these conditions than the amounts provided by the feeding in question. Utilizing this approach with a formula in which soy protein supplied 7 per cent of caloric intake, rates of gain in length and weight and relation of retention of nitrogen to intake of nitrogen were similar to those recorded with breast-fed infants (Fomon et al., 1964). Intakes of methionine, valine and isoleucine by infants receiving the soy formula were less than the requirements for these amino acids estimated by Snyderman et al. In that study concentrations of proteins in sera of the infants were not determined and, therefore, an important criterion of protein nutritional status is lacking. Thus, a conclusion about requirements for essential amino acids does not seem justified on the basis of the data presented.

An estimate of average requirements for essential amino acids can be obtained by utilizing data on volumes of intake by normal infants (Chapter Four) and average concentrations of essential amino acids in human milk (Chapter Eleven). Such values may serve as rough guides in those instances in which it seems desirable to restrict intakes of one or more essential amino acids.

APPENDIX

Terms Employed in Discussion of Protein Quality

Protein Efficiency Ratio (PER)

Formula: $\dfrac{\text{weight gain (gm)}}{\text{protein consumed (gm)}}$

Among the factors known to influence rate of growth of rats are amount of food consumed, level of protein in the diet, age, sex, strain of rat, and length of assay period. Methods most commonly employed (Chapman et al., 1959; A.O.A.C., 1960) utilize 21-day-old male rats fed ad libitum a diet containing 9 or 10 per cent protein by weight for a period of four weeks. The test is standardized by use of rats fed casein as a control protein. See text for comment about limitations of the method.

Biologic Value (BV)

Formula: $\dfrac{\text{retained N} \times 100}{\text{absorbed N}}$

$$= \frac{(\text{food N} - \text{urine N} - \text{fecal N} + \text{endogenous N}) \times 100}{\text{food N} - \text{fecal N} + \text{endogenous N}}$$

where endogenous N is the amount of nitrogen excreted in urine and feces by animals receiving a protein-free diet.

True Digestibility (D)

Formula: $\dfrac{\text{absorbed N} \times 100}{\text{food N}}$

$$= \frac{(\text{food N} - \text{fecal N} + \text{fecal endogenous N}) \times 100}{\text{food N}}$$

Net Protein Utilization (NPU)

Formula: $\text{BV} \times \text{D}$

$$= \frac{\text{retained N} \times 100}{\text{food N}}$$

$$= \frac{C_p - C_o}{\text{food N}}$$

where C_p is the amount of nitrogen in the carcass of an animal fed the protein containing diet and C_0 is the amount of nitrogen in the carcass of an animal fed the protein-free diet. NPU is defined as the difference in carcass content of nitrogen* between animals receiving the protein-containing test diet and those receiving a protein-free control diet, divided by the amount of nitrogen consumed by the test animals (Bender and Miller, 1953a; Miller and Bender, 1955). It is assumed that nitrogen content of the carcass of animals fed the protein-free diet decreases during the course of the assay in proportion to the requirements of the animal for maintenance and therefore the result is interpreted in relation to requirements of the test animals for growth rather than for growth plus maintenance. However, body turnover of proteins is almost certainly less for animals receiving a protein-free diet than for animals receiving appreciable amounts of protein. The major advantage of NPU over PER is that the former takes an aspect of body composition into account while the latter merely concerns change in weight.

Chemical Score

$$\text{Formula:} \quad \frac{\% \text{ limiting amino acid}}{\% \text{ of that amino acid in egg}} \times 100$$

Nitrogen Balance

Formula: $I - U - F$

where I is nitrogen in ingested food, U is nitrogen in excreted urine and F is nitrogen in feces. True accretion of nitrogen by the subject will always be less than the apparent nitrogen retention estimated by this formula (see text).

REFERENCES

A.O.A.C.: Official Methods of Analysis. 9th ed. Washington, D. C., Assoc. Off. Agr. Chemists, 1960.

Barness, L. A., Baker, D., Guilbert, P., Torres, F. E., György, P.: Nitrogen metabolism of infants fed human and cow's milk. J. Pediat. 51:29, 1957.

Barness, L. A., Omans, W. B., Rose, C. S., and György, P.: Progress of premature infants fed a formula containing demineralized whey. Pediatrics 32:52, 1963.

Bender, A. E., and Doell, B. H.: Biological evaluation of proteins: a new aspect. Brit. J. Nutr. 11:140, 1957.

Bender, A. E., and Miller, D. S.: A new brief method of estimating net protein value. Biochem. J. 53:VII, 1953a.

---

*Since the ratio of nitrogen to water in the carcass has been found to be fairly constant, it has been suggested that dry weight rather than nitrogen content of the carcass could also be utilized (Bender and Miller, 1953b).

Bender, A. E., and Miller, D. S.: Constancy of the N/H_2O ratio of the rat and its use in the determination of the net protein value. Biochem. J. 53:VII, 1953b.

Bressani, R., Wilson, D. L., Béhar, M., and Scrimshaw, N. S.: Supplementation of cereal proteins with amino acids. III. Effect of amino acid supplementation of wheat flour as measured by nitrogen retention of young children. J. Nutr. 70: 176, 1960.

Carpenter, K. J.: Chemical methods of evaluating protein quality. Proc. Nutrition Soc. (Eng. Scot.) 17:91, 1958.

Carpenter, K. J.: The estimation of the available lysine in animal-protein foods. Biochem. J. 77:604, 1960.

Caspani, R., Negri, M., and Sticca, C.: L'elettroforesi su carta delle siero-proteine. Osservazione nal bambini sano con particalone riguardo all'etta del lattanta. Minerva paediat. (Torino) 5:198, 1953.

Chapman, D. G., Castillo, R., and Campbell, J. A.: Evaluation of protein in foods. I. A method for the determination of protein efficiency ratios. Can. J. Biochem. Physiol. 37:679, 1959.

Cox, W. M., Jr., Mueller, A. J., Elman, R., Albanese, A. A., Kemmerer, K. S., Barton, R. W., and Holt, L. E., Jr.: Nitrogen retention studies on rats, dogs and man; the effect of adding methionine to an enzymic casein hydrolysate. J. Nutrition 33:437, 1947.

Droese, W., and Stolley, H.: Daily nitrogen balance and urinary organic acid studies in 40 healthy infants from the 4th to the 86th day of life fed acidified and non-acidified milk-formulas. Presented at Seventh International Congress of Nutrition, Hamburg, Germany, August 3–10, 1966.

Ewerbeck, H., and Levens, H. E.: Die Bildung der Serumeiweisskörper des kindlichen Organismus bis zur Geburt und ihre Beziehung zum mütterlicher serumeiweisspektrum während der Schwangerschaft. Mschr. Kinderheilk. 98:436, 1950.

Fomon, S. J.: Comparative study of human milk and a soya bean formula in promoting growth and nitrogen retention by infants. Pediatrics 24:577, 1959.

Fomon, S. J.: Comparative study of adequacy of protein from human milk and cow's milk in promoting nitrogen retention by normal full-term infants. Pediatrics 26:51, 1960.

Fomon, S. J.: Nitrogen balance studies with normal full-term infants receiving high intakes of protein. Comparisons with previous studies employing lower intakes of protein. Pediatrics 28:347, 1961.

Fomon, S. J., and May, C. D.: Metabolic studies of normal full-term infants fed pasteurized human milk. Pediatrics 22:101, 1958.

Fomon, S. J., and Owen, G. M.: Comment on metabolic balance studies as a method of estimating body composition of infants. Pediatrics 29:495, 1962a.

Fomon, S. J., and Owen, G. M.: Retention of nitrogen by normal full-term infants receiving an autoclaved formula. Pediatrics 29:1005, 1962b.

Fomon, S. J., Owen, G. M., and Thomas, L. N.: Methionine, valine and isoleucine. Am. J. Dis. Child. 108:487, 1964.

Gordon, H. H., Levine, S. Z., Wheatley, M. A., Marples, E.: Respiratory metabolism in infancy and childhood. XX. The nitrogen metabolism in premature infants — comparative studies of human and cow's milk. Am. J. Dis. Child. 54:1030, 1937.

Hansen, J. D. L., and Freesemann, C.: The use of the nitrogen balance technique in the assessment of the nutritive value of proteins for children. Proc. Nutrition Soc. (S. Afr.) 1:47, 1960.

Harper, A. E.: Amino acid toxicities and imbalances. In Munro, H. N., and Allison, J. B. (eds.): Mammalian Protein Metabolism. New York, Academic Press, Inc., 1964a, vol. 2., p. 87.

Harper, A. E., Leung, P., Yoshida, A., and Rogers, Q. R.: Some new thoughts on amino acid imbalance. Fed. Proc. 23:1087, 1964b.

Holt, L. E., Jr., and Snyderman, S. E.: The amino acid requirements of infants. J.A.M.A. 175:100, 1961.

Imperato, C.: Ricerche elettroforetiche sulle proteine seriche nel lattante sano e immaturo. Lattante 22:449, 1951.

Knapp, E. L., and Routh, J. I.: Electrophoretic studies of plasma proteins in normal children. Pediatrics 4:508, 1949.

Levin, B., Mackay, H. M. M., Neill, C.A., Oberholzer, V. G., and Whitehead, T. P.: Weight Gains, Serum Protein Levels, and Health of Breast Fed and Artificially Fed Infants. Privy Council-Medical Research Council, Special Report Series, No. 296. London, Her Majesty's Stationery Office, 1959.

Levin, B., Oberholzer, V. G., and Whitehead, T. P.: Serum protein fractions: A comparison of precipitation methods with electrophoresis. J. Clin. Path. 3:260, 1950.

Longsworth, L. G., Curtis, R. M., and Pembroke, R. H., Jr.: The electrophoretic analysis of maternal and fetal plasmas and sera. J. Clin. Invest. 24:46, 1945.

McCance, R. A., and Widdowson, E. M.: The Composition of Foods. Med. Res. Council, Spec. Rept. Ser. 296, 1960.

Miller, D. S., and Bender, A. E.: The determination of the net utilization of proteins by a shortened method. Brit. J. Nutr. 9:382, 1955.

Mitchell, H. H.: Determination of the nutritive value of the proteins of food products. Ind. Eng. Chem., Anal. Ed. 16:696, 1944.

Mueller, A. J., and Cox, W. M., Jr.: Comparative nutritive value of casein and lactalbumin for man. J. Nutrition 34:285, 1947a.

Mueller, A. J., and Cox, W. M., Jr.: Comparative nutritive value of casein and lactalbumin for man. Science 105:580, 1947b.

Munro, H. N., and Allison, J. B. (eds.): Mammalian Protein Metabolism. New York, Academic Press, Inc., 2 volumes, 1964.

Norton, P. M., Kunz, H., and Pratt, E. L.: Electrophoretic analysis of serum proteins in premature infants. Pediatrics 10:527, 1952.

Omans, W. B., Barness, L. A., Rose, C. S., György, P.: Prolonged feeding studies in premature infants. J. Pediat. 59:951, 1961.

Rice, H. L., and Flodin, N. W.: Nitrogen balance response of young men to changes in quality of dietary protein. Fed. Proc. 19:13, 1960.

Rogers, R. R., Filer, L. J., Jr., and Fomon, S. J.: Concentrations of protein in serum of 112-day-old infants in relation to diet. 1967. To be published.

Rose, W. C.: The nutritive significance of the amino acids. Physiol. Rev. 18:109, 1938.

Scrimshaw, N. S., Bressani, R., Béhar, M., and Viteri, F.: Supplementation of cereal proteins with amino acids I. Effect of amino acid supplementation of corn-massa at high levels of protein intake on the nitrogen retention of young children. J. Nutrition 66:485, 1958.

Snyderman, S. E., Roitman, E. L., Boyer, A., and Holt, L. E., Jr.: Essential amino acid requirements of infants: leucine. Am. J. Dis. Child. 102:157, 1961a.

Snyderman, S. E., Boyer, A., Phansalkar, S. V., and Holt, L. E., Jr.: Essential amino acid requirements of infants: tryptophan. Am. J. Dis. Child. 102:163, 1961b.

Snyderman, S. E., Holt, L. E., Jr., Dancis, J., Roitman, E., Boyer, A., and Balis, M. E.: "Unessential" nitrogen: A limiting factor for human growth. J. Nutrition 78:57, 1962.

Snyderman, S. E., Boyer, A., Roitman, E., Holt, L. E. Jr., and Prose, P. H.: The histidine requirement of the infant. Pediatrics 31:786, 1963.

Snyderman, S. E., Boyer, A., Norton, P. M., Roitman, E., and Holt, L. E., Jr.: The essential amino acid requirements of infants. IX. Isoleucine. Am. J. Clin. Nutr. 15:313, 1964a.

Snyderman, S. E., Boyer, A., Norton, P. M., Roitman, E., and Holt, L. E., Jr.: The essential amino acid requirements of infants. X. Methionine. Am. J. Clin. Nutr. 15:322, 1964b.

Wallace, W. M.: Nitrogen content of the body and its relation to retention and loss of nitrogen. Fed. Proc. 18:1125, 1959.

Waterlow, J. C., and Wills, V. G.: Balance studies in malnourished Jamaican infants. I. Absorption and retention of nitrogen and phosphorus. Brit. J. Nutr. 14:183, 1960.

Williams, C. M.: Effect of different feedings on blood urea levels in prematurity. Med. J. Australia. 2:698, 1963.

Chapter Six

Fats and Fatty Acids

Concern over the incidence of atherosclerosis in most of the technically advanced countries of the world has in recent years led to discussion concerning the merits of preventive measures that might be instituted during infancy. For reasons mentioned later in this chapter, no general recommendations for modifying patterns of dietary fat intake (quantitatively or qualitatively) seem appropriate at the present time. Therefore, choice of fat for infant feeding may be based on more immediate consequences such as extent of fecal loss of fat and related losses of minerals. Data from studies of normal infants will be presented.

With the exception of the essential fatty acids, linoleic and arachidonic, which must be present in the diet at least in small amounts for normal growth and integrity of the skin, it is not absolutely necessary to include fat in the diet. However, fat-free diets prove relatively unpalatable even for infants and, as will be discussed, diets exceptionally high in protein and carbohydrate may give rise to diarrhea and dehydration in some infants. The high caloric density of fat appears to be a particular asset during the early months of life when energy requirements per unit of body weight are exceptionally great. The function of fat as a carrier of fat-soluble vitamins is well recognized, but water miscible forms of most of the fat-soluble vitamins are now available and have been shown to be well absorbed even in the absence of dietary fat.

Terminology and Chemistry

Fats (or lipids) include an array of rather dissimilar organic compounds that have been grouped together on the basis of their solubility in such "fat solvents" as chloroform, ether, benzene and acetone. Most separated (visible) natural fats are made up of about 98 to 99 per cent triglycerides (A.M.A. Council on Foods and Nutrition, 1962).* The remaining 1 or 2 per cent includes phospholipids, free fatty acids, monoglycerides, diglycerides, cholesterol and other nonsaponifiable matter.

Triglycerides

The triglyceride molecule consists of about 95 per cent (by weight) fatty acids and 5 per cent glycerol (Fig. 6–1). Triglycerides usually contain at least two and commonly three different fatty acids. Ordinarily, both saturated and unsaturated fatty acids are included, most fats containing at least eight to ten fatty acids attached in various positions to the glyceride molecule.

Trace amounts of the mono- and diglycerides and of free fatty acids are present in natural fats, and within the body these lipids are found during digestion and absorption and are present in the circulating lipids of the plasma.

Phospholipids

Although visible or "separated" fat contains only small amounts of phospholipids, these compounds are essential components of cell membranes and various other cellular components, form a large percentage of lipids of serum, and are important in absorption and transport of fatty acids. Phospholipids contain phosphoric acid esterified with glycerol or sphingosine. In animal tissues the most prevalent compounds in this group are glycerides in which two of the hydroxyl groups of the glycerol molecule are combined with fatty acids and the third with phosphoric acid.

Nonsaponifiable Lipids

When lipids are treated with alkali, fatty acids and phosphoric acid are split from the glycerol molecule — a process known as saponification. Sterols and a few compounds of relatively little nutritional interest may then be separated from the saponified components and

---

*Several other reviews have also been consulted frequently in preparing the section on terminology and chemistry of fats and fatty acids. These include Food and Nutrition Board (1958), Hilditch (1956) and Hilditch and Jasperson (1959).

are termed "nonsaponifiable lipids." The nonsaponifiable fraction makes up only about 1 per cent of dietary fat but may comprise a considerably higher percentage of fecal fat.

Fatty Acids

Naturally occurring fatty acids may contain from four to about 24 carbon atoms in a molecule; most prevalent are long-chain fatty acids, which contain 12 or more carbon atoms; of these, fatty acids with 16 or 18 carbon atoms predominate. About 55 per cent of the fatty acids of human milk and 65 per cent of the fatty acids of cow milk have 18 carbons in the chain. Long-chain fatty acids yield 9 kcal/gm. Medium-chain fatty acids, containing eight or ten carbon atoms in the chains, yield only 8.3 kcal/gm and are not prevalent in food fats but are nevertheless of considerable interest because such triglycerides are more readily absorbed than those of longer chain fatty acids. Short-chain fatty acids, containing four to six carbon atoms are not abundant in food fats and yield only 5.3 kcal/gm.

Fatty acids are classified according to the number of reactive (unsaturated or "double-bond" linkages) between the carbon atoms. *Saturated fatty acids,* those devoid of double bonds, are rather stable chemically and account for much of the firmness of fats at room temperature. The most common saturated fatty acids in natural fats are palmitic (16 carbon atoms) and stearic (18 carbon atoms).

Monosaturated fatty acids (monoenoic) are those with one reactive, unsaturated ("double-bond") linkage, which has two hydrogen atoms missing. Oleic acid, with one double-bond linkage and 18 carbon atoms, furnishes approximately one-third of all the fatty acids in human milk and cow milk (Table 6–1). *Polyunsaturated fatty acids* are classed as dienoic, trienoic and tetraenoic, depending on the number of double-bond linkages. Of greatest interest are linoleic acid (18 carbon atoms, two double bonds), arachidonic (20 carbon atoms, four double bonds) and linolenic (18 carbon atoms, three double bonds). The position of unsaturation influences the point of breakup of the chain in metabolism and the ability of the body to metabolize the remaining fragments. In addition, the shape of the molecule is of nutritional significance. As polyunsaturated fatty acids normally occur in unprocessed foods, the fatty acid molecule is folded upon itself at each of the double bonds (called the cis configuration). During the course of processing, the cis form may be converted to the trans (unfolded) form, thereby acquiring different nutritional properties. For example, when linoleic acid is converted from the cis to the trans form it becomes ineffective as an essential fatty acid. Positions of the carbon atoms in fatty acids are numbered successively beginning at the carboxyl (acid) end of the chain, which

Table 6-1. *Fatty Acid Composition and Estimated Triglyceride Structure of Some Fats Used in Infant Feeding*

	Human Milk	Cow Milk	Goat Milk	Beef	Lamb	Oleo Oils	Coco-nut	Corn	Palm	Pea-nut	Soy	Saf-flower
Fatty acids° (% of total)												
Saturated												
Butyric (C–4)	—	3	3			—	—	—	—	—	—	—
Caproic (C–6)	—	1	2			—	tr	—	—	—	—	—
Caprylic (C–8)	—	2	3	1	2	—	6	—	—	—	—	—
Capric (C–10)	1	3	10			—	6	—	—	—	—	—
Lauric (C–12)	6	4	6			—	47	—	—	—	—	—
Myristic (C–14)	8	14	12			—	18	tr	3	tr	tr	—
Palmitic (C–16)	23	25	28	28	29	22	10	13	42	8	12	6
Stearic (C–18)	7	9	6	19	25	10	2	3	4	4	2	3
C–20 and above	1	1	tr	—	—	—	tr	—	—	7	tr	tr
Unsaturated												
C–14 and below	1	2	1	—	—	—	—	—	—	—	—	—
Palmitoleic (C–16)	5	4	2	—	—	—	tr	—	—	1	tr	—
Oleic (C–18)	36	30	21	44	36	66	8	31	42	53	29	13
Linoleic (C–18)	8	4	4	2	3	—	1	53	9	26	51	77
Linolenic (C–18)	—	—	—	tr	1	—	—	—	—	—	—	—
C–20 and above	4	tr	2	—	—	—	—	—	—	—	—	—
Estimated triglyceride structure†												
S₃	9	35	39	14	5	0	82	0	6	0	0	0
S₂U	40	36	46	51	42	0	18	2	38	9	0	0
SU₂	43	29	15	35	53	100	0	41	48	49	58	23
U₃	8	0	0	0	0	0	0	57	8	42	42	77

°Values for beef and lamb from Home Economics Research Report #7, (1959); all other values from Hilditch and Jasperson (1959) or Hilditch (1956).

†Molar per cent of triglycerides that contain 3 saturated fatty acids (S_3), two (S_2U), one (SU_2) or none (U_3).

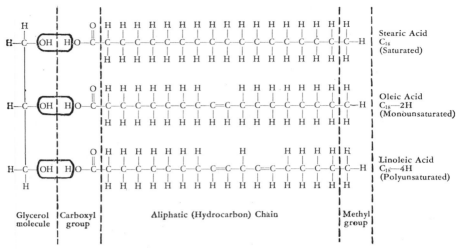

Figure 6–1. Structure of a mixed triglyceride. (From Coons, C. M.: Fats and fatty acids. *In* Food, the Yearbook of Agriculture, 1959. Washington, D. C., United States Department of Agriculture.)

attaches to the glycerol (Fig. 6–1). The position of linkage carries the number of the lower or first of the two carbons that it joins. Most common fatty acids with a single unsaturated linkage, including oleic, have this double bond in the 9 position, that is, between the ninth and tenth carbons. Unsaturated linkages of linoleic acid are in the 9 and 12 positions.

Essential Fatty Acids

The term, essential fatty acid, is reserved for those active in promotion of growth as well as in maintenance of dermal integrity, namely, linoleic and arachidonic acids. When weanling rats receive diets devoid of fat, they develop scaliness of the skin, loss of hair, emaciation, impairment of growth and reproductive capacity, increase in intake of food and water, increase in metabolic rate, and death at a relatively early age (Aaes-Jørgensen, 1961). These conditions can be prevented or ameliorated by daily administration of small quantities of linoleic acid. Generally similar manifestations of deficiency of essential fatty acids have been produced experimentally in the young of a variety of other animals, and in the human infant (Hansen et al., 1962). All manifestations of deficiency of essential fatty acids can be relieved by administration of small amounts of linoleic or arachidonic acids; these are the only fatty acids with a specific effect on growth. Some of the manifestations of fatty acid deficiency, notably the skin changes, can be relieved by administration of linolenic acid.*

---

*Only gamma-linolenic acid (double bonds at 6, 9 and 12 positions) is effective in this regard.

Studies by several investigators have demonstrated that evidences of essential fatty acid deficiency can be produced experimentally in the human infant when linoleic acid accounts for less than 0.1 per cent of total caloric intake (Hansen et al., 1962). There is as yet no explanation for the more rapid development of skin manifestations by infants receiving diets nearly devoid of fat than by infants receiving a diet equally deficient in essential fatty acids but supplying 18 per cent of calories as fat.

When linoleic acid comprises about 1 per cent of caloric intake of normal infants, skin manifestations of essential fatty acid deficiency do not appear and rates of growth are as rapid as those of infants receiving higher intakes of linoleic acid. However, infants receiving 1 per cent of the calories as linoleic acid may voluntarily ingest more calories than do infants receiving 4 to 5 per cent of the calories as linoleic acid, and the ratio of concentrations of triene to diene fatty acids in serum is elevated (Hansen et al., 1962). Although this ratio is elevated in essential fatty acid deficiency in animals, it may be merely a manifestation of dietary intake and is not necessarily an indication of deficiency.

In summary, when linoleic and/or arachidonic acid accounts for 1 per cent of caloric intake, health appears normal. Whether greater intakes afford additional benefit is a matter of speculation. Unfortunately, studies have not been carried out to indicate whether growth and dermal integrity are different when 0.5 or 0.7 per cent of the calories are supplied as linoleic acid than when 1 per cent of the calories are so supplied.

The suggestion that atopic eczema in infancy may be related to deficiency of essential fatty acids is based on several reports published more than 20 years ago which stated that this condition is more common in infants fed formulas of cow milk than in breast-fed infants, and from the observation that concentrations of polyunsaturated fatty acids are lower in sera of infants with eczema than in sera of normal infants (Hansen et al., 1962). However, more recent studies have failed to demonstrate a greater incidence of infantile eczema in the formula-fed than in the breast-fed infant, and administration of linoleic acid has not regularly resulted in improvement of eczema. It seems unlikely that atopic eczema is related to deficiency of essential fatty acids.

Desirable Intakes of Fat

Although it is possible to manage infants with diets providing 1 per cent of caloric intake from essential fatty acids and otherwise free of fat, such a regimen is rarely advisable. When less than 20 per cent of caloric intake is derived from fat, protein content of the diet may be so high that renal solute load is excessive (Chapter Nine), or disaccharide content of the diet may exceed the ability of the disaccharidases to split these sugars (Chapter Seven), with resultant diarrhea.

As is true of diets nearly free of fat, diets exceptionally high in fat content are relatively unpalatable. Rarely is it desirable to provide more than 50 per cent of caloric intake from fat. Most commercially available formulas for infants provide 35 to 50 per cent of calories from fat. Such formulas are generally well tolerated.

Animal Fats and Vegetable Oils

As indicated in Table 6–1, the fatty acid composition of common food fats is extremely variable. Most vegetable fats are rich in polyunsaturated fatty acids, although coconut oil consists primarily of saturated fatty acids and remains liquid at room temperature primarily because of its high content of medium- and short-chain fatty acids. Palm oil contains a high percentage of palmitic acid (saturated, C-16) and is a poor source of polyunsaturated fatty acids. Most animal fats are relatively poor sources of polyunsaturated fatty acids, although poultry may contain as much as 25 per cent linoleic acid. The fatty acid composition of fat in nonruminant animals is markedly influenced by diet; linoleic acid content of lard, for example, varies from a few per cent to more than 30 per cent of total fatty acids. Fish oils are rich in polyunsaturated fatty acids but are poor sources of the essential fatty acids, linoleic and arachidonic.

Digestion and Absorption

Digestion of fats consists of hydrolysis of triglycerides to diglycerides, monoglycerides, free fatty acids and glycerol. Although some of this hydrolysis may occur in the stomach, most requires the action of bile or of intestinal or pancreatic enzymes. Shorter chain fatty acids and unsaturated fatty acids are split from the glyceride molecule more readily than are the longer, saturated fatty acids. Longer chain fatty acids with two or more unsaturated linkages (e.g., linoleic or linolenic) are more readily split than are fatty acids with only one unsaturated linkage (e.g., oleic). In general, the fatty acids in the 1 and 3 positions on the glycerol molecule are more easily split off than are those in the 2 position. Thus, not only the fatty acid composition of a fat but also the pattern of arrangement of fatty acids on the triglyceride molecule influences digestibility.

As may be seen from Figure 6–2, absorption of lipid occurs primarily in the form of fatty acids and monoglycerides (Isselbacher, 1965). These lipid moieties, in association with conjugated bile salts, enter the intestinal mucosal cells. Fatty acids and monoglycerides are then esterified to triglycerides, either with or without intermediate formation of phospholipids.

Triglycerides of short- or medium-chain fatty acids (10 carbon atoms or less) can enter mucosal cells without prior hydrolysis and are then hydrolyzed and transported in an unesterified form to the portal blood (Playoust and Isselbacher, 1964). Lymphatic transport is not required. Studies by several investigators in the past few years have suggested that medium-chain triglycerides may be valuable in treatment of chyluria (Hashim et al., 1964), intestinal lymphangiectasia (Holt, 1964) and various steatorrheas (Fernandes et al., 1962; Iber, 1963; Cancio and Menéndez-Corrada, 1964; Pinter et al., 1964; Kuo and Huang, 1965; Holt et al., 1965; Winawer et al., 1966; Zurier et al., 1966). Infants who have had major segments of the bowel removed, those with hyperlipemia and infants of low birth weight may be expected to benefit from medium-chain triglycerides. The product, Portagen (Mead Johnson Company), has recently been marketed (Table 11–9).

Triglycerides with short-chain fatty acids, though readily absorbed (Snyderman et al., 1955), provide only slightly more calories per gram than does carbohydrate (5.3 vs 4.0 kcal/gm) and are, therefore, likely to be of less practical value than medium-chain triglycerides.

Triglyceride Composition of Some Fats Used in Infant Feeding

The estimated triglyceride composition of some fats used in infant feeding is indicated in Table 6–1. A relatively high percentage of the triglycerides in animal fats have two or three saturated fatty acids. In cow milk, for example, 35 per cent of the triglycerides contain only saturated fatty acids (S_3) and 36 per cent contain two saturated fatty acids (S_2U). Oleo oils (destearinated beef fat) is an exception since triglycerides with S_3 and S_2U structure are removed in the process of destearination. With the exception of coconut and palm oils, triglycerides with the S_3 and S_2U structure generally account for relatively small percentages of total triglycerides in vegetable oils.

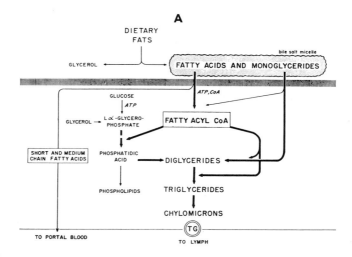

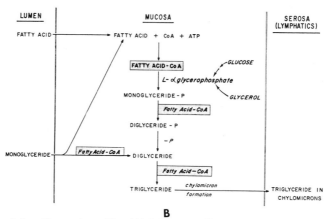

Figure 6–2. Absorption of fat. *(A)* Schematic illustration of pathways involved in absorption of fatty acids and monoglycerides across epithelial cell of intestinal mucosa. *(B)* Major biochemical reactions in transport of long-chain fatty acids and monoglycerides by intestinal mucosa. (From Isselbacher, K. J.: Fed. Proc. 24:16, 1965.)

In general, triglycerides with the S$_3$ and S$_2$U structure are less easily digested than those with the SU$_2$ or U$_3$ structure. However, even an S$_3$ triglyceride is readily absorbed if it includes only medium-chain or short-chain fatty acids. Table 6–2 provides an estimate of the triglyceride structure of fats and fat mixtures commonly employed in infant feeding. An indication of the number of saturated fatty acids with 14 or more carbon atoms is also included. By studying the triglyceride structure and noting the percentage of total fatty acids accounted for by long-chain saturated fatty acids, a reasonable prediction can be made concerning relative digestibility of various fats.

Such an approach to prediction of digestibility of various fats is an oversimplification that may be expected to lead to some discrepancies between predicted and observed digestibility. Saturated fatty acids of 18 carbon-chain length are less well absorbed than those with 14 carbon-chain length, although this distinction is ignored in Table 6–2. In addition, the digestibility of two S_2U triglycerides may vary considerably. Even when the same fatty acids are involved, a triglyceride with the structure SSU will differ in digestibility from one with the structure SUS.

Extent of Absorption of Various Fats

In spite of these limitations, it will be seen that data in Table 6–2 are of some value in predicting digestibility of various fat mixtures. The studies summarized in this table concern full-size infants during the first two weeks of life, a time when the ability to absorb many fats is sharply limited.

As would be expected, human milk fat was found to be more readily digested than cow milk fat since it contains fewer long-chain fatty acids, more triglycerides of the SU_2 and U_3 type and fewer triglycerides of the S_3 type. Corn and soy oils are readily absorbed because relatively few of the saturated fatty acids contain 14 or more carbon atoms and because few of the triglycerides are of the relatively poorly digested S_3 or S_2U type. Coconut oil, with only slightly more long-chain saturated fatty acids than corn oil, is less well absorbed because these fatty acids exist exclusively as S_3 or S_2U triglycerides. The mixture of corn and coconut oils is, therefore, slightly less well absorbed than corn oil alone.

Differences in digestibility of human milk fat and the mixture of palm, peanut and coconut oils with rather similar triglyceride and fatty acid composition are difficult to explain on the basis of this oversimplified approach to prediction of digestibility.

After the newborn period, extent of fat absorption generally increases but, as may be seen from Table 6–3, appreciable losses of fat may occur even in older infants. For example, when infants 31 to 60 days of age received homogenized cow milk as the only food, fecal excretion of fat averaged 34 per cent of intake. Since 50 per cent of calories provided by whole cow milk are derived from fat, fecal loss of fat equal to 34 per cent of fat intake amounts to a loss of 17 per cent of caloric intake. With an intake of 120 kcal/kg, this equals a loss of 20 kcal/kg/day. It is therefore clear that calculated caloric intakes may be misleading with respect to energy actually available

(Text continued on page 93.)

Table 6-2. *Average Daily Metabolic Balance Values for Infants Four to Ten Days of Age*

A. Composition of Feeding

Fat	Protein		Triglyceride Structure				Saturated Fatty Acids
	Source	% of Cal	S_3	S_2U	SU_2	U_3	(% C-14 or higher)
Human milk	human milk	6–7	9	40	43	8	39
Butterfat	cow milk	14	35	36	29	0	49
Coconut oil	cow milk	10	82	18	0	0	30
Peanut oil	cow milk	10	0	9	49	42	54
Medium-chain triglyceride	cow milk	15	100	0	0	0	0
Corn + coconut (1:1)	cow milk	10	41	10	20	29	23
Peanut + corn + coconut (2:1:1)	cow milk	9	20	10	35	35	22
Butterfat + corn + coconut (2:1:1)	cow milk	10	38	23	25	14	38
Palm + peanut + coconut (2:1:1)	cow milk	9	14	26	36	14	37
Soy	soy	15	0	0	58	42	14
Corn + coconut (1:1)	soy	11	41	41	20	29	23
Partially hydrogenated soy	soy	{ 6 15	isomeric forms				14?

Table 6–2. *Average Daily Metabolic Balance Values for Infants Four to Ten Days of Age (Continued)*

B. Fat and Mineral Balances

Fat	Number of Subjects	Mean Body Weight (gm)	Intake of Formula (ml)	Carmine Passage Time (hr)	Nitrogen I (mg/kg)	Nitrogen R	Fat I (gm/kg)	Fat R (%)	Ca I (mg/kg)	Ca R	Mg I (mg/kg)	Mg R	P I (mg/kg)	P R
Human milk	6†	3165	493		439		2.87	87	44	20	4.4	1.9	24	21
	10‡	3522					4.91	92						
Butterfat	5	3084	495	8	547	227	4.14	61	137	-23	13.8	-1.6	107	28
Coconut oil	5	2976	511	23	362	176	6.11	79	111	-27	10.4	3.4	57	8
Peanut oil	5	3497	504	9	311	139	5.00	83	92	26	8.6	3.7	48	3
Medium-chain triglyceride	7	3186	386	18	547	189	3.18	96	69	26	5.4	-0.8	71	24
Corn + coconut (1:1)	15	3488	526	7	401	199	5.13	90	99	36	9.1	1.9	79	33
Peanut + corn + coconut (2:1:1)	12	3390	574	8	410	199	6.08	85	95	32	9.5	2.3	79	25
Butterfat + corn + coconut (2:1:1)	6	3206	470	21	431	203	5.18	83	99	25	9.6	1.3	89	36
Palm + peanut + coconut (2:1:1)	13	3375	535	18	394	180	5.67	76	90	13	9.2	0.9	77	22
Soy	4	3182	455	9	611	231	4.87	90	102	6	9.1	1.6	104	20
Corn + coconut (1:1)	8	3276	526	8	441	156	5.80	79	102	39	8.9	0.9	71	30
Partially hydrogenated soy	6	3139	572	6	282	125	6.82	61	117	17	10.4	0.3	72	10
	5	3238	563	6	668	246	5.98	66	131	4	15.3	3.3	133	23

*All data are those of Filer and Fomon except as noted.
†Data of Welsch et al. (1965).
‡Data of Widdowson (1965).

Table 6–3. *Influence of Age on Excretion of Fat (% of Intake) by Normal Infants Receiving Various Feedings Ad Libitum*

Dietary Fat		Age (days)								Investigators[*]
		8–30		31–60		61–90		91–182		
Type	(% of total kcal)	Number of Studies	Mean	Number of Studies	Mean	Number of Studies	Mean	Number of Studies	Mean	
Human milk	50	10	13	14	7	11	5	39	5	Fomon and May, 1958a
Corn	36	–	11	6	3	5	4	10	4	Fomon, 1961
Corn, coconut (1:1)	48	6	11	11	7	7	8	28	7	Fomon and May, 1958b
Cow milk (evaporated)	50	3	17	3	19	5	15	14	15	Fomon, 1961
Cow milk (homogenized)	50	4	21	8	34	9	37	5	28	Fomon, 1961
Soy (partially hydrogenated)		9	21	9	15	2	11	9	7	Fomon and Filer, to be published

[*]Descriptions of subjects and diets are given in the reports indicated. With the exception of data on excretion of fat by infants between 31 and 60 days of age (Fomon, 1961), the data included in this table have not previously been published.

for maintenance and for growth. For this reason, when an infant fails to gain weight normally in spite of an apparently adequate caloric intake, one should consider the possibility that fecal losses of fat may be appreciable. As may be seen from Table 6–2, losses of calcium, phosphorus and magnesium in the feces are generally roughly proportional to losses of fat.

Fecal losses of fat are frequently high in the infant of low birth weight, especially when fats of relatively poor digestibility are fed (Tidwell et al., 1935; Morales et al., 1950; Davidson and Bauer, 1960). Discussion of the significance of these findings in relation to management of infants of low birth weight is included in Chapter Thirteen.

Tests for Fat Absorption

In the Pediatric Metabolic Unit of the University of Iowa the extent of fat absorption is determined by metabolic balance studies as described in Appendix II (p. 282). In arriving at a quantitative estimation of fat absorption, such an approach is believed to be preferable to various other absorption tests. However, other absorption tests have the obvious advantages of speed (hours rather than days to complete the test) and more simple methodology.

The author has had no experience with the Lipiodol absorption test as described by Neerhout et al. (1964) or the measurement of serum turbidity after ingestion of butterfat as described by Goldbloom et al. (1964). These tests would appear to be useful in establishing the diagnosis of steatorrhea. They are almost certainly superior to tests of vitamin A absorption.

Serum and Tissue Concentrations of Lipids

Concentrations of total lipids, phospholipids and cholesterol in serum of infants have been demonstrated by a number of investigators to be significantly correlated with diet (Rafstedt, 1955; Pomeranze et al., 1958; Méndez et al., 1959; Fomon and Bartels, 1960; Lindquist and Malmcronai, 1960; Sweeney et al., 1961; György et al., 1963; Woodruff et al., 1964). Concentrations of cholesterol and total lipids in serum are relatively high when fat is derived primarily from human milk or cow milk and are usually considerably lower when mixtures containing vegetable fats are fed. With continued feeding of a diet, fatty acid composition of adipose tissue comes to resemble to some extent the fatty acid composition of serum (Fig. 6–3) (Sweeney et al., 1963).

Atherosclerosis

That fatty streaking of the intima of arteries makes its appearance early in infancy has now been amply documented (Zinserling, 1925; Kube and Ssolowjew, 1930; Albert, 1939; Field, 1946; Minkowski, 1947; Fangman and Hellwig, 1947; Moon, 1957; Holman et al., 1958). It is, therefore, not surprising that concern over the incidence

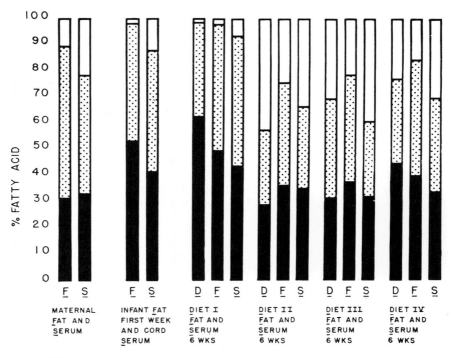

Figure 6–3. Total saturated, monounsaturated, and diunsaturated fatty acid percentage distributions from C12:0 through C18:2 in the test diets, subcutaneous fat of mothers, and subcutaneous fat of test infants during the first week of life and at six to eight weeks of age, and in the cholesterol-triglyceride fraction of the sera of mothers, cord blood, and six- to eight-week-old infants. (From Sweeney, M. J., et al.: J. Clin. Invest. 42:1, 1963.)

of atherosclerosis in most of the technically advanced countries of the world has led to the suggestion that preventive measures be instituted during infancy (Holman, 1961).

Since dietary measures (i.e., substitution of various mixtures of vegetable oils for butterfat) are effective in reducing concentrations of lipids in serum, it would, in fact, be relatively simple to maintain low concentrations of serum lipids throughout infancy. In this regard, studies of children with cystic fibrosis of the pancreas are of interest since such individuals may be assumed to have lost through fecal excretion most long-chain saturated fatty acids in the diet. Serum concentrations of lipids and cholesterol have been shown to be low (Luzzatti and Hansen, 1944). Aortas of such children dying between six and 12 years of age demonstrate much less atherosclerotic change than do aortas of children of similar age who die from other causes (Holman et al., 1959).

Maintaining a relatively low concentration of lipids in serum during infancy may eventually be demonstrated to be desirable, but several considerations suggest that any general recommendation to this effect is at present premature and unwarranted. Among the points that seem worthy of special review in this regard are the following: (1) Concentrations of lipids in sera of breast-fed infants are at least as great as those in sera of infants receiving commonly employed formulas containing butterfat. Thus, if feeding of butterfat during infancy is to be considered hazardous because it promotes cardiovascular morbidity and mortality later in life, it would seem likely that breast feeding is equally hazardous. (2) Studies in which monkeys were fed a diet with butterfat or one with a mixture of vegetable oils demonstrated significant differences in serum concentrations of lipids but at one year of age did not demonstrate a difference in degree of fatty streaking of the blood vessels (Pickering et al., 1961). Rate of incorporation of labeled acetate and mevalonate into cholesterol in the liver was actually less in the animals fed butterfat than in those fed vegetable oils, suggesting a lower rate of cholesterol synthesis (Van Bruggen et al., 1962). (3) Even if fatty streaking of the intima of arteries could be minimized by avoidance of butterfat and/or avoidance of breast feeding, and even though no unfavorable consequences resulted from maintaining consistently low concentrations of total lipids and cholesterol in serum and tissues, this effect might well prove to be insignificant in relation to dietary history during the remainder of life.

Thus, our understanding of the importance of serum concentrations of lipids and fatty streaking of arteries during infancy is considered to be so meager at present that it seems unreasonable to consider these factors in making recommendations for infant feeding.

REFERENCES

Aaes-Jørgensen, E.: Essential fatty acids. Physiol. Rev. 41:1, 1961.

Albert, Z.: Die Veränderungen der Aorta bei Kindern und ihr Verhältnis zur Atherosklerose. Virchow's Arch. path. Anat. 303:265, 1939.

A.M.A. Council on Foods and Nutrition: The regulation of dietary fat. J.A.M.A. 181: 411, 1962.

Cancio, M., and Menéndez-Corrada, R.: Absorption of medium chain triglycerides in tropical sprue. Proc. Soc. Exp. Biol. & Med. 117:182, 1964.

Coons, C. M.: Fats and fatty acids. In Stefferud, A. (ed.): Food. The Yearbook of Agriculture. Washington, D. C., U. S. Government Printing Office, 1959, p. 74.

Davidson, M., and Bauer, C. H.: Patterns of fat excretion in feces of premature infants fed various preparations of milk. Pediatrics 25:375, 1960.

Fangman, R. J., and Hellwig, C. A.: Histology of coronary arteries in newborn infants. Am. J. Path. 23:901, 1947.

Fernandes, J., van de Kamer, J. H., and Weijers, H. A.: Differences in absorption of the various fatty acids studied in children with steatorrhea. J. Clin. Invest. 41:488, 1962.

Field, M. H.: Medical calcification of arteries of infants. Arch. Path. 42:607, 1946.

Filer, L. J., Jr., and Fomon, S. J.: Excretion of fat by normal full-size infants during the first two weeks of life. To be published.

Fomon, S. J.: Nitrogen balance studies with normal full-term infants receiving high intakes of protein. Pediatrics 28:347, 1961.

Fomon, S. J., and Bartels, D. J.: Concentrations of cholesterol in serum of infants in relation to diet. Am. J. Dis. Child. 99:27, 1960.

Fomon, S. J., and May, C. D.: Metabolic studies of normal full-term infants fed pasteurized human milk. Pediatrics 22:101, 1958a.

Fomon, S. J., and May, C. D.: Metabolic studies of normal full-term infants fed a prepared formula providing intermediate amounts of protein. Pediatrics 22: 1134, 1958b.

Food and Nutrition Board: The Role of Dietary Fat in Human Health. Washington, D. C., National Academy of Sciences–National Research Council, Publication 575, 1958.

Goldbloom, R. B., Blake, R. M., and Cameron, D.: Assessment of three methods for measuring intestinal fat absorption in infants and children. Pediatrics 34:814, 1964.

György, P., Rose, C., and Chu, E.: Serum cholesterol and lipoproteins in premature infants. Am. J. Dis. Child. 106:165, 1963.

Hansen, A. E., Stewart, R., Hughes, G., and Soderhjelm, L.: The relation of linoleic acid to infant feeding. Acta Paediatrica Suppl. 137, 1962.

Hashim, S. A., Roholt, H. B., Babayan, V. K., and Van Itallie, T. B.: Treatment of chyluria and chylothorax with medium-chain triglyceride. New England J. Med. 270:756, 1964.

Hilditch, T. P.: The Chemical Constitution of Natural Fats. 3rd ed. New York, John Wiley & Sons, Inc., 1956.

Hilditch, T. P., and Jasperson, H.: Lipids in Relation to Arterial Disease. A Summary of Current Biochemical Evidence. Liverpool, England, J. Bibby and Sons, Ltd., 1959.

Holman, R. L.: Atherosclerosis – a pediatric nutrition problem? Am. J. Clin. Nutr. 9:565, 1961.

Holman, R. L., Blanc, W. A., and Andersen, D.: Decreased aortic atherosclerosis in cystic fibrosis of the pancreas. Pediatrics 24:34, 1959.

Holman, R. L., McGill, H. C., Jr., Strong, J. P., and Geer, J. C.: The natural history of atherosclerosis. The early aortic lesions as seen in New Orleans in the middle of the 20th century. Am. J. Path. 34:209, 1958.

Holt, P. R.: Dietary treatment of protein loss in intestinal lymphangiectasia. Pediatrics 34:629, 1964.

Holt, P. R., Hashim, S. A., and Van Itallie, T. B.: Treatment of malabsorption syndrome and exudative enteropathy with synthetic medium chain triglycerides. Am. J. Gastroenterol. 43:549, 1965.

Home Economics Research Report #7: Fatty Acids in Food Fats. Washington, D. C., U. S. Department of Agriculture, 1959.

Iber, F. L., Hardoon, E., and Sangree, M. H.: Use of eight and ten carbon fatty acids as neutral fat in the management of steatorrhea. Clin. Res. 11:185, 1963.

Isselbacher, K. J.: Metabolism and transport of lipid by intestinal mucosa. Fed. Proc. 24:16, 1965.

Kube, N., and Ssolowjew, A.: Über die Lipoidablagerung in der Aorta von Kindern im fruhen Säuglingsalter. Frankfurter Ztschr. Path. 40:302, 1930.

Kuo, P. T., and Huang, N. N.: The effect of medium chain triglyceride upon fat absorption and plasma lipid and depot fat of children with cystic fibrosis of the pancreas. J. Clin. Invest. 44:1924, 1965.

Lindquist, B., and Malmcrona, R.: Dietary fat in relation to serum lipids in the normal infant. Am. J. Dis. Child. 99:39, 1960.

Luzzatti, L., and Hansen, A. E.: Study of the serum lipids in the celiac syndrome. J. Pediat. 24:417, 1944.

Méndez, J., Savits, B. S., Flores, M., and Scrimshaw, N. S.: Cholesterol levels of maternal and fetal blood at parturition in upper and lower income groups in Guatemala City. Am. J. Clin. Nutr. 7:595, 1959.

Minkowski, W. L.: The coronary arteries of infants. Am. J. Med. Sci. 214:623, 1947.

Moon, H. D.: Coronary arteries in fetuses, infants and juveniles. Circulation 16:263, 1957.

Morales, S., Chung, A. W., Lewis, J. M., Messina, A., and Holt, L. E., Jr.: Absorption of fat and vitamin A in premature infants. I. Effect of different levels of fat intake on the retention of fat and vitamin A. Pediatrics 6:86, 1950.

Neerhout, R. C., Lanzkowsky, P., Kimmel, J. R., Lloyd, E. A., Wilson, J. F., and Lahey, M. E.: A new test for fat absorption which employs an iodinated triglyceride. J. Pediat. 65:701, 1964.

Pickering, D. E., Fisher, D. A., Perley, A., Basinger, G., and Moon, H. D.: Influence of dietary fatty acids on serum lipids. Studies of the immature rhesus monkey (Macaca mulatta). Am. J. Dis. Child. 102:42, 1961.

Pinter, K. G., McCracken, B. H., Lamar, C., Jr., and Goldsmith, G. A.: Fat absorption studies in various forms of steatorrhea. Am. J. Clin. Nutr. 15:293, 1964.

Playoust, M. R., and Isselbacher, K. J.: Studies on the intestinal absorption and intramucosal lipolysis of a medium chain triglyceride. J. Clin. Invest. 43:878, 1964.

Pomeranze, J., Goalwin, A., and Slobody, L. B.: The effect of a corn oil-evaporated milk mixture on serum cholesterol levels in infancy. Am. J. Dis. Child. 95: 622, 1958.

Rafstedt, S.: Studies on serum lipids and lipoproteins in infancy and childhood. Acta Paediatrica 44: Suppl. 102, 1955.

Snyderman, S. E., Morales, S., and Holt, L. E., Jr.: The absorption of short-chain fats by premature infants. Arch. Dis. Childhood 30:83, 1955.

Sweeney, M. J., Etteldorf, J. N., Dobbins, W. T., Somervill, B., Fisher, R., and Ferrell, C.: Dietary fat and concentrations of lipid in the serum during the first six to eight weeks of life. Pediatrics 27:765, 1961.

Sweeney, M. J., Etteldorf, J. N., Throop, L. J., Timma, D. L., and Wrenn, E. L.: Diet and fatty acid distribution in subcutaneous fat and in the cholesterol-triglyceride fraction of serum of young infants. J. Clin. Invest. 42:1, 1963.

Tidwell, H. C., Holt, L. E., Jr., Farrow, H. L., and Neale, S.: Studies of Fat Metabolism. II. Fat absorption in premature infants and twins. J. Pediat. 6:481, 1935.

Van Bruggen, J. T., Elwood, J. C., Marcó, A., and Bernards, W. C.: In vitro studies on oxidative and lipid metabolism in the immature Macaque monkey. J. Atheroscler. Res. 2:388, 1962.

Welsch, H., Heinz, F., Lagally, G., and Stahlfauth, K.: Fettresorption aus Frauenmilch bei Neugeborenen. Klin. Wschr. 43:60, 1965.

Widdowson, E. M.: Absorption and excretion of fat, nitrogen, and minerals from "filled" milks by babies one week old. Lancet 2:1099, 1965.

Winawer, S. J., Broitman, S. A., Wolochow, D. A., Osborne, M. P., and Zamcheck, N.: Successful management of massive small-bowel resection based on assessment of absorption defects and nutritional needs. New England J. Med. 174:72, 1966.

Woodruff, C. W., Bailey, M. C., Davis, J. T., Rogers, N., and Coniglio, J. G.: Serum lipids in breastfed infants and in infants fed evaporated milk, Am. J. Clin. Nutr. 14:83, 1964.

Zinserling, W. D.: Untersuchungen Über Atherosklerose. I. Über die Aortaverfettung bei Kindern. Virchow's Arch. path. Anat. 255:677, 1925.

Zurier, R. B., Campbell, R. G., Hashim, S. A., and Van Itallie, T. B.: Use of medium-chain triglyceride in management of patients with massive resection of the small intestine. New England J. Med. 274:490, 1966.

Chapter Seven

Carbohydrate

A tremendous surge of interest in carbohydrate metabolism has resulted from identification in recent years of primary and secondary disaccharidase deficiencies. In South Africa, lactase deficiency has been found in approximately 60 per cent of infants and children with kwashiorkor (Bowie et al., 1965). Whether acquired disaccharidase deficiency is also frequent in various other diseases is unknown. Newer studies have improved our understanding of hypoglycemia in early infancy. These developments, together with satisfactory progress of properly treated infants with galactosemia, have been responsible for the current high level of interest in carbohydrates in the infant's diet.

Absorption

Only a brief résumé concerning current knowledge of carbohydrate absorption will be presented. For a more detailed discussion the reader is referred to the excellent monograph of Cornblath and Schwartz (1966). Carbohydrates fed to infants may include all those present in the diet of the adult (Table 7–1), although during early infancy most infants receive their carbohydrate intake in the form of disaccharides and monosaccharides while the adult ingests a much larger percentage of his carbohydrate as polysaccharide (starch). Chemical relationships between starch, disaccharides and mono-

(Text continued on page 103.)

Table 7-1. *Carbohydrate Content of Some Foods Consumed by Infants*[*]
(gm carbohydrate per 100 gm edible food)

	Fructose	Glucose	Reducing Sugars	Sucrose	Other[†]
Apple	5.0	1.7	8.3	3.1	Cellulose, hemicellulose, pectin, starch
Apple juice	0.4		8.0	4.2	
Apricots	0.4	1.9		5.5	Cellulose, hemicellulose, pectin
Banana					
yellow	3.5	4.5	8.4	8.9	Starch
flecked				11.9	Starch
powder			32.6	33.2	9.6% Dextrins, 7.8% starch
Orange					
composite values	1.8	2.5	5.0	4.6	Cellulose, hemicellulose, pectin, pentosans
fresh juice	2.4	2.4	5.1	4.7	
frozen, reconstituted			4.6	3.2	
Peaches	1.6	1.5	3.1	6.6	Dextrins, pectin
Pear, Bartlett	5.0	2.5	8.0	1.5	Pectin
Pineapple, ripened on plant	1.4	2.3	4.2	7.9	
Prunes, uncooked	15.0	30.0	47.0	2.0	2.8% Cellulose, 10.7% hemicellulose, pectin, 2.0% pentosans, starch
Tomatoes	1.2	1.6	3.4		Cellulose, hemicellulose, pectin

Table 7-1. Carbohydrate Content of Some Foods Consumed by Infants* (gm carbohydrate per 100 gm edible food) (Continued)

	Fructose	Glucose	Reducing Sugars	Sucrose	Other†
Beans, snap, fresh			1.7	0.5	Cellulose, dextrins, hemicellulose, pectin, pentosans, 2.0% starch
Beets, sugar				12.9	Cellulose, hemicellulose
Carrots, raw			5.8	1.7	Cellulose, 1.7% hemicellulose, pectin
Corn, fresh		0.5		0.3	Cellulose, dextrins, hemicellulose, 1.3% pentosans, 14.5% starch
Peas, green				5.5	Cellulose, 2.2% hemicellulose, 4.1% starch
Potatoes, white	0.1	0.1	0.8	0.1	Cellulose, hemicellulose, 17.0% starch
Spinach	0.2		0.2		Cellulose, hemicellulose
Squash, butternut		0.1		0.4	2.6% Starch
Sweet potato, baked			14.5	7.2	4% Starch
Soybean flour				6.8	4.2% Galactans, 1.9% raffinose†, 5.2% stachyose‡
Peanut butter			0.9		5.9% Starch
Barley flour				3.1	Pentosans, 69% starch

Table 7-1. *Carbohydrate Content of Some Foods Consumed by Infants** *
(gm carbohydrate per 100 gm edible food) (Continued)

	Fructose	Glucose	Reducing Sugars	Sucrose	Other†
Corn, yellow					4.5% Cellulose, 4.9% hemicellulose, 6.2% pentosans, 62.0% starch
Oats, hulled					6.4% Pentosans, 56.4% starch
Rice, polished, raw		2.0	trace	0.4	Cellulose, dextrins, 1.8% pentosans, 72.9% starch
Rye flour					4.1% Pentosans, 71.4% starch
Wheat flour			2.0	0.2	5.5% Dextrins, 2.1% pentosans, 68.8% starch
Corn syrup high conversion medium conversion		21.2 33.0 26.0			34.7% Dextrins, 26.4% maltose 19.0% Dextrins, 23.0% maltose 23.0% Dextrins, 21.0% maltose
Corn sugar		87.5			3.5% Maltose, dextrins
Honey	40.5	34.2		1.9	Dextrins
Invert sugar	8.0		74.0	6.0	
Molasses		8.8		53.6	

* Abstracted from data of Hardinge et al., 1965.
† Less than 1.5 per cent unless noted otherwise.
‡ Content of dry soybeans.

saccharides are indicated in Figure 7–1. Starch and glycogen are digested to maltose (primarily) and isomaltose through the action of amylase in saliva and pancreatic juice (Fig. 7–2). The disaccharides — maltose, isomaltose, sucrose and lactose — are absorbed into the brush border of the small intestine, where they are split by appropriate disaccharidases and then absorbed into the blood. The monosaccharides — galactose, glucose and fructose — are absorbed through the brush border of the intestinal tract into the blood. Galactose and glucose, whether provided as such in the diet or produced by the action of disaccharidases within the brush border, are absorbed actively against concentration gradients, while fructose appears to be passively absorbed. Absorption of D-xylose, a nonmetabolizable sugar, has been employed as a measure of absorptive capacity of the small intestine.

Of the monosaccharides that are absorbed intact into the portal circulation, almost all the galactose and much fructose are removed by the liver. The extent of hepatic uptake of glucose varies greatly and depends upon the nutritional status of the individual, the quantity of glucose absorbed, the amount of potassium available and a variety of hormonal factors. Disaccharides may be absorbed without hydrolysis, and trace quantities not infrequently appear in the urine of young infants.

A key intermediate for a variety of metabolic pathways is glucose-6-phosphate, a substance that can be formed from glucose by all the tissues of the body. Energy requirements of the cell, availability of other substrates, and concentrations of oxygen and certain hormones determine whether glucose-6-phosphate is then converted to glycogen for storage, metabolized by way of the glycolytic pathway to provide glycerol for fat synthesis and high energy phosphates

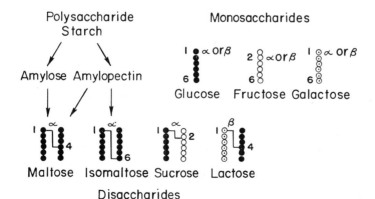

Figure 7–1. Chemical relationships of starch, disaccharides and monosaccharides. (Adapted from Prader, A., Auricchio, S., and Semenza, G.: Mschr. Kinderheilk. *112*: 177, 1964.)

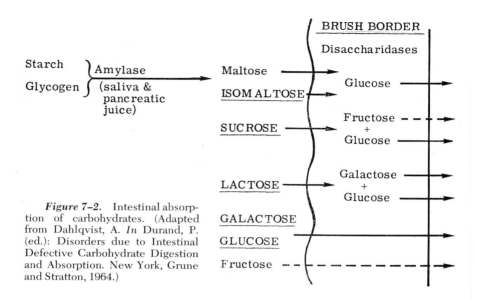

Figure 7-2. Intestinal absorption of carbohydrates. (Adapted from Dahlqvist, A. *In* Durand, P. (ed.): Disorders due to Intestinal Defective Carbohydrate Digestion and Absorption. New York, Grune and Stratton, 1964.)

(ATP), or oxidized by way of the pentose phosphate cycle to provide reduced cofactors (TPNH) for synthesis of fatty acids and pentose.

Quantitative Aspects of Disaccharide Hydrolysis in Newborn Infants

Capacity of the infant to split disaccharides is presumably related to disaccharidase activity per unit of small intestinal mucosa and to the length of the small intestine. In studies of three full-term newborn infants who died after one day of age, Auricchio et al. (1965) have estimated the maximal velocities of hydrolysis of various disaccharides in vitro. The maximal rate of hydrolysis of lactose, ranging from 57 to 67 gm in 24 hours, probably exceeds by a considerable margin the actual capacity of the intestinal mucosa to split lactose in vivo. It may be noted, for example, that the rate of passage of a carmine marker from time of feeding to appearance of carmine in the stool is frequently three to four hours. Presumably, the greater portion of the feeding reaches the small intestine in a relatively short period of time, and carbohydrate is either hydrolyzed and absorbed or passes into the colon.

When disaccharides are not hydrolyzed and absorbed, their presence in the colon exerts an osmotic effect that leads to passage of frequent, loose stools. In the case of lactase deficiency, the presence of lactose in the ileocecal region leads to fermentation of the carbohydrate by intestinal bacteria with resultant production of carbon dioxide and lactic acid (Fig. 7–3). These products of bacterial activity exert an irritative effect on the colon, further aggravating the diarrhea and being responsible for the acid pH of the stools. As concluded by Haemmerli et al. (1965), it seems likely that the relatively large quantities of lactose ingested by the breast-fed infant may exceed the capacity of the small intestinal mucosa for hydrolysis. Several formulas commercially prepared for infants contain lactose as the only carbohydrate in concentration similar to that of human milk. Infants receiving these feedings during the early weeks of life have frequent, rather loose stools of acid pH, thus resembling breast-fed infants in stool pattern (Barbero et al., 1952; Pratt and Read, 1955).

Much additional information will be required for a full understanding of the relation between the load of disaccharide ingested and the ability to hydrolyze the load. It seems probable that the most efficient utilization of the disaccharide mechanism would result from ingestion of relatively small amounts of milk or formula in equally spaced feedings throughout the 24-hour period.

Because maltase activity of the intestinal mucosa is relatively high at birth, moderate amounts of starch can probably be tolerated even by the newborn infant (Auricchio et al., 1965). This conclusion appears to be supported by clinical observation, since introduction of cereal into the diet at or before one month of age does not usually result in any major change in stool pattern.

Carbohydrate Content of Milks and Formulas

Human milk provides 37 per cent of calories from carbohydrate and cow milk provides 29 per cent of calories from this dietary com-

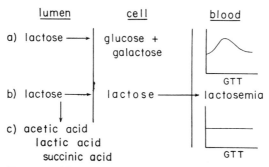

Figure 7–3. Diagram of fate of lactose in the small intestine in presence of lactase (a) and in absence of lactase (b). (From Sunshine, P., and Kretchmer, N.: Pediatrics 34:38, 1964.)

ponent. With few exceptions, commercially prepared formulas for infants provide from 32 to 51 per cent of calories from carbohydrate, and the great majority of such formulas provide from 40 to 45 per cent (see Chapters Eleven and Twelve). Infants grow normally and generally seem to tolerate a feeding of evaporated milk and water without additional carbohydrate (Fomon et al., 1966), although, as discussed in Chapter Six, fecal excretion of fat may be quite high.

Studies have not been carried out to determine whether normal infants will grow normally and remain free of symptoms when receiving diets providing less than 20 per cent of calories from carbohydrate. Such formulas will present the infant with substantially more than 20 per cent of calories from protein and/or more than 60 per cent of calories from fat. As discussed in Chapters Five and Six, some infants do not tolerate formulas of this nature.

When more than 50 per cent of calories are derived from carbohydrate, there is increased likelihood of exceeding the ability of the intestinal mucosal cells to hydrolyze the load of disaccharides. A diet in which 84 per cent of calories were derived from carbohydrate, 15 per cent from protein and 1 per cent from fat was found by Hansen et al. (1963) to be tolerated poorly. Fourteen of 20 full-size infants and seven of 12 infants of low birth weight were reported to have loose stools. "Growth and development" were judged to be "exceptionally poor" in six of 20 full-size infants and in two of 12 infants of low birth weight. Although the authors were inclined to attribute the relatively poor performance to deficiency of linoleic acid, excessive carbohydrate content of the diet may have been of greater significance.

In management of certain premature infants, infants with severe congenital heart disease and other conditions in which volume of food intake is limited, it is often desirable to increase the energy content of the formula above 67 kcal/100 ml. Either of two methods is employed: the formula is supplemented with carbohydrate or it is increased in concentration by alteration of the ratio of concentrated liquid (or powder) to water. The former method is more likely to result in excessive disaccharide load than is the latter.

Acquired Disaccharidase Deficiency

Bowie et al. (1963, 1965, 1966) have shown that the diarrhea associated with protein-calorie malnutrition in infants and children in South Africa is due to a specific lactase deficiency in intestinal mucosal cells. The lactose intolerance demonstrated by these infants may persist for months after the apparent cure of protein-calorie malnutrition. Further study is required to determine the frequency of acquired disaccharidase deficiency among infants in technically advanced countries. The diagnosis should be suspected in every instance in which diarrhea persists for more than two or three weeks.

Symptoms and Diagnosis of Disaccharidase Deficiency

Manifestations of disaccharidase deficiency occur only after ingestion of the specific disaccharide to which the patient is intolerant. Abdominal pain and passage of voluminous, watery, foamy stools of low pH is characteristic. Severe and, at times, life-threatening malnutrition may be present in infants. Manifestations subside when the disaccharide is excluded from the diet.

The diagnosis of disaccharide intolerance is made by history, examination of the stool, and demonstration of enzyme deficiency either directly by in vitro assay of disaccharidase activity in intestinal mucosa or indirectly by sugar tolerance tests. Since peroral biopsy of small infants is hazardous except in the hands of highly experienced individuals, demonstration of enzyme deficiency will generally be based on history, examination of the stool and results of tolerance tests with the disaccharide in question.

The infant should be treated with a diet free of the suspected disaccharide for several days before testing and diarrhea must be absent at the time of the test (Dahlqvist, 1966). After a fast of four to eight hours, the sugar to be tested is given in water in a dosage of 2 gm/kg of body weight or 50 gm/m² of body surface area.

Carbohydrate Intake and Body Content of Fat

Studies of rats have raised the possibility that the choice of carbohydrate may influence body composition. It has long been known that an excessive intake of lactose is toxic for the young rat, leading to diarrhea, enlargement of the cecum, failure to thrive and reduced body content of fat. Presumably the cause is failure of hydrolysis of lactose, since administration of glucose and galactose in the same amounts does not give rise to these manifestations.

Rats fed lactose-containing diets gain less weight and have less body fat than those fed diets containing equal amounts of other sugars (Sarett and Snipper, 1956; Tomarelli et al., 1960). When the food intake of rats fed glucose-containing diets was restricted to an amount that promoted weight gain equal to that of the lactose-fed rats, body content of fat was significantly greater than that of the rats fed lactose (Tomarelli et al., 1960).

The rather frequent, loose stools of low pH characteristic of the breast-fed infant may reflect lactose intake greater than can be handled by the lactase of the intestinal mucosa. Whether the type of carbohydrate in the diet of the human infant influences body composition is unknown.

Effect of Sugars on Absorption of Calcium, Magnesium and Strontium

Many reports document the beneficial effect of lactose on the absorption of calcium from the gastrointestinal tract of experimental animals, although relatively few studies have been performed with the human (Mills et al., 1940; Greenwald et al., 1963). Interpretation of animal studies is difficult because of differences in species, in the age of the animals, in the amounts of lactose given and in the experimental procedures. Wasserman and Comar (1959) have demonstrated that absorption of calcium by rats is not enhanced by administration of sugars that are rapidly absorbed from the intestinal tract (glucose, fructose, galactose and sucrose), while carbohydrates that are more slowly absorbed (lactose, cellobiose and several others) do enhance calcium absorption. Studies of isolated intestinal loops have demonstrated that in the rat many sugars promote absorption of calcium in the lower end of the gut (Vaughan and Filer, 1960). The favorable effect of lactose may be related to its relatively slow absorption, thus providing amounts of sugar in the lower intestinal tract which promote calcium absorption. The mechanism by which lactose promotes absorption of calcium is unknown. Absorption of magnesium and strontium is probably influenced by factors similar to those influencing absorption of calcium.

Hypoglycemia of the Newborn

Hypoglycemia in the full-size newborn infant is defined as concentration of glucose in blood less than 30 mg/100 ml between birth and 72 hours of age or concentration less than 40 mg/100 ml thereafter (Cornblath and Schwartz, 1966). In the infant of low birth weight, hypoglycemia is defined as concentration of glucose in the blood less than 20 mg/100 ml. The finding of low concentration of glucose should be confirmed by repeating the determination with a second specimen of the infant's blood, although it will usually be wise to begin therapy before the report of the second specimen is received. With this definition of hypoglycemia, the incidence will be found to be between 1 and 3 per 1000 births.

Symptoms frequently associated with hypoglycemia are tremors, cyanosis, convulsions, apnea, apathy, high-pitched or weak cry, refusal to feed, eye-rolling and irregular respirations. Differential diagnosis of these symptoms and of neonatal hypoglycemia has been discussed in detail by Cornblath and Schwartz (1966).

Studies of infants of low birth weight have demonstrated that concentrations of sugar in the blood are correlated significantly with the age at which feedings are instituted. In general, the earlier a group of infants is fed, the greater will be the mean concentration of sugar in the blood during the early days of life. Studies currently in progress in several centers concern the relation between the age of initiation of feedings, the concentration of sugar in the blood and mortality.

The age at which feedings are instituted is clearly only one feature of management requiring study. Equally important are caloric intake and composition of the diet.

When a diagnosis of symptomatic hypoglycemia is made, Cornblath and Schwartz (1966) have recommended rapid intravenous administration of 1 to 2 ml/kg of a solution of glucose in water (50 gm/100 ml), followed by continuous infusion, 75 to 110 ml/kg/day, of a 15 gm/100 ml solution of glucose in water. Oral feedings are instituted as soon as clinical manifestations subside, but the intravenous infusion is continued for 48 hours after concentration of glucose returns to normal. Concentration of glucose in the infusion solution is reduced to 5 gm/100 ml before being discontinued.

Choice of feeding in management of hypoglycemia of the newborn has not been a subject of study. Whether a 15 gm/100 ml solution of glucose or a milk formula is to be preferred is unknown but, at least after 48 hours of life, a milk formula seems preferable because of its provision of various nutrients other than carbohydrate. Frequent small feedings are probably preferable to larger feedings at greater intervals. Feedings by gavage at intervals of 2 to 3 hours will generally be found to be practical.

Lactosuria and Lactulosuria

Presence of lactose in urine in small amounts (less than 100 mg/100 ml) was found by Gryboski and Boehm (1965) in four of 26 infants fed evaporated milk, 19 of 88 infants fed Similac and two of seven breast-fed infants. Lactulose, a synthetic disaccharide containing fructose and galactose, is formed during heat processing of milk by converting the glucose portion of the lactose molecule to fructose. This sugar, for which no disaccharidase is present in the human, was not excreted in urine of breast-fed infants but was present to the extent of 50 to 200 mg/100 ml in urine of four of 26 infants fed evaporated milk and 34 of 88 infants fed Similac (Gryboski and Boehm, 1965).

Galactosemia and Galactose-free Diet

Galactosemia is a disorder of carbohydrate metabolism resulting from deficiency of the enzyme, galactose-1-phosphate uridyl transferase, that normally converts galactose-1-phosphate to glucose-1-phosphate. Because of impairment of this conversion, dietary galactose, including that resulting from splitting of the disaccharide, lactose, cannot be metabolized and accumulates within the body. Manifestations are failure to thrive, hepatosplenomegaly, cirrhosis, cataracts and mental retardation. Concentration of galactose in the blood is elevated, galactose-1-phosphate uridyl transferase activity in erythrocytes can be demonstrated to be deficient, and urine contains galactose, amino acids and albumin. Frequency of the disorder has been estimated as one in 18,000 births (Hansen et al., 1964).

Since glucose can be converted by the body to galactose in sufficient quantities to fulfill the requirements for galactose, dietary management can be based on the goal of eliminating galactose from the diet. All symptoms and signs of the disorder can be prevented by elimination of galactose from the diet. Even when manifestations of galactosemia are advanced, much improvement may result from consumption of a galactose-free diet.

In infancy it is relatively easy to provide a galactose-free diet since parental control of food intake is almost absolute. A galactose-free diet consists of a milk substitute and avoidance of all foods containing physiologically available galactose. Milk substitutes of three types are available: Nutramigen, a casein hydrolysate; meat-based formulas and soy-based formulas. These products are discussed in Chapter Twelve. Nutramigen contains approximately 16 mg of lactose (equivalent to 8 mg of galactose) in 67 kcal (Committee on Nutrition, 1963), but this amount appears to be too small to constitute a hazard and the formula has been used successfully in management of galactosemia (Isselbacher, 1959; Donnell et al., 1961).

Meat Base Formula* contains a trace of galactose, presumably arising from a galactoside in beef heart muscle. Reports of use of this formula or of Lambase* formula (these are the only two commercially

---

*Gerber Products Co.

available formulas in the United States based on meat) in the management of patients with galactosemia have not been published.

Soy-based formulas contain appreciable amounts of the alpha-galactosides, stachyose and raffinose, which contain galactose. Gitzelmann and Auricchio (1965) have calculated that a protein intake of 3 gm/kg/day from soy would provide a daily intake of stachyose and raffinose of 0.32 and 0.07 gm/kg/day, respectively, equivalent to 0.18 gm/kg/day of galactose. If this quantity of galactose could be released from the stachyose and raffinose, it would surely be harmful and several authors have warned against use of soy-based formulas for management of infants with galactosemia (Schwarz, 1966; Cornblath and Schwartz, 1966). However, recent investigations support clinical observations that soy-based formulas are satisfactory in management of galactosemia (Gitzelmann and Auricchio, 1965; Gitzelmann, 1966).

Gitzelmann and Auricchio point out that ingestion of alpha-galactosides could be hazardous for a galactosemic patient by three possible mechanisms: they could be hydrolyzed by intestinal mucosal cells with absorption of galactose; they could be absorbed as alpha-galactosides and transported to other tissues where hydrolysis might occur; they could be acted upon by intestinal bacteria with liberation of galactose, which might then be absorbed. It has now been shown that alpha-galactosidases are absent in the human intestinal mucosa (Gitzelmann and Auricchio, 1965). Small amounts of raffinose do appear in the urine after feeding of this sugar, indicating that it can be absorbed, but erythrocyte content of galactose-1-phosphate does not increase and evidence of hydrolysis in various body tissues is therefore lacking. During diarrhea, hydrolysis of alpha-galactosides occurs, as demonstrated by the finding of free hexoses in the stools. However, absorption from the colon appears to be extremely limited. It therefore appears safe to utilize soy-based formulas for treatment of galactosemia.

REFERENCES

Auricchio, S., Rubino, A., and Mürset, G.: Intestinal glycosidase activities in the human embryo, fetus, and newborn. Pediatrics 35:944, 1965.
Barbero, G. J., Runge, G., Fischer, D., Crawford, M. N., Torres, F. E., and György, P.: Investigations on the bacterial flora, pH, and sugar content in the intestinal tract of infants. J. Pediat. 40:152, 1952.
Bowie, M. D., Brinkman, G. L., and Hansen, J. D. L.: Diarrhoea in protein-calorie malnutrition. Lancet 2:550, 1963.
Bowie, M. D., Brinkman, G. L., and Hansen, J. D. L.: Acquired disaccharide intolerance in malnutrition. J. Pediat. 66:1083, 1965.
Bowie, M. D., Hansen, J. D. L., and Barbezat, G. O.: Disaccharide intolerance in protein-calorie malnutrition. Presented at 7th Internat. Congress Nutr., Hamburg, Germany, Aug. 3–10, 1966.
Committee on Nutrition, American Academy of Pediatrics: Appraisal of nutritional

adequacy of infant formulas used as cow milk substitutes. Pediatrics *31*:329, 1963.

Cornblath, M., and Schwartz, R.: Disorders of Carbohydrate Metabolism in Infancy. Philadelphia, W. B. Saunders Company, 1966.

Dahlqvist, A.: *In* Durand, P. (ed.): Disorders due to Intestinal Defective Carbohydrate Digestion and Absorption. New York, Grune & Stratton, 1964.

Dahlqvist, A.: Disaccharide intolerance. J.A.M.A. *195*:225, 1966.

Donnell, G. N., Collado, M., and Koch, R.: Growth and development of children with galactosemia. J. Pediat. *58*:836, 1961.

Fomon, S. J., Younoszai, M. K., and Thomas, L. N.: Influence of vitamin D on linear growth of normal full-term infants. J. Nutrition *88*:345, 1966.

Gitzelmann, R.: (Letter to Editor) The handling of soya α-galactosides by a normal and a galactosemic child. Pediatrics *37*:532, 1966.

Gitzelmann, R., and Auricchio, S.: The handling of soya α-galactosides by a normal and a galactosemic child. Pediatrics *36*:231, 1965.

Greenwald, E., Samachson, J., and Spencer, H.: Effect of lactose on calcium metabolism in man. J. Nutrition *79*:531, 1963.

Gryboski, J. D., and Boehm, J. J.: Lactulosuria in the neonate: A preliminary report. Pediatrics *35*:340, 1965.

Haemmerli, U. P., Kistler, H., Ammann, R., Marthaler, T., Semenza, G., Auricchio, S., and Prader, A.: Acquired milk intolerance in adult caused by lactose malabsorption due to a selective deficiency of intestinal lactase activity. Am. J. Med. *38*:7, 1965.

Hansen, A. E., Wiese, H. F., Boelsche, A. N., Haggard, M. E., Adam, D. J. D., and Davis, H.: Role of linoleic acid in infant nutrition. Clinical and chemical study of 428 infants fed on milk mixtures varying in kind and amount of fat. Pediatrics *31*:171, 1963.

Hansen, R. G., Bretthauer, R. K., Mayes, J., and Nordin, J. H.: Estimation of frequency of occurrence of galactosemia in the population. Proc. Soc. Exper. Biol. & Med. *115*:560, 1964.

Hardinge, M. G., Swarner, J. B., and Crooks, H.: Carbohydrates in foods. J. A. Dietet. Ass. *46*:197, 1965.

Isselbacher, K. J.: Galactose metabolism and galactosemia. Am. J. Med. *26*:715, 1959.

Mills, R., Breiter, H., Kempster, E., McKey, B., Pickens, M., and Outhouse, J.: The influence of lactose on calcium retention in children. J. Nutrition *20*:467, 1940.

Prader, A., Auricchio, S., and Semenza, G.: Die Hereditäre Saccharose- und Isomaltose-malabsorption. Monatsschrift Kinderheilk. *112*:177, 1964.

Pratt, A. G., and Read, W. T., Jr.: Influence of type of feeding on pH of stool, pH of skin, and incidence of perianal dermatitis in the newborn infant. J. Pediat. *46*:539, 1955.

Sarett, H. P., and Snipper, L. P.: Effect of adding carbohydrate to milk diets. I. Growth and body composition. J. Nutrition *58*:529, 1956.

Schwarz, V.: (Letter to Editor) The handling of soya α-galactosides by a normal and a galactosemic child. Pediatrics *37*:531, 1966.

Sunshine, P., and Kretchmer, N.: Studies of small intestine during development. III. Infantile diarrhea associated with intolerance to disaccharides. Pediatrics *34*:38, 1964.

Tomarelli, R. M., Hartz, R., and Bernhart, F. W.: The effect of lactose feeding on the body fat of the rat. J. Nutrition *71*:221, 1960.

Vaughan, O. W., and Filer, L. J., Jr.: The enhancing action of certain carbohydrates on the intestinal absorption of calcium in the rat. J. Nutrition *71*:10, 1960.

Wasserman, R. H., and Comar, C. L.: Carbohydrates and gastrointestinal absorption of radiostrontium and radiocalcium in the rat. Proc. Soc. Exper. Biol. Med. *101*:314, 1959.

Chapter Eight

Vitamins

In technically advanced countries, vitamin deficiency diseases in infancy are relatively uncommon. For example, in the United States during the past 20 years, deficiencies of riboflavin and niacin in infancy have not been reported; vitamin A deficiency has been reported only in infants with steatorrhea or those receiving milk-free diets (or diets based on skim milk) not fortified with vitamin A; and thiamine deficiency has been reported in only two infants, both of whom had received a soy-based formula which was not fortified with thiamine. During this period, reports of vitamin A intoxication outnumbered reports of deficiency, suggesting the need for reappraisal of current practices in infant feeding. Publicity about a possible causal relation between mild overdosage of vitamin D and infantile hypercalcemia has called attention to the need for caution in vitamin administration to infants, although the number of children potentially at risk from such mild overdosage is undoubtedly small.

Deficiency diseases related to certain other vitamins have by no means been eliminated. Mild deficiency of vitamin K in the newborn is relatively common. In the United States rickets due to vitamin D deficiency continues to occur sporadically and scurvy occurs in certain geographic areas. The frequency of iron deficiency anemia may mask manifestations of folic acid deficiency so that the true incidence of folic acid deficiency in infancy may be considerably higher than is now appreciated.

113

As emphasized previously (Chapter Three), requirements for essential nutrients vary considerably with the circumstances of their determination. Nowhere is this more evident than with respect to the vitamins (Gershoff, 1964). As the carbohydrate content of the diet increases, the requirement for thiamine increases. As protein content of the diet increases, requirement for vitamin B_6 increases while that for pantothenic acid decreases. Increased dietary intake of polyunsaturated fatty acids results in increased requirement for vitamin E. Methionine may have a sparing effect with respect to requirement for folic acid and vitamin B_{12}. Tryptophan can replace all or part of the requirement for niacin. Abundant evidence indicates that composition of the diet influences synthesis of B vitamins by microorganisms of the gastrointestinal tract, but whether these vitamins are then absorbed to a sufficient extent to be of practical value is uncertain.

Chemistry and physiologic functions have been well summarized for the fat-soluble vitamins by Dam and Søndergaard (1964) and for the water-soluble vitamins by Goldsmith (1964), Chow (1964) and Woodruff (1964).

Vitamin A

Preformed vitamin A, a fat-soluble vitamin, occurs only in the animal kingdom, being present in high concentrations in livers of fish and of most land vertebrates, in eggs and in the fat of milks. At least ten different carotenoids exhibit provitamin A activity but only alpha- and beta-carotene and cryptoxanthine are of importance in human nutrition (Dam and Søndergaard, 1964).

One international unit of vitamin A activity is equivalent to 0.344 μg of vitamin A_1 acetate, 0.30 μg of vitamin A_1 alcohol or 0.60 μg of the provitamin, beta-carotene.

Deficiency

Deficiency of vitamin A ranks among the most prevalent of nutritional deficiency diseases throughout technically underdeveloped countries of the world.

In technically advanced countries this deficiency is rare for three main reasons: first, intake of dairy products and meat is relatively large and these foods provide rather generous amounts of preformed vitamin A; second, carotenes, the precursors of vitamin A, are present in many commonly ingested foods, particularly yellow and green vegetables; third, the amount of fat in the diet is sufficient to assure adequate absorption of vitamin A and carotenes. By contrast, in countries in which vitamin A deficiency is prevalent, consumption of dairy products and meat is usually slight; if carotenes are present in adequate amounts in commonly ingested foods, dietary intake of fat is usually so low that absorption of carotenes is slight.

In vitamin A deficiency, young animals cease to grow and, especially in prolonged deficiency, nearly all organs are affected. The human infant manifests failure to thrive, apathy, mental retardation, dry and scaly skin and corneal changes that may progress to a stage of ulceration. Cartilage and bone are often involved in addition to other epithelial and connective tissues.

Requirement and Advisable Intake

The requirement of the infant for vitamin A is unknown. Requirements for various mammalian species range from 20 to 100 I.U./kg/day (Rubin and deRitter, 1954) and requirements of human adult volunteers were found to be 1300 I.U./day (Hume and Krebs, 1949) or approximately 20 I.U./kg/day. On the basis of this estimate, the human infant would require 70, 170 and 200 I.U./day at ages one, six and 12 months, respectively.

Because we do not know whether the vitamin A requirement of the adult is applicable to the infant on a body weight basis, the advisable intake during the first year of life is listed in Table 8–1 as 600 I.U./day or three times the estimated requirement of an infant weighing 10 kg. It is therefore recommended that supplementation of an infant's diet with vitamin A should be restricted to instances in which average daily intakes are less than 600 I.U./day. Since the human liver is able to store vitamin A effectively, *average* daily intakes are probably of more significance than intakes on individual days. There is, therefore, no justification for supplementation of the diet with vitamin A merely because daily intake occasionally falls below 600 I.U.

As may be seen from the tables included in Chapters Eleven and Twelve, human milk, cow milk and most commercially available formulas for infants are relatively rich sources of vitamin A. In addition, many strained or chopped foods commercially prepared for infants supply abundant amounts of carotene. Therefore, supplementation of the diet of normal infants is rarely indicated except in the case of an infant receiving skim milk or a milk-free formula to which no vitamins have been added. Even in such instances, strained foods commercially prepared for infants will ordinarily provide an adequate intake of vitamin A (Table 8–2).

Because water-miscible preparations of vitamin A are better absorbed than oily preparations, it is recommended that only the

Table 8-1. *Requirements and Advisable Intakes of Vitamins*

	Estimated Daily Requirement			Advisable Intake		
	Age 1 mo	Age 6 mo	Age 12 mo	Age 1 mo	Age 6 mo	Age 12 mo
A (I.U.)	70	170	200	600	600	600
D (I.U.)	100–200	100–200	100–200	400	400	400
E (mg)*	?	?	?	1.3	1.8	1.8
C (mg)	10	10	10	20	20	20
Thiamine (mg)	——— ? 0.2 mg/1000 kcal ———			0.12	0.16	0.21
Riboflavin (mg)	——— ? 0.3 mg/1000 kcal ———			0.27	0.34	0.44
Niacin equivalents (mg)	——— ? 4.4 mg/1000 kcal ———			3.7	4.7	6.2
B$_6$ (μg/gm protein)	9	9	9	18	18	18

*Expressed as milligrams of alpha-tocopherol. When the diet is relatively low in polyunsaturated fats, as in the feeding of cow milk, lower intakes are adequate (see text).

Table 8–2. *Carotene Content of Some Strained Foods for Infants*

Food	Carotene (Vitamin A equivalence*) (I.U./100 gm food)
Carrots	12,000–14,000
Vegetable soup ⎫ Garden vegetables ⎬ Mixed vegetables ⎭	3500–5700
Sweet potatoes	3500–4100
Creamed spinach	2700–3200
Vegetables and beef ⎫ Vegetables and bacon ⎬ Vegetables and lamb ⎭	2300–2700
Squash	1900
Plums ⎫ Prunes ⎬ Apricots ⎭	400–2000
Vegetables and meat (except those mentioned above	400–1100
Peas	300–500
Most vegetables not listed above	100–300
Most fruits not listed above	50–150

*0.6 μg beta carotene = 1 I.U. vitamin A

former be used for supplementation of the infant's diet. Infants with chronic steatorrhea should receive about 2000 I.U. daily of a water-miscible preparation of vitamin A.

Toxicity

For the reasons mentioned, it seems unlikely that any normal infant in North America receiving an otherwise adequate diet will benefit from supplementary administration of vitamin A. In fact, the hazards of vitamin A overdosage exceed the dangers of deficiency. It is unfortunate that American physicians have not acted upon the thoughtful warnings of several writers about overdosage of vitamin A. These warnings have been aptly summarized by Caffey (1961): "Hazards of vitamin A poisoning from the routine prophylactic feeding of vitamin concentrates A and D to healthy infants and children on good diets are considerably greater than the hazards of vitamin A deficiency in healthy infants and children not fed vitamin concentrates."

Manifestations of vitamin A toxicity include anorexia, irritability, increased intracranial pressure, desquamation of the skin, roentgenographically demonstrable changes in the long bones and increased concentration of vitamin A in serum. Until recently, chronic poisoning with vitamin A had been reported only in the case of prolonged gross overdosage (e.g., ingestion of teaspoonful amounts of a vitamin preparation containing the recommended daily allowance in a fraction of a milliliter). Generally, the individual had received 75,000 to 500,000 I.U. daily for three to 12 months before overt signs of toxicity were recognized (Caffey, 1950).

Since aqueous suspensions of vitamin A have become commercially available, the dosage of vitamin A and the time required to produce manifestations of toxicity seem to have been markedly reduced. Persson et al. (1965) have reported five cases of vitamin A toxicity developing in infants less than six months of age. In one instance 18,500 I.U. of vitamin A daily for three months and in three instances 22,500 I.U. of vitamin A daily for one to one and one half months resulted in manifestations of toxicity.

Presumably, the greater ease of absorption of vitamin A in aqueous suspension than in an oily medium (Kramer et al., 1947; Lewis et al., 1947) results in greater toxicity. In the future we must consider that daily ingestion of 20,000 I.U. of vitamin A for one or two months is likely to be toxic (compared to about 75,000 I.U. daily for four to six months when oily preparations were used). In discussing vitamin A toxicity, it is necessary to distinguish between ingestion of vitamin A and ingestion of carotenes. Although carotenes can fulfill the requirement for vitamin A, excessive ingestion of carotenes results in the benign disorder, carotenemia, and not in hypervitaminosis A.

Vitamin D

Most vertebrates require vitamin D, a group of fat-soluble vitamins, for optimal absorption of calcium and phosphorus. The vitamin may be supplied through the diet or by suitable irradiation of the body.

Vitamin D is represented by a group of steroid alcohols of which vitamins D_2 and D_3 are most important. The international unit of vitamin D is equivalent to 0.025 μg of vitamin D_3. The provitamins

D, including ergosterol, 7-dehydrocholesterol and several related compounds, may originate from food or be synthesized in the body (Dam and Søndergaard, 1964).

Determination of vitamin D content of foods is carried out primarily by a bioassay based on healing of rickets in rats. Because the method is difficult and lacks precision, manufacturers who fortify foods with vitamin D have ordinarily added an excess in order to be certain that the label claim was met. The extent of this "overage" in various products is not specified.

Deficiency

Vitamin D deficiency of infants is manifested by clinical, biochemical (especially decreased inorganic phosphorus concentration and increased alkaline phosphatase activity in the serum) and roentgenographic evidence of scurvy. During the years 1956 through 1960, 843 cases of rickets were recognized among approximately 2,350,000 infants and children admitted to 226 teaching hospitals in the United States (Committee on Nutrition, 1962). Because some cases of rickets were probably not recognized, because not all children with rickets were admitted to hospitals, and because the survey mentioned was limited to relatively few hospitals, it seems likely that nutritional rickets is not uncommon in the United States.

The requirement for vitamin D during infancy is between 100 and 200 I.U./day (Committee on Nutrition, 1963b). In contrast to the situation with respect to vitamin A, little storage of vitamin D occurs and regular ingestion of the advisable intake is important. An intake of 400 I.U. represents at least twice the requirement and is suggested as the advisable daily intake.

Although casual exposure to sunlight will ordinarily fulfill the need for vitamin D after one year of age, it seems reasonable to ignore the contribution of sunlight during the first year of life and to provide the advisable intake of 400 I.U. of vitamin D daily from foods and, when necessary, a vitamin supplement. Administration of a supplement of vitamin D is inadvisable when dietary sources provide 400 I.U. daily.

Sources of Vitamin D

In the United States, evaporated milk, most commercially prepared formulas for infants and approximately 85 per cent of fresh whole milk sold by dairies (but only 1 per cent of fresh milk sold in Canada) are fortified with vitamin D so as to provide at least 400 I.U. per quart.

Foods other than milk that are commonly fortified with vitamin

D include breakfast drinks, breakfast cereals, milk flavorings, margarine and some breads. None of these foods is commonly ingested in large amounts by infants. Among commercially available strained foods for infants, egg yolk and tuna fish provide approximately 200 I.U. per 100 gm, but amounts of vitamin D in other strained foods are extremely low. Therefore, when an infant's average daily intake of vitamin D from milk or formula remains below 400 I.U., it is reasonable to administer a supplement sufficient to raise the daily intake to 400 I.U.

The vitamin D content of human milk is less than 100 I.U. per liter and the advisable intake of 400 I.U. daily should therefore be provided as a supplement.

Toxicity or Hypersensitivity

Concern regarding excessive intakes of vitamin D arises primarily from the possible but unproven etiologic role of vitamin D in producing infantile idiopathic hypercalcemia. The severe form of this disorder is characterized by failure to thrive, vomiting, mental retardation, bony changes, elevated concentration of calcium in serum, and, in some cases, aortic stenosis and/or progressive renal failure and hypertension. The facies have been described as elflike.

In 1953 and 1954 approximately 100 new cases of idiopathic hypercalcemia were diagnosed annually in Great Britain, and an extensive survey of infant feeding practices revealed that many infants were receiving 3000 to 4000 I.U. of vitamin D daily (British Paediatric Association, 1956). Major sources of vitamin D in infants' diets were powdered milks, cereals and vitamin supplements. On the basis of recommendations made in 1956 and 1957, the extent of fortification of foods with vitamin D in Great Britain was reduced to the extent that relatively few infants received as much as 1500 I.U. daily. The incidence of idiopathic hypercalcemia in infants in Great Britain has since decreased. However, the decrease did not occur immediately but only after several years, and thus the sequence of events does not offer strong support for the conclusion that excessive intake of vitamin D is etiologically related to infantile hypercalcemia (British Paediatric Association, 1964).

When the extent of vitamin D fortification of foods for infants was reduced in Great Britain in 1957, there was some concern that this measure, undertaken for the benefit of relatively few infants who might be unusually sensitive to moderate overdosage of vitamin D, would result in an increased incidence of rickets. Thus, the over-all effect of reduction of vitamin D intake by the infant population would prove to be detrimental rather than beneficial. However, no increase in incidence of rickets has been noted (Editorial, Brit. M. J., 1964; British Paediatric Association, 1964; Bransby et al., 1964).

Therefore, in spite of the still dubious nature of the relation between intake of vitamin D and infantile hypercalcemia, there would appear to be no hazard but some possible benefit from restricting intake of vitamin D to approximately 400 I.U. daily for all infants and avoiding greater intakes. To achieve this goal, all milks and formulas commercially available for feeding of infants should be fortified to the extent of 400 I.U. per liter. Other foodstuffs should not be fortified with vitamin D. Vitamin D supplements should provide 400 I.U. per daily dose and should not be prescribed for infants whose intakes from other sources amount to 400 I.U. daily.

Vitamin E

Vitamin E represents a group of fat-soluble substances required by many species for normal reproduction, normal development of muscles, normal resistance of erythrocytes to hemolysis and a series of other biochemical and physiologic functions (Dam and Søndergaard, 1964). There is no longer reason for doubt that this vitamin is essential for the human infant.

Seven clinically related compounds — alpha-, beta-, gamma-, delta-, epsilon-, zeta- and eta-tocopherol — exert vitamin E activity. Of these, alpha-tocopherol is most potent. Although the only rich sources of tocopherols are some vegetable oils, smaller quantities are present in a wide variety of foods. Tocopherols are important natural antioxidants in foods and are especially effective in preventing oxidation of fats (Vasington et al., 1960).

In the past few years, use of paper or column chromatography and/or gas chromatography has permitted more accurate determination of the alpha-tocopherol content of biologic fluids, tissues and foods. These newer methods are specific for alpha-tocopherol and do not, as was true in the past, also detect some non-alpha-tocopherol reducing substances. Values are somewhat lower than those previously reported. Table 8–3 indicates normal values for alpha-tocopherol in human milk, cow milk and several infant formulas.

Evidences of Vitamin E Deficiency

Human infants who receive low intakes of vitamin E and children who fail to absorb vitamin E because of steatorrhea, especially those with cystic fibrosis of the pancreas or biliary atresia, demonstrate biochemical and pathologic findings similar to those seen in experimentally produced vitamin E deficiency in animals. Children with chronic steatorrhea, infants of low birth weight and, at times and to a lesser extent, full-size infants whose intakes of tocopherol have been

Table 8–3. Concentration of Alpha-Tocopherol in Human Plasma,
Human Milk and Cow Milk

Material	Mean Value by Older Methodology	Mean Revised Value
Plasma, adult (mg/100 ml)		
Harris et al., 1961	1.01 (S.D. 0.24)	
Herting and Drury, 1965a		
Rochester, N.Y.		0.36 (S.D. 0.08)
Syracuse, N.Y.		0.51 (S.D. 0.09)
Plasma, newborn, full size, (mg/100 ml)		
Nitkowsky et al., 1962a	0.45 (S.D. 0.14)	
Assumed value°		0.22
Plasma, newborn, low birth weight (mg/100 ml)		
Nitkowsky et al., 1962b	0.39 (S.D. 0.10)	
Assumed value°		0.20
Human milk (µg/gm lipid)		
Harris et al., 1952	80 (range 25–107)	
Herting and Drury, 1965b		40
Cow milk (µg/gm lipid)		
Harris et al., 1952	(range 23–40)	
Herting and Drury, 1965b		16 (range 4–30†)

°Alpha-tocopherol assumed to account for approximately one-half of value determined by older methodology.

†Lower value in early spring; higher value mid fall.

low, demonstrate low concentrations of tocopherol in plasma, increased hemolysis of erythrocytes in dilute solutions of hydrogen peroxide and excessive creatinuria. All these findings are reversed by administration of alpha-tocopherol (Nitowsky et al., 1962a). In addition, the creatine content of muscle of patients with cystic fibrosis of the pancreas has been shown to increase after administration of alpha-tocopherol (Nitowsky et al., 1962b).

Pathologic manifestations, including focal necrosis of skeletal muscle (Oppenheimer, 1956; Weinberg et al., 1958; Landing, 1960) and deposition of ceroid pigment in smooth muscle (Blanc et al., 1958; Kerner and Goldbloom, 1960), have been demonstrated in patients with cystic fibrosis of the pancreas or biliary atresia. It seems likely that these manifestations are, in fact, evidences of vitamin E deficiency.

Requirements and Advisable Intakes

Requirements of the infant for vitamin E are still somewhat

uncertain. Probably the amounts provided by formulas based on cow milk unfortified with alpha-tocopherol are about at the level of requirement for the full-size infant and somewhat less than the requirement for infants of low birth weight.

FULL-SIZE INFANT. It has been demonstrated that serum concentrations of alpha-tocopherol, which are characteristically low at birth, rise rapidly in the breast-fed infant but may remain low for many months when formulas based on cow milk are fed (Gordon et al., 1958). Nevertheless, other biochemical and pathologic evidences of tocopherol deficiency have not been detected in these infants, and extensive clinical experiences with such formulas suggest that intakes from them are adequate.

Assuming that the average concentration of alpha-tocopherol in cow milk is 16 μg per gram of lipid (Table 8–3) and that lipid content of most formulas containing fat from cow milk is 2.8 gm/100 ml (Chapter Eleven, Table 11–6), alpha-tocopherol content will be approximately 45 μg/100 ml. Because average volumes of milk or formula consumed by infants receiving their sole caloric intakes from this source are approximately 750 ml/day at age one month (Chapter Four), and perhaps 1000 ml/day at age six months, intakes of alpha-tocopherol are estimated as 0.34 mg/day at age one month and 0.45 mg/day at age six months. Intakes by 12-month-old infants are probably not much greater than those by six-month-old infants. For infants receiving butterfat as the major source of dietary lipid, intakes of 0.34, 0.45 and 0.45 mg/day of alpha-tocopherol are considered adequate for ages one, six and 12 months of age, respectively.

When dietary lipid provides greater amounts of polyunsaturated fatty acids, average amounts of alpha-tocopherol consumed by the breast-fed infant are advisable: 1.3, 1.8 and 1.8 mg/day, respectively, at ages one, six and 12 months (calculated in a manner similar to that described for cow milk formulas). These values are listed in Table 8–1 as advisable intakes.

PREMATURE INFANT. Body stores of tocopherol of the premature infant are lower at birth than those of the full-term infant (Dju et al., 1952), and the biochemical and pathologic findings mentioned previously provide at least a suggestion that tocopherol deficiency exists. Furthermore, Dyggve and Probst (1963) demonstrated that average concentrations of bilirubin were lower and concentrations of hemoglobin higher in premature infants who had received 100 mg of alpha-tocopherol intramuscularly at birth than in those who had not received tocopherol. Presumably, the premature infant is somewhat handicapped in achieving normal concentrations of tocopherol in plasma and tissues because of relatively low body stores at birth, relatively rapid rate of gain in weight and somewhat diminished ability to absorb fat. For these reasons it seems desirable to accept the recommendation of several authors (Mackenzie, 1954; Nitowsky et al., 1956, 1962a and b; Goldbloom, 1963; Committee on Nutrition, 1963a) that a supplement of tocopherol be given to premature infants. A daily dose of alpha-tocopherol of 0.5 mg/kg would seem to be a reasonable recommendation (Nitowsky et al., 1962b).

STEATORRHEA. Infants with chronic steatorrhea of any cause should receive daily supplementation with a water-miscible preparation of tocopherol. For such infants a dosage of 200 to 300 mg/day has been recommended by Nitowsky et al. (1962b) and 100 mg/day by Goldbloom (1963).

Vitamin K

Vitamin K is a group of fat-soluble methylnaphthoquinone derivatives required for biosynthesis of several factors necessary for normal clotting of the blood. Vitamin K_1 is present in green plants, and a series of substances referred to as vitamin K_2 are synthesized by bacteria. Laboratory confirmation of vitamin K deficiency and of its correction after treatment is readily made by determining one-stage prothrombin time. This test is sensitive to three of the vitamin K-dependent clotting factors—prothrombin, and factors VII and IX (Committee on Nutrition, 1961).

Synthetic as well as natural compounds have vitamin K activity. Water-soluble vitamin K compounds (i.e., synthetic water-soluble analogues of menadione) have been extensively utilized in the past for the treatment and prophylaxis of hemorrhagic disease of the newborn. The choice of these vitamin K compounds was made because they could be administered subcutaneously or intramuscularly whereas preparations of vitamin K_1 (phytonadione) available at that time could be administered only by the oral or intravenous routes. During the past few years it has become clear that attempts to prevent hemorrhagic disease of the newborn by administration of large doses of water-soluble analogues of menadione to the woman in labor or to the newborn infant may be followed by hemolytic anemia, hyperbilirubinemia, kernicterus and death of the infant (Committee on Nutrition, 1961). Susceptibility of individual infants to the influence of water-soluble analogues of menadione probably varies widely.

Requirement and Advisable Intake

Intakes of human milk, cow milk or various formulas commercially prepared for infants provide more than 1 mg of vitamin K daily although the requirement is believed to be no greater than 5 μg daily (Committee on Nutrition, 1961). Vitamin K is also present in a wide variety of foods other than milk.

NEWBORN INFANT. Most infants develop a mild deficiency of vitamin K two to three days after birth. In approximately 1 in 400 infants, the deficiency is associated with clinical manifestations of bleeding and is then termed "hemorrhagic disease of the newborn" (Smith, 1966). The coagulation abnormality can be corrected by administration of compounds with vitamin K activity (Aballi et al., 1957; Vietti et al., 1960).

Water-miscible preparations of vitamin K_1 now available (Aqua-Mephyton, Konakion, Mono-Kay) may be administered orally, intramuscularly, subcutaneously or intravenously. Since the margin of safety with vitamin K_1 is great, it seems unwise to administer water-soluble vitamin K preparations (Hykinone, Synkayvite) known to have a small margin of safety during the newborn period. *It is recommended that every newborn infant receive a single parenteral dose of 1.0 mg of vitamin K_1 soon after birth.*

A particular problem may arise in management of infants born to women who have been receiving coumarin drugs in anticoagulant therapy. Such infants may demonstrate severe clotting defects (Gordon and Dean, 1955) and may require repeated doses of vitamin K.

It is obvious that no program of vitamin K administration begun after birth will protect the infant from bleeding at the time of birth. A recent study by Owen et al. (1967) has demonstrated that oral administration of 5 mg of vitamin K_1 daily to women for several days before delivery resulted in significant improvement in prothrombin time of the newborn infant. Serum concentrations of bilirubin were not affected. Additional studies will be necessary to determine whether clinical advantage results from this improvement in prothrombin time. In the current state of our knowledge, it is probably desirable to combine a program of prenatal prophylaxis (5 mg of vitamin K_1 daily beginning two weeks before the anticipated date of delivery) with a single parenteral dose of 1 mg given to the infant soon after birth.

OLDER INFANTS. For normal infants it is unncessary to supplement the diet with vitamin K after the newborn period. When infants are unable to ingest a normal diet as, for example, when gastrointestinal surgery is required, vitamin K_1 should be given parenterally in a dosage of 1 mg each week. Hepatic injury or inadequate intestinal absorption of lipids, such as occurs in obstructive jaundice, biliary fistula, insufficient production of bile acids or pancreatic insufficiency, may lead to vitamin K deficiency. After the newborn period, water-soluble analogues of menadione can be safely used in the management of infants with these disorders. Oral doses of 2 to 5 mg weekly are recommended.

Ascorbic Acid

Ascorbic acid, a water-soluble vitamin, is a strong reducing substance both in vitro and in biologic systems. It is important for the normal development of fibroblasts, osteoblasts and odontoblasts, although the mechanism of its action is poorly understood (Woodruff, 1964). In addition, it functions in intermediary metabolism of a number of substances, including the 5-hydroxylation of tryptophan and the oxidation of tyrosine. It may also be important in formation of adrenal steroids (Woodruff, 1964).

Deficiency

Earliest clinical evidences of ascorbic acid deficiency are apathy, irritability and anorexia. As the illness progresses, irritability increases, tenderness of the lower extremities is prominent and pseudo-paralysis develops. Costochondral beading, hemorrhages of skin and mucous membranes, especially about the erupting teeth, also appear. Iron deficiency anemia is a frequent accompaniment.

Serum concentrations of ascorbic acid are less than 0.1 mg/100 ml and roentgenograms demonstrate characteristic changes at the cartilage-shaft junctions of the long bones, especially the distal end of the femur.

INCIDENCE OF SCURVY. Failure of infants to receive adequate amounts of ascorbic acid can be traced primarily to faulty nutritional education of parents or to failure of physicans to realize that certain milks and formulas are deficient in content of ascorbic acid. In the United States, scurvy is no less prevalent in Florida than in states where citrus fruits are less readily available.

In the five-year period, 1956–1960, 226 teaching hospitals in the United States reported admission of 713 infants and children with scurvy. The incidence was greatest in the southeastern portion of the country despite the ready availability of citrus fruits in much of that area. Among an estimated 58,400 infants and children admitted to hospitals in Louisiana during the five-year period, 128 cases of scurvy were identified, or 1 case of scurvy in every 460 infants and children admitted. Reports of scurvy in Canada in 1958 and 1959 (Whelen et al., 1958; Grewar, 1958 and 1959) were of sufficient concern to result in legislation permitting the addition of ascorbic acid to evaporated milk.

The age of occurrence of infantile scurvy may be seen from Figure 8–1. Caffey (1961) has stated that neither clinical nor roentgenographic evidence of scurvy has been verified in infants younger than three months of age. Roentgenographic manifestations of congenital syphilis have occasionally been interpreted as those of scurvy. Grewar (1965) found that infants over 12 months of age developed scurvy only in instances of severe feeding difficulties, as in mental retardation.

Requirements and Advisable Intakes

Requirements for human subjects are a matter of considerable controversy since evidence of capillary fragility, bony abnormalities and other early manifestations of scurvy are prevented by daily ingestion of much smaller doses than those required for tissue saturation. Until some advantage of tissue saturation is demonstrated, it seems unreasonable to assume that maximal concentrations of ascorbic acid in tissues indicate optimal nutritional status.

Concentrations of ascorbic acid in serum reflect dietary intake during the preceding weeks or few months. Tissue concentrations (e.g., concentrations in leukocytes) reflect more remote intake. Concentration of ascorbic acid both in serum and in leukocytes of breast-fed infants may average 0.6 mg in 100 ml (or 100 gm). If the infant is then given a diet free of ascorbic acid, serum concentration will decrease to about 0.1 mg/100 ml in two to three months and to undetectable levels thereafter. Concentrations will remain at detectable levels for a month or so longer in leukocytes than in serum. Evidences of scurvy develop only when concentrations in leukocytes are no longer detectable. Thus, concentrations of 0.2 to 0.3 mg/100 ml in serum indicate a considerable margin of safety with respect to prevention of scurvy. Such serum concentrations can be maintained in adults by intakes of 10 mg of ascorbic acid daily (Bartley et al., 1953).

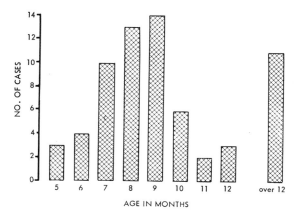

Figure 8–1. Age incidence of scurvy. (Grewar, D.: Clin. Pediat. 4:82, 1965.)

Table 8-4. *Ascorbic Acid Content of Fruit Juices and of Strained Fruits and Vegetables*

	mg per 100 ml or 100 gm
Strained fruit juice, commercially prepared for infants	40–55
Strained bananas	7–40
Other strained fruit	1–7
Strained potato, creamed spinach, creamed peas	7–12
Other strained vegetables	1–7

Requirement for the infant for prevention of scurvy probably ranges between 5 and 10 mg daily (Woodruff, 1964). Hamil et al. (1938) found that 10 mg daily was sufficient to prevent the earliest roentgenographic evidences of disease. This value has therefore been listed as the requirement and twice this value as the advisable intake.

Ascorbic Acid Content of Foods

As indicated in Chapters Eleven and Twelve, human milk is a rich source of ascorbic acid but cow milk in any form, unless it has been fortified, is a poor source by the time it reaches the consumer. Although most commercially prepared formulas are now fortified with ascorbic acid, this is not uniformly so (Tables 11–4 and 12–1). The physician must be clearly aware of the vitamin content of infant formulas he prescribes, relying on the label declaration rather than on published tables since manufacturers are prone to make changes in their products.

Processing of strained foods commercially prepared for infants results in appreciable loss of ascorbic acid so that few such foods provide adequate amounts unless they have been fortified. Fruit juices commercially prepared for infants and strained bananas are fortified with ascorbic acid, the latter to prevent color change from oxidation once the jar is opened. Other strained fruits are poor sources of ascorbic acid (Table 8–4). Scurvy has been reported in a mentally retarded child whose diet for the preceding year had consisted almost entirely of chopped ("junior") vegetables with meat (LoPresti et al., 1964).

Thiamine, Riboflavin and Niacin

Although deficiencies of thiamine, riboflavin and niacin remain important causes of disease in technically underdeveloped countries, few cases of such deficiencies in infants have been recognized in technically advanced countries during the past 20 years. In the United States and Canada, the author is aware of two case reports of infantile beriberi since 1945 and no cases of riboflavin or niacin deficiency. Except when milk-free diets unsupplemented with these vitamins provide the major source of nutrients, deficiency is unlikely. Supplementation of the infant's diet with thiamine, riboflavin and niacin is unnecessary when the infant is breast fed or receives milk-based formulas or equivalent amounts of the vitamins from other sources. Supplementation of the diet in excess of the requirement is merely wasteful and not hazardous, the unneeded amount being excreted in the urine.

THIAMINE

Metabolism of carbohydrate, with eventual liberation of carbon dioxide and water, requires the presence of decarboxylating enzymes, usually consisting of thiamine pyrophosphate and magnesium linked to a substrate-specific protein. Participation of thiamine in mammalian metabolism has been discussed in detail by Handler (1958).

Because of this key role in carbohydrate metabolism, thiamine requirements are considered to be proportional to carbohydrate content of the diet: approximately 0.2 mg/1000 kcal (Food and Nutrition Board, 1964). Since the mean concentration of thiamine in human milk is 0.16 mg/liter (or about 0.16 mg per 740 kcal), human milk provides approximately 0.22 mg/1000 kcal. Using the mean concentration of thiamine in human milk and data from Chapter Four (Fig. 4–1) on volume of intake by normal infants fed milk or formula as sole source of calories, the 50th percentile value for intake of thiamine by breast-fed infants is estimated as 0.12 mg daily at age one month and 0.16 mg daily at age six months. In view of the absence of reports of thiamine deficiency in breast-fed infants in technically developed countries, such intakes must be well above the average requirement, being adequate for virtually all infants. These values have therefore been accepted tentatively as "advisable intakes" for infants receiving diets providing no more than 50 per cent of calories from carbohydrate. Greater intake of thiamine may be desirable when diets high in carbohydrates are fed, but such diets are not generally recommended. Advisable intakes by one-year-old infants have been assumed to be 130 per cent of those of six-month-old infants since caloric intakes are approximately 30 per cent greater.

As already mentioned, thiamine deficiency has been reported in only two infants in the United States and Canada during the past 20 years (Davis and Wolf, 1958; Cochrane et al., 1961). These infants had received soy-based formulas not supplemented with thiamine as the major source of calories for prolonged periods. Mull-Soy powder as currently marketed is deficient in thiamine and amounts supplied by Soyalac powder may be insufficient for some infants (Tables 12-1 and 13-1). Thiamine supplementation is desirable for infants receiving most of their caloric intake from one of these sources.

RIBOFLAVIN

Amino acid oxidases, succinic dehydrogenases, xanthine and aldehyde oxidases and a number of other enzymes important in cellular oxidation reactions require riboflavin as a part of the coenzyme.

Although requirement for riboflavin is commonly considered to be proportional to rate of protein synthesis, Bro-Rasmussen (1958) has concluded that requirements are more closely dependent on energy metabolism. The requirement for human adults is believed to be 0.3 mg/1000 kcal (Food and Nutrition Board, 1964). The average concentration of riboflavin in human milk is 0.36 mg/liter (Chapter Eleven) or approximately 0.5 mg/1000 kcal.

By the utilization of data from Chapter Four (as described for calculations of intakes of thiamine), 50th percentile values for riboflavin intakes by breast-fed infants can be calculated to approximate 0.27, 0.34 and 0.44 mg/day at ages one, six and 12 months, respectively. These figures have been accepted as advisable intakes (Table 8-1).

Rich sources of riboflavin are meats, milk, eggs, green leafy vegetables, legumes and whole grains. Since several of these are likely to be included in an infant's diet in the United States, the absence of riboflavin deficiency is not surprising.

NIACIN

Niacin or one of its derivatives is an essential component of coenzymes involved in glycolysis, protein and amino acid metabolism, pentose biosynthesis, lipid metabolism and the process by which high-energy phosphate bonds are synthesized. These coenzymes, diphosphopyridine nucleotide or coenzyme I (niacin adenine dinucleotide) and triphosphopyridine nucleotide or coenzyme II (niacin adenine dinucleotide phosphate) have been shown to be involved in more than 40 biochemical reactions (Goldsmith, 1964). As is true of thiamine and riboflavin, requirement is related to energy metabolism.

Under suitable conditions, which include an adequate dietary intake of vitamin B_6, niacin can be synthesized from tryptophan in mammalian tissues. Approximately 60 mg of tryptophan are required for synthesis of 1 mg of niacin. The minimum amount of niacin that will prevent pellagra, including that formed from tryptophan, is 4.4 mg/1000 kcal. At low caloric intakes, at least 8.8 mg/1000 kcal is required (Food and Nutrition Board, 1964). Human milk provides approximately 5 mg of niacin equivalents per liter, 50th percentile intakes of the breast-fed infant therefore being 3.7, 4.7 and 6.2 mg/day at ages one, six and 12 months, respectively. These values have been accepted as advisable intakes (Table 8–1).

Niacin deficiency is most likely to occur in patients with cirrhosis of the liver, chronic diarrheal diseases, diabetes mellitus, neoplasia, prolonged febrile illnesses and after parenteral feeding without niacin supplements (Goldsmith, 1964). Hartnup disease, an hereditary disorder of amino acid metabolism in which tryptophan metabolism is severely disturbed, is characterized by reversible cerebellar ataxia and a pellagra-like rash. The skin manifestations can be cured by administration of niacin, and supplementation of the diets of such patients is desirable.

Vitamin B_6

Three chemically related compounds—pyridoxine, pyridoxal and pyridoxamine—together comprise vitamin B_6. These substances are readily phosphorylated and readily converted from one form to another in the body. The physiologically active form, pyridoxal-5-phosphate, is important in protein, carbohydrate and lipid metabolism, serving as a coenzyme for nearly all enzymatic reactions involving nonoxidative degradation and interconversion of amino acids. It forms one component of the phosphorylase responsible for breakdown of glycogen to glucose-1-phosphate, and serves in lipid metabolism, among other functions in conversion of linoleic to arachidonic acid.

In 1953 and 1954 several investigators reported convulsive seizures in infants receiving a commercially prepared formula subjected to a new type of heat processing (Committee on Nutrition, 1966). The findings were similar to those previously described in an infant in whom vitamin B_6 deficiency had been produced experimentally (Snyderman et al., 1950). The seizures observed in 1953 and 1954 and the other manifestations suggesting vitamin B_6 deficiency (abnormal electroencephalogram, abnormal tryptophan load test) disappeared after administration of pyridoxine.

Table 8–5.   *Vitamin B$_6$ Content of Strained and Junior Foods*
Packed in Three Geographically Separated Areas
*of the United States**

Product	Michigan	New York	California
	(mg vitamin B$_6$/100 gm)		
Soups:			
Junior vegetables and beef	0.08	0.06	0.09
Strained vegetables and beef	0.07	0.06	0.08
Strained chicken noodle dinner	0.06	0.06	0.05
Junior chicken noodle dinner	0.05	0.05	0.05
Egg Products:			
Strained egg yolks	0.19	–	0.17
Vegetables:			
Strained peas	0.10	0.10	0.10
Strained carrots	0.08	0.10	0.10
Junior carrots	0.08	0.10	0.10
Strained and junior creamed spinach	0.06	0.08	0.08
Fruits:			
Strained applesauce	0.03	0.03	0.03
Junior applesauce	0.03	0.03	0.03
Fruit Juices:			
Orange-pineapple	0.03	–	0.03
Apple juice	0.02	–	0.03
Pineapple-grapefruit	0.02	–	0.03

*Hurley and Stewart, 1960.

Most of the vitamin B$_6$ in milk and other products of animal
origin is in the form of pyridoxal or pyridoxamine, both of which
are quite sensitive to heat, and it was shown that the formula contained only 60 μg of vitamin B$_6$ compounds. Subsequently, it has
been demonstrated that a physiologically inactive disulfide of pyridoxal phosphate may also be formed on exposure to heat (Wendt
and Bernhart, 1960). Commercially prepared formulas marketed at
present commonly are fortified with the relatively heat-stable pyridoxine. Concentrations of vitamin B$_6$ in various strained foods are
presented in Table 8–5.

Requirement and Advisable Intake

Requirement for pyridoxine is probably related more to protein
content than to caloric content of the diet. Breast-fed infants rarely
develop clinical manifestations of vitamin B$_6$ deficiency, although

excretion of xanthurenic acid is high after administration of trypto-phan (i.e., "abnormal" result of tryptophan load test). Thus, the average concentration of vitamin B_6 in mature human milk (100 $\mu g/100$ ml) is presumably adequate for handling the relatively small protein load (1.1 gm/100 ml) presented by this feeding and an intake of 9 $\mu g/gm$ of protein is an approximation of the requirement. Bessey et al. (1957) have reported that infants receiving human milk con-taining less than 100 μg of vitamin B_6 per liter developed convul-sions. The ratio of vitamin B_6 to protein in cow milk is approximately 19 $\mu g/gm$ and thus considerably greater than the ratio in human milk.

Because administration of isoniazid increases the requirement for vitamin B_6, it is recommended that infants receiving isoniazid be given 10 to 25 mg of pyridoxine daily. Other infants who may bene-fit from large daily doses of pyridoxine are those with myoclonic epilepsy (100 to 200 mg daily), phenylketonuria and congenital or acquired vitamin B_6 dependency (Committee on Nutrition, 1966). The extent to which administration of pyridoxine may benefit patients with phenylketonuria remains to be determined (Loo and Ritman, 1964; Heeley, 1965; Editorial, 1966).

VITAMIN B_6 DEPENDENCY. Infants with vitamin B_6 dependency, an abnormality of heredofamilial incidence, typically are meconium-stained at birth and develop respiratory distress, although prenatal course and delivery have been uneventful. At three to seven hours of age they demonstrate hyperirritability, rolling of the eyes, grimac-ing, brief periods of apnea, distressed cry and tonic and clonic con-vulsions (Scriver and Hutchison, 1963; Robins, 1966; Committee on Nutrition, 1966; Scriver, 1967). A few infants have demonstrated hematologic manifestations rather than those involving the central nervous system (Hines and Harris, 1964).

Therapy other than vitamin B_6 is ineffective. Without specific therapy, death may occur, and with late therapy permanent neuro-logic damage may result. Treatment consists of 10 to 100 mg of pyridoxine hydrochloride administered intravenously or intramuscu-larly. Daily maintenance therapy of 4 to 10 mg orally for an indefinite period is necessary.

Vitamin B_{12}

Vitamin B_{12} (cyanocobalamin, cobalamin) functions in such trans-methylations as synthesis of choline from methionine, serine from glycine and methionine from homocysteine. It is also involved in pyrimidine and purine metabolism and in the synthesis of the deoxy-riboside moiety of deoxyribonucleic acid. Vitamin B_{12} affects, directly or indirectly, the metabolism of folic acid and may be essential for the formation of the folinic acid coenzyme. The manner in which the vitamin is involved in metabolism of nervous tissue is unknown. The most commonly detected manifestation of vitamin B_{12} deficiency is megaloblastic anemia.

Although there has been considerable controversy about the role of vitamin B_{12} deficiency on appetite and growth retardation in childhood (Howe, 1958a and b; Committee on Nutrition, 1958), this controversy applies primarily to the child beyond infancy. There is little evidence to suggest that deficiency of vitamin B_{12} is an important cause of decreased appetite or growth retardation during the first year of life.

The requirement of adults for vitamin B_{12} is thought to be 1 to 2 μg daily, and the requirement for infants is probably less than 1 μg. In contrast to the situation with respect to many water-soluble vitamins, vitamin B_{12} is rather well stored and infants born to well nourished mothers may receive diets deficient in vitamin B_{12} for several months without development of deficiency manifestations.

Folic Acid

Folic acid (folacin, pteroylglutamic acid) is converted in the presence of ascorbic acid to the more active folinic acid, which probably functions as a coenzyme in such reactions as methylation of homocysteine to methionine, conversion of glycine to serine and the formation of creatine, thymine deoxyriboside, ribose nucleic acids, and porphyrin compounds. From a clinical standpoint, the most important activity of folates is the role they play in the synthesis of the purine and pyrimidine compounds which are utilized for the formation of nucleoproteins. In the absence of an adequate supply of nucleoproteins, normal maturation of primordial erythrocytes fails to occur and hematopoiesis is arrested at the megaloblastic stage.

Not only folic acid but several other compounds in foods exhibit folic acid activity. Unfortunately, folates available to the microorganisms used in assay procedures may differ considerably from folates available to the human subject (Ghitis, 1966). Thus, only a human assay is valid for determining the available folate in food for man. However, the commonly employed *L. casei* assay provides information on the *apparent* folate content, and as our information increases we may anticipate that for specified foods it will be possible to relate apparent folate content to folic acid activity for man.

The requirement for folic acid for the adult has been estimated to be about 50 μg/day (Herbert, 1962). Requirements for infants and children have been estimated by Vélez et al. (1963) to be 5 to 20 μg/day and by Sullivan et al. (1966) to be 20 to 50 μg/day.

Major sources of folates are meats and leafy green vegetables. Megaloblastic anemia responsive to folic acid has been reported in infants of low birth weight fed formulas of cow milk, suggesting that the amounts of folates provided by these formulas, although presumably adequate for most full-size infants, may be inadequate for low birth weight infants (Strelling, 1966).

Table 8–6. Folate Content of Milks and Formulas[*]

	Number of Samples	Range (μg/l)
Cow milk	7	62–100
	7	27–55[†]
	5	43–70[‡]
	4	40–65[§]
Goat milk	6	7–13
	9	2–20[†]
	8	<5[§]
Milk-based formulas, powdered		
Similac	5	36–88
Lactum	7	31–100
Bremil	5	30–70
Baker's infant formula	2	>100
Milk-based formulas, liquid		
Modilac	5	>100
Enfamil	5	35–68
Meat-based (liquid)	5	28–64
Soy-based formulas		
Mull-Soy (liquid)	4	>100
Sobee (powder)	2	>100
Soyalac (powder)	2	>100
Nutramigen (powder)	2	>100
Lofenalac (powder)	2	>100

[*]Data of Naiman and Oski (1964), except as noted.
[†]Data of Sullivan et al. (1966).
[‡]Data of Ghitis (1966).
[§]Data of Becroft and Holland (1966).

Concentrations of folates in goat milk are less than those in cow milk (Table 8–6) and megaloblastic anemia is likely to develop in infants fed goat milk unless other sources of folates are provided (Naiman and Oski, 1964; Sullivan et al., 1966; Becroft and Holland, 1966).

REFERENCES

Aballi, A. J., Banús, V. L., de Lamerens, S., and Rozenguaig, S.: Coagulation studies in the newborn period. Alterations of thromboplastin generation and effects of vitamin K in full-term and premature infants. Am. J. Dis. Child. 94:589, 1957.

Bartley, W., Krebs, H. A., and O'Brien, J. R. P.: Vitamin C requirement of human adults. Report by Vitamin C Subcommittee of Accessory Food Factors Committee. Med. Res. Coun., Spec. Rep. Lond. (#280), 1953.

Becroft, D. M. O., and Holland, J. T.: Goat's milk and megaloblastic anaemia of infancy: A report of three cases and a survey of the folic acid activity of some New Zealand milks. New Zealand M. J. 65:303, 1966.

Bessey, O. A., Adam, D. J. D., and Hansen, A. E.: Intake of vitamin B_6 and infantile convulsions: A first approximation of requirements of pyridoxine in infants. Pediatrics 20:33, 1957.

Blanc, W. A., Reid, J. D., and Andersen, D. H.: Avitaminosis E in cystic fibrosis of the pancreas. Pediatrics 22:494, 1958.

Bransby, E. R., Berry, W. T. C., and Taylor, D. M.: Study of vitamin D intakes of infants in 1960. Brit. M. J. 1:1661, 1964.

British Paediatric Association, Committee on Hypercalcaemia: Hypercalcaemia in infants and vitamin D. Brit. M. J. 2:149, 1956.

British Paediatric Association: Infantile hypercalcaemia, nutritional rickets, and infantile scurvy in Great Britain. Brit. M. J. 1:1659, 1964.

Bro-Rasmussen, F.: The riboflavin requirement of animals and man and associated metabolic relations. Nutr. Abst. Rev. 28:369, 1958.

Caffey, J.: Chronic poisoning due to excess of vitamin A. Pediatrics 5:672, 1950.

Caffey, J.: Pediatric X-ray Diagnosis. 4th ed., Chicago, Year Book Publishers, Inc., 1961.

Chow, B. F.: The B vitamins: B_6, B_{12}, folic acid, pantothenic acid, and biotin. In Beaton, G. H., and McHenry, E. W. (eds.): Nutrition. New York, Academic Press, Inc., 1964, Vol. II, p. 207.

Cochrane, W. A., Collins-Williams, C., and Donohue, W. L.: Superior hemorrhagic polioencephalitis (Wernicke's disease) occurring in an infant—probably due to thiamine deficiency from use of a soya bean product. Pediatrics 28:771, 1961.

Committee on Nutrition, American Academy of Pediatrics: Appraisal of the use of vitamin B_1 and B_{12} as supplements promoted for the stimulation of growth and appetite in children. Pediatrics 21:860, 1958.

Committee on Nutrition, American Academy of Pediatrics: Vitamin K compounds and the water-soluble analogues. Pediatrics 28:501, 1961.

Committee on Nutrition, American Academy of Pediatrics: Infantile scurvy and nutritional rickets in the United States. Pediatrics 29:646, 1962.

Committee on Nutrition, American Academy of Pediatrics: Vitamin E in human nutrition. Pediatrics 31:324, 1963a.

Committee on Nutrition, American Academy of Pediatrics: The prophylactic requirement and the toxicity of vitamin D. Pediatrics 31:512, 1963b.

Committee on Nutrition, American Academy of Pediatrics: Vitamin B_6 requirements in man. Pediatrics 38:1068, 1966.

Dam, H., and Søndergaard, E.: Fat-soluble vitamins. *In* Beaton, G. H., and McHenry, E. W. (eds.): Nutrition. New York, Academic Press, Inc., 1964, Vol. II, pp. 1-107.

Davis, R. A., and Wolf, A.: Infantile beriberi associated with Wernicke's encephalopathy. Pediatrics 21:409, 1958.

Dju, M. Y., Mason, K. E., and Filer, L. J., Jr.: Vitamin E (tocopherol) in human fetuses and placentae. Études Néo-Natales 1:49, 1952.

Dyggve, H. V., and Probst, J. H.: Vitamin E to premature infants. Acta paediat. 48: (Suppl. 146), 1963.

Editorial: Vitamin D as a public health problem. Brit. M. J. 1:1654, 1964.

Editorial: Pyridoxine and phenylketonuria. J.A.M.A. 196:361, 1966.

Food and Nutrition Board: Recommended Dietary Allowances, 6th ed. Washington, D. C., National Academy of Sciences–National Research Council, Publication 1146, 1964.

Gershoff, S. N.: Effects of dietary levels of macronutrients on vitamin requirements. Fed. Proc. 23:1077, 1964.

Ghitis, J.: The labile folate of milk. Am. J. Clin. Nutr. 18:452, 1966.

Goldbloom, R. B.: Studies of tocopherol requirements in health and disease. Pediatrics 32:36, 1963.

Goldsmith, G. A.: The B vitamins: thiamine, riboflavin, niacin. *In* Beaton, G. H., and McHenry, E. W. (eds.): Nutrition. New York, Academic Press, Inc., 1964, Vol. II, pp. 109-206.

Gordon, H. H., Nitowsky, H. M., Tildon, J. T., and Levin, S.: Studies of tocopherol deficiency in infants and children: V. An interim summary. Pediatrics 21:673, 1958.

Gordon, R. R., and Dean, T.: Foetal deaths from antenatal anticoagulant therapy. Brit. M. J. 2:719, 1955.

Grewar, D.: Infantile scurvy in Manitoba. Canad. M. A. J. 78:675, 1958.

Grewar, D.: Scurvy and its prevention by vitamin C fortified evaporated milk. Canad. M. A. J. 80:977, 1959.

Grewar, D.: Infantile scurvy. Clin. Pediat. 4:82, 1965.

Hamil, B. M., Reynolds, L., Poole, M. W., and Macy, I. G.: Minimal vitamin C requirement of artificially fed infants. Am. J. Dis. Child. 55:561, 1938.

Handler, P.: Beriberi. Part V. Metabolism of thiamine. Fed. Proc. 17:31, 1958.

Harris, P. L., Hardenbrook, E. G., Dean, F. P., Cusack, E. R., and Jensen, J. L.: Blood tocopherol values in normal human adults and incidence of vitamin E deficiency. Proc. Soc. Exp. Biol. & Med. 107:381, 1961.

Harris, P. L., Quaife, M. L., and O'Grady, P.: Tocopherol content of human milk and of cows' milk products used for infant feeding. J. Nutrition 46:459, 1952.

Heeley, A. F.: The effect of pyridoxine on tryptophan metabolism in phenylketonuria. Clin. Sci. 29:465, 1965.

Herbert, V.: Minimal daily adult folate requirements. Arch. Int. Med. 110:649, 1962.

Herting, D. C., and Drury, E. J. E.: Plasma tocopherol levels in man. Am. J. Clin. Nutr. 17:351, 1965a.

Herting, D. C., and Drury, E. J. E.: Vitamin E content of milk and simulated milks. Fed. Proc. 24:720, 1965b. (Abstract.)

Hines, J. D., and Harris, J. W.: Pyridoxine-responsive anemia. Description of three patients with megaloblastic erythropoiesis. Am. J. Clin. Nutr. 14:137, 1964.

Howe, E. E.: Effect of vitamin B_{12} on growth-retarded children: A review. Am. J. Clin. Nutr. 6:818, 1958a.

Howe, E. E.: Letter to Editor. Vitamin B_{12} supplementation. Pediatrics 22:1202, 1958b.

Hume, E. M., and Krebs, H. A.: Vitamin A requirements of human adults: An experimental study of vitamin A deprivation in man. Med. Res. Coun. Spec. Rept. Ser. 264, 1949.

Hurley, N. A., and Stewart, R. A.: The vitamin B_6 content of infant foods. Pediatrics 26:679, 1960.

Kerner, I., and Goldbloom, R. B.: Investigation of tocopherol deficiency in infancy and childhood. Am. J. Dis. Child. 99:597, 1960.

Kramer, B., Sobel, A. E., and Gottfried, S. P.: Serum levels of vitamin A in children: a comparison following the oral and intramuscular administration of vitamin A in oily and aqueous medium. Am. J. Dis. Child. 73:543, 1947.

Landing, B. H.: *In* McIntosh, R. (ed.): Transactions of the International Research Conference on Cystic Fibrosis. Baltimore, French-Bray, 1960, p. 139.

Lewis, J. M., Bodansky, O., Birmingham, J., and Cohlan, S. Q.: Comparative absorption, excretion, and storage of oily and aqueous preparations of vitamin A. J. Pediat. 31:496, 1947.

Loo, Y. H., and Ritman, P.: New metabolites of phenylalanine. Nature 203:1237, 1964.

LoPresti, J. M., Gutelius, M.F., and Lefkowicz, L.: Grand rounds: scurvy. Clin. Proc. Child. Hosp. Dist. Columbia. 20:119, 1964.

Mackenzie, J. B.: Relation between serum tocopherol and hemolysis in hydrogen peroxide of erythrocytes in premature infants. Pediatrics 13:346, 1954.

Naiman, J. L., and Oski, F. A.: The folic acid content of milk: Revised figures based on an improved assay method. Pediatrics 34:274, 1964.

Nitowsky, H. M., Gordon, H. H., and Tildon, J. T.: Studies of tocopherol deficiency in infants and children: IV. The effect of alpha tocopherol on creatinuria in patients with cystic fibrosis of the pancreas and biliary atresia. Bull. Johns Hopkins Hosp. 98:361, 1956.

Nitowsky, H. M., Hsu, K. S., and Gordon, H. H.: Vitamin E requirements of human infants. Vitamins Hormones. 20:559, 1962a.

Nitowsky, H. M., Tildon, J. T., Levin, S., and Gordon, H. H.: Studies of tocopherol deficiency in infants and children: VII. The effect of tocopherol on urinary, plasma and muscle creatine. Am. J. Clin. Nutr. 10:368, 1962b.

Oppenheimer, E. H.: Focal necrosis of striated muscle in an infant with cystic fibrosis of the pancreas and evidence of lack of absorption of fat-soluble vitamins. Bull. Johns Hopkins Hosp. 98:353, 1956.

Owen, G. M., Nelsen, C. E., Baker, G. L., and Jacobs, J. P.: Use of vitamin K in pregnancy: Effect on bilirubin metabolism and coagulation mechanisms in the newborn. Am. J. Obst. & Gynec. In press.

Persson, B., Tunell, R., and Ekengren, K.: Chronic vitamin A intoxication during the first half year of life. Description of 5 cases. Acta Paediat. Scandinav. 54:49, 1965.

Robins, M. M.: Pyridoxine dependency convulsions in a newborn. J.A.M.A. 195:491, 1966.

Rubin, S. H., and deRitter, E.: Vitamin A requirements of animal species. Vitamins Hormones 12:101, 1954.

Scriver, C. R.: Vitamin B_6 deficiency and dependency in man. Am. J. Dis. Child. 113: 109, 1967.

Scriver, C. R., and Hutchison, J. H.: Vitamin B_6 deficiency syndrome in human infancy: Biochemical and clinical observations. Pediatrics 31:240, 1963.

Smith, C. H.: Blood Diseases of Infancy and Childhood. 2nd ed. St. Louis, The C. V. Mosby Co., 1966, p. 655.

Snyderman, S. E., Carretero, R., and Holt, L. E., Jr.: Pyridoxine deficiency in the human being. Fed. Proc. 9:371, 1950.

Strelling, M. K., Blackledge, G. D., Goodall, H. B., and Walker, C. H. M.: Megaloblastic anemia and whole blood folate levels in premature infants. Lancet 1:898, 1966.

Sullivan, L. W., Luhby, A. L., and Streiff, R. R.: Studies of the daily requirement for folic acid in infants and the etiology of folate deficiency in goat's milk megaloblastic anemia. Am. J. Clin. Nutr. 18:311, 1966.

Vasington, F. D., Reichard, S. M., and Nason, A.: Biochemistry of vitamin E. Vitamins Hormones 18:43, 1960.

Vélez, H., Ghitis, J., Pradilla, A., and Vitale, J. J.: Cali-Harvard nutrition project. I. Megaloblastic anemia in kwashiorkor. Am. J. Clin. Nutr. 12:54, 1963.

Vietti, T. J., Murphy, T. P., James, J. A., and Pritchard, J. A.: Observations on the prophylactic use of vitamin K in the newborn infant. J. Pediat. 56:343, 1960.

Weinberg, T., Gordon, H. H., Oppenheimer, E. H., and Nitowsky, H. M.: Myopathy in association with tocopherol deficiency in cases of congenital biliary atresia and cystic fibrosis of the pancreas. Am. J. Pathol. 34:565, 1958.

Wendt, G., and Bernhart, F. W.: The structure of a sulfur-containing compound with vitamin B_6 activity. Arch. Biochem. Biophys. 88:270, 1960.

Whelen, W. S., Fraser, D., Robertson, E. C., and Tomczak, H.: The rising incidence of scurvy in infants. Canad. M. A. J. 78:177, 1958.

Woodruff, C. W.: Ascorbic acid. *In* Beaton, G. H., and McHenry, E. W. (eds.): Nutrition. New York, Academic Press, Inc., 1964, Vol. II, p. 265.

Chapter Nine

Major
Minerals
and Water

Because of their relative abundance in the human body, the major minerals are considered to be sodium, chloride, potassium, calcium, phosphorus, magnesium and sulfur. These minerals* and water, which are considered in the present chapter, occur in generous amounts in human milk, cow milk and many other foods commonly fed to infants. Standard textbooks of pediatrics provide adequate review of their many functions in the human body and discuss pathogenesis, diagnosis and treatment of acute and chronic excesses and deficiencies. The present chapter is primarily devoted to consideration of requirements, advisable intakes, factors influencing absorption of calcium and phosphorus, the significance of renal solute load in relation to intake of water, and possible implications of amounts of salt consumed by normal infants.

Requirements and Advisable Intakes of Major Minerals

As discussed in Chapter Three, the requirement for any nutrient strictly applies only to the exact circumstances under which it was

---

*Sulfur is unique among the major minerals in that it probably functions as a trace element except for the appreciable requirement for sulfur-containing amino acids. The requirement for sulfur is therefore not considered.

determined. With respect to requirement for a specified major mineral, important variables influencing requirement are the amounts of other major minerals in the diet (e.g., requirement for magnesium is increased when amounts of calcium and phosphorus in the diet are increased), the chemical form of the mineral (e.g., certain phosphorus salts are better absorbed than others) and the nonmineral constituents of the diet (e.g., certain poorly absorbed fats are responsible for relatively large fecal losses of calcium).

Although there is clearly a need for extreme caution in interpreting any estimate of requirement, it is nevertheless necessary that some estimate be available. The infant with severe congenital heart disease and congestive cardiac failure may be managed for a few days or even a week or two with a diet free of sodium. It will then be necessary to add some sodium to the diet. Twice the requirement may be well tolerated, but ten times the requirement may once again precipitate congestive cardiac failure. In this situation an estimate of requirement might be extremely useful even if it were not exactly applicable to the particular clinical problem being considered.

Approach to Estimation of Requirement

With the precautions in interpretation just mentioned, the requirement for a mineral may be considered in relation to the amount necessary for normal growth plus obligatory losses through such routes as skin and urinary tract. To achieve an intake sufficient to meet these needs, the extent of absorption of the minerals must be taken into account. Unfortunately, there are as yet insufficient data for confident estimates to be made by this approach. Requirements for growth may be calculated and information concerning extent of absorption is available for at least most of the minerals. However, knowledge of obligatory losses is scant.

Estimated Requirement for Growth

On the basis of the assumed rate of growth of fat-free body mass and estimated concentrations of minerals per unit of fat-free body mass, the requirements of these minerals for growth may be calculated as indicated in the Appendix to this chapter. Results of these calculations are presented in Tables 9–1 and 9–2.

Requirements and Advisable Intakes

SODIUM, CHLORIDE AND POTASSIUM. Obligatory losses of minerals occur from skin (sweat and desquamated epithelium), from mucous membranes, in urine and in feces. However, losses in feces

Table 9–1. *Estimated Requirements and Advisable Intakes of Sodium, Chloride and Potassium*

	Birth to Age 4 Months				Age 4 Months to Age 12 Months			
	Needed for Tissue Synthesis	Loss through Skin*	Estimated Requirement†	Advisable Intake‡	Needed for Tissue Synthesis	Loss through Skin	Estimated Requirement	Advisable Intake
Sodium (meq/day)	1.4	1.0	>2.6	8	1.0	1.0	>2.2	7
Chloride (meq/day)	0.8	1.4	>2.5	8	0.5	1.4	>2.1	6
Potassium (meq/day)	1.1	1.1	>2.5	8	0.8	1.1	>2.1	6

*Cooke et al., 1950.

†Assuming 90 per cent absorption. This estimated requirement is less than the true requirement because obligatory losses in urine have been ignored.

‡Approximately three times the estimated requirement.

Table 9-2. *Estimated Requirements for Growth and Advisable Intakes of Calcium, Phosphorus and Magnesium from Birth to Age 12 Months*

| | Requirement for Growth | | Advisable Intake† |
	Tissue Increment	Estimated Requirement°	
Calcium (mg/day)	148	250	500
Phosphorus (mg/day)	89	110	220
Magnesium (mg/day)	4	7	21

°On the basis of data summarized in Table 9-3, it is assumed that approximately 60 per cent of the intake of calcium and magnesium and 80 per cent of the intake of phosphorus will be absorbed.

†Advisable intake is tentatively set as twice the estimated requirement for calcium and phosphorus and three times the estimated requirement for magnesium (see text).

may be ignored because a value for "absorption" is utilized in the calculation of requirement. By combining amounts needed for growth and to replace losses through skin, and by increasing this total to account for the amount of unabsorbed mineral, an estimate of requirement is made (Table 9-1). The estimate is less than the true requirement because obligatory urinary losses of these minerals have been ignored. For this reason, the advisable intake is considered, tentatively, to be three times (rather than twice) the estimated requirement.

CALCIUM. In contrast to the situation that obtains with sodium, chloride and potassium, in which obligatory losses are relatively high in relation to requirement for growth, obligatory losses of calcium are much less. Therefore, on the basis of the calculated requirements for growth and data on extent of absorption, total requirements can be estimated (Table 9-2). As indicated in Table 9-3, average absorption of calcium during the first six months of life ranged from 50 to 67 per cent of intake for four normal male infants fed human milk. The ability of the male reference infant to absorb calcium from human milk is therefore assumed to average 60 per cent of intake, and the calcium requirement for the male reference infant is assumed to be 270 mg/day (148 mg/day ÷ 0.6), an amount supplied by 800 ml of human milk.

Because absorption of calcium may be quite different with feedings other than human milk, the calculated calcium requirement of the male reference infant when he is fed human milk is of limited value. Extent of absorption is influenced not only by the concentration of calcium in the diet and its chemical form but also, as will be discussed subsequently, by the type of fat in the diet.

Table 9-3. Calcium and Phosphorus Balance Studies with Normal Male Infants Fed Human Milk during the First Six Months of Life*

Subject	Number of Studies	Calcium Balance			Phosphorus Balance		
		Intake (mg/day)	Absorption (% of intake)	Retention (% of intake) (mg/day)	Intake (mg/day)	Absorption (% of intake)	Retention (% of intake) (mg/day)
M.R.	8	348	67	59 210	109	87	66 88
L.M.	11	338	54	45 161	110	82	40 45
M.Ew.	9†	332	50	44 150	109	81	32 28
M.Ev.	9	271	54	41 111	104	75	59 61

*Data of Fomon et al., 1963.
†Absorption figure based on seven balance studies.

The advisable intake when the infant is not fed human milk is tentatively set at twice the requirement of the reference infant: 500 mg/day.

PHOSPHORUS. With phosphorus, as with calcium, obligatory losses are small in relation to requirement for growth. As indicated in the chapter appendix, the tissue increment of phosphorus is approximately 89 mg/day; the requirement to achieve this tissue increment, assuming that 80 per cent of intake is absorbed, is 110 mg/day (Table 9–2). This amount of phosphorus is provided by approximately 790 ml of human milk.

Advisable intakes of phosphorus by infants not receiving human milk are tentatively set at twice the estimated requirement: 220 mg/day.

MAGNESIUM. As discussed in the chapter appendix, approximately 4 mg of magnesium daily are required for tissue synthesis. Assuming that absorption of magnesium is similar to that of calcium when human milk is fed (i.e., 60 per cent of intake), the requirement is estimated as 7 mg/day (4 mg/day ÷ 0.6). The advisable intake is tentatively set at three times (rather than twice) the estimated requirement because of uncertainty regarding the extent of obligatory losses.

Calcium and Phosphorus Balance Studies

As was discussed in relation to nitrogen balance studies (Chapter Five), calcium and phosphorus balance studies are of limited value as a means of estimating growth. From Table 9–4 it may be seen that retention of calcium (mg/kg) is found to be two to three times as great when high intakes of calcium (cow milk and added carbohydrate) are fed as when lower intakes (human milk) are given. Mineralization of bone may, in fact, proceed more rapidly with relatively high intakes of calcium and phosphorus than with lower intakes, but it seems quite unlikely that the magnitude of the differences approaches that suggested by balance studies.

Although metabolic balance studies probably do not indicate the rate of deposition of these minerals in the body, they are of considerable value in assessing the adequacy of the diet. Errors inherent in metabolic balance studies are likely to lead to overestimation of true retention. Therefore, any feeding that results in apparent retentions of calcium and phosphorus consistently less than those recorded for infants fed human milk (Tables 9–3 and 9–4) should be considered inadequate.

The commonly held belief that the ratio of calcium to phosphorus in human milk is particularly advantageous for the infant is not sup-

Table 9-4. Calcium and Phosphorus Balance Studies at Various Ages*

	Human Milk			Similac			Cow Milk and Carbohydrate		
	Intake (mg/kg)	Retention (mg/kg)	Retention (% of intake)	Intake (mg/kg)	Retention (mg/kg)	Retention (% of intake)	Intake (mg/kg)	Retention (mg/kg)	Retention (% of intake)
Calcium									
8–30	72.9 (12.0)†	23.7 (12.3)	32.6 (16.7)	140.7 (27.9)	36.3 (17.5)	25.2 (8.2)			
31–60	67.8 (22.3)	28.6 (17.6)	40.5 (17.8)	145.2 (34.7)	32.9 (32.3)	23.0 (11.1)			
61–90	50.4 (6.7)	24.0 (9.9)	47.4 (16.6)	142.7 (21.7)	64.5 (27.6)	40.5 (15.3)	158.7 (11.3)	66.2 (10.0)	40.8 (7.8)
91–120	55.0 (10.8)	30.3 (12.4)	54.1 (14.3)	123.9 (16.5)	54.8 (15.2)	44.2 (11.3)	149.3 (15.6)	63.2 (12.4)	43.0 (9.3)
121–150	46.0 (5.1)	21.2 (4.4)	47.1 (12.2)	105.9 (16.5)	38.8 (16.4)	37.0 (25.3)	141.9 (4.9)	53.7 (11.2)	37.8 (7.9)
151–180	45.5 (8.7)	22.1 (9.5)	46.9 (12.5)	105.9 (18.1)	40.9 (16.3)	39.1 (16.7)	138.1 (4.3)	63.6 (17.3)	46.3 (8.8)
Phosphorus									
8–30	27.4 (2.5)	13.4 (3.8)	49.5 (20.7)	109.5 (17.9)	27.3 (10.5)	24.8 (7.6)			
31–60	23.0 (5.5)	13.2 (6.2)	58.6 (21.0)	116.8 (32.1)	32.3 (20.0)	27.5 (18.1)			
61–90	18.0 (2.5)	11.6 (4.5)	63.2 (21.3)	108.5 (17.6)	40.5 (22.4)	36.7 (18.9)	124.7 (8.0)	36.2 (6.1)	29.2 (5.4)
91–120	18.5 (3.0)	11.7 (5.1)	60.7 (19.1)	98.6 (15.6)	31.2 (11.3)	31.3 (9.1)	113.4 (12.7)	34.0 (5.9)	30.2 (5.2)
121–150	16.2 (2.0)	9.5 (3.5)	58.0 (17.0)	82.0 (9.7)	22.8 (13.8)	26.4 (17.7)	107.0 (7.9)	33.6 (6.4)	31.6 (7.2)
151–180	16.4 (2.8)	8.0 (1.7)	46.6 (27.0)	83.9 (16.8)	27.8 (12.8)	32.5 (13.2)	110.3 (7.0)	33.2 (8.7)	29.9 (6.3)

*Data on human milk and Similac from Fomon et al. (1963); data on cow milk and carbohydrate from Nelson (1931).
†Values in parentheses are standard deviations.

ported by data from metabolic balance studies. Thus, Widdowson et al. (1963) have demonstrated that the addition of moderate amounts of phosphate to the diet of five- to eight-day-old breast-fed infants enhanced rather than hindered absorption of calcium and magnesium.

Negative balances of calcium and magnesium may be associated with high fat excretion in the newborn period (Widdowson, 1965). However, it seems unlikely that transiently negative balances of this sort are of clinical significance for normal infants. When steatorrhea persists (either because a poorly absorbed fat has been included in the diet or because of metabolic abnormality), development of mineral deficiency may result.

Concentrations of Calcium and Inorganic Phosphorus in Serum

As has been shown by Bruck and Weintraub (1955) (Table 9–5), concentrations of calcium in serum are less in the newborn infant than in the adult and are less in the infant of low birth weight than in the full-size infant. Concentrations decrease with increasing time before onset of the first feeding. The minimum concentration of cal-

Table 9–5. Concentrations of Calcium and Phosphorus of Newborn Infants in Relation to Birth Weight*

	Low Birth Weight	Full Size
Calcium		
Number of subjects	51	21
Number of determinations	154	43
Mean (mg/100 ml)	8.3 (1.3)†	9.1 (0.8)
Mean of lowest value of each subject (mg/100 ml)	7.4 (1.2)	8.9 (0.9)
Phosphorus		
Number of subjects	51	20
Number of determinations	145	39
Mean (mg/100 ml)	7.7 (1.7)	7.5 (1.8)
Mean of highest value of each subject (mg/100 ml)	8.7 (1.4)	8.4 (1.7)

*Data of Bruck and Weintraub (1955).
†Values in parentheses are standard deviations.

cium recorded for each infant during the first three weeks of life is shown in Figure 9-1 in relation to type of feeding. With full-size infants beyond the newborn period, concentrations of calcium are similar to those of the adult whether the infant is breast fed or receives evaporated milk and water without added carbohydrate (Table 9-6). The latter feeding provides a relatively high intake of calcium.

During the newborn period, concentrations of inorganic phosphorus in serum of full-size infants and infants of low birth weight are considerably higher than those of adults (Table 9-5). Maximum serum concentrations of inorganic phosphorus in relation to birth weight and feeding are indicated in Figure 9-2. As discussed by Owen et al. (1963), beyond the newborn period concentrations of inorganic phosphorus continue to be considerably greater than those of adults. From 56 to 168 days of age (Table 9-6), mean serum concentration of inorganic phosphorus of breast-fed infants is 6.2 mg/100 ml, with approximately 16 per cent of normal breast-fed infants demonstrating concentrations less than 5.7 mg/100 ml, and 16 per cent demonstrating concentrations greater than 6.7 mg/100 ml. When dietary intakes of phosphorus are greater, serum concentrations are also greater. Infants receiving evaporated milk and water without additional carbohydrate have a mean serum concentration of approximately 7.2 mg/100 ml between 56 and 168 days of age (Table 9-6), with 16 per cent of values below 6.6 mg/100 ml and 16 per cent above 7.8 mg/100 ml.

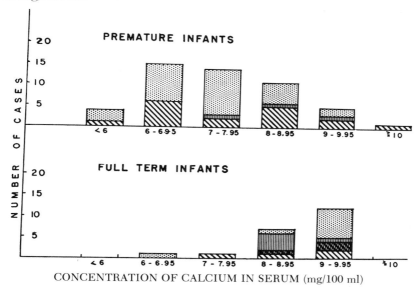

CONCENTRATION OF CALCIUM IN SERUM (mg/100 ml)

Figure 9-1. Minimum serum calcium concentration in 51 infants of low birth weight ("premature infants") and 21 full-size ("full term") infants during the first three weeks of life. The type of feeding when the minimum level was attained is indicated: stippled area, no feeding; diagonal hatching, cow milk formulas; vertical hatching, human milk. (From Bruck and Weintraub: A.M.A. J. Dis. Child. 90:653, 1955.)

Table 9–6. *Concentrations of Calcium and Inorganic Phosphorus in Sera of Normal Full-Size Infants during the First Five and One-Half Months of Life**

Age (days)	Breast Fed			Evaporated Milk and Water		
	Number of Infants	Calcium (mg/100 ml)	Phosphorus (mg/100 ml)	Number of Infants	Calcium (mg/100 ml)	Phosphorus (mg/100 ml)
28	24	10.1† (0.6)	6.8 (0.7)	19	9.9 (0.6)	7.4 (0.7)
56	23	9.8 (0.3)	6.3 (0.7)	17	10.1 (0.5)	7.4 (0.5)
84	23	10.1 (0.6)	6.2 (0.5)	21	10.1 (0.5)	7.1 (0.7)
112	24	10.1 (0.5)	6.2 (0.7)	14	10.0 (0.5)	7.5 (0.5)
140	20	9.9 (0.4)	6.1 (0.6)	20	9.9 (0.6)	7.1 (0.7)
168	18	9.7 (0.5)	6.3 (0.2)	20	9.8 (0.7)	7.0 (0.5)

*Data of Fomon et al., 1966.
†Values in parentheses are standard deviations.

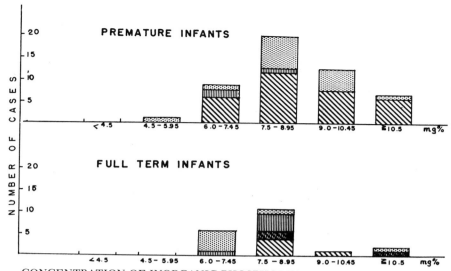

CONCENTRATION OF INORGANIC PHOSPHORUS IN SERUM (mg/100 ml)

Figure 9–2. Maximum serum concentration of inorganic phosphorus during the first three weeks of life. (See legend of Fig. 9–1). (From Bruck and Weintraub: A.M.A. J. Dis. Child. 90:653, 1955.)

Water

The requirement for water consists of the amount necessary for growth, that lost through skin and lungs, and obligatory excretion in urine and feces. As may be calculated from values given in Figure 2–8, the amount necessary for growth of the male reference infant is small in relation to usual intakes: 1480 ml between birth and four months of age and 2060 ml between four and 12 months of age or approximately 13 and 9 ml/day, respectively, in the two age intervals. Losses from skin and lungs are relatively great, ranging from 30 to 70 ml/kg/day in normal infants (Pratt et al., 1948; Cooke et al., 1950; Drescher et al., 1962), and perhaps averaging 175, 350 and 500 ml/day for the "male reference infant" at birth and at ages four and 12 months, respectively.

Fecal losses of water are generally less than 10 ml/kg/day (Pratt et al., 1948; Cooke et al., 1950).

As will be discussed, obligatory urinary losses depend largely on the renal solute load provided by metabolism of the infant's own tissue and by his diet. Under circumstances of minimal renal solute load, the amount of water necessary for urinary excretion may be approximately 40, 70 and 100 ml/day at birth, four months and 12 months of age, respectively.

The requirement for water is therefore the sum of those components previously mentioned, or about 250 ml/day during the first few weeks of life and 600–700 ml/day at age 12 months.

Table 9–7.   Calculation of Approximate Renal Solute Load of Diet

$$\text{Urea (mosmol)} = \text{nitrogen (mg)} \times \frac{1 \text{ mosmol *}}{28 \text{ mg nitrogen}}$$

Sodium: 1 mosmol = 1 meq = 23 mg
Chloride: 1 mosmol = 1 meq = 35 mg
Potassium: 1 mosmol = 1 meq = 39 mg

Renal solute load assumed to consist of urea, sodium, chloride and potassium (see text).

---

*Nitrogen calculated as protein ÷ 6.25; two nitrogen atoms (atomic weight 14) per molecule of urea.

Renal Solute Load

Renal solute load consists of metabolic end-products, especially nitrogenous compounds and electrolytes, that must be excreted by the kidneys. These solutes arise from endogenous sources (i.e., through normal or abnormal catabolism) and from diet. An approximation of the size of renal solute load presented by a diet may be made by assuming that all dietary protein is excreted as urea (1 gm of dietary protein yields approximately 5.7 mosmol of urea), and that all the sodium, chloride and potassium of the diet is excreted (Table 9–7).*

With usual diets consumed during infancy, sodium, chloride, potassium and urea account for 75 to 80 per cent of urinary solutes. Calcium is present in relatively large amounts in the diet but little is excreted in the urine, and the contribution of calcium to the renal solute load can be ignored. Phosphorus accounts for approximately 10 per cent of renal solute load from milk, but for most other foods its contribution is considerably less (Appendix I, p. 280), † and it has been ignored in calculations presented in Tables 9–7 and 9–8.

Although some of the nitrogen, sodium, chloride and potassium

---

*As pointed out by Drescher et al. (1962), urea does not appear to obligate water unless the ratio of urea to other solutes (both expressed as milliosmols) exceeds 0.8. With many diets, the ratio of urea to other solutes will not, in fact, exceed 0.8. Nevertheless, data concerning renal concentrating ability at various ages is based largely on measurements of effective osmolality of the urine as measured by freezing point depression and, if such osmolalities are utilized in calculations of water required for renal excretion, the contribution of urea must be included.

†Assuming that all dietary phosphorus is excreted in the urine, 1 mosmol of phosphorus in the urine will be derived from each 31 mg of phosphorus in the diet.

of the diet is utilized for growth or is excreted in the feces or through the skin (Table 9–1), the amounts thus subtracted from the renal solute load presented by the diet are to some extent balanced by excretion of phosphorus and other minerals, creatinine, and ammonia or bicarbonate. Thus, a reasonable approximation of the renal solute load may be calculated on the assumption that all dietary nitrogen is excreted in the urine as urea, that all dietary sodium, chloride and potassium are excreted in the urine and that the contribution of other solutes to the renal solute load is negligible. Such calculations are not precise and actually will lead to an overestimation of renal solute load, especially when renal solute loads are relatively low. At high renal solute loads – the only circumstances under which this consideration is ordinarily important in infant feeding – the estimate will be sufficiently accurate for practical use and more cumbersome calculations do not seem warranted.

Calculations employed in determining renal solute load are indicated in Table 9–7. Renal solute loads presented by milks and formulas may be seen from Table 9–8, those for strained foods from Table 9–9. Also included in Tables 9–8 and 9–9 are the calculated amounts of water required for excretion of the renal solute load if urine concentrating ability is 1000 mosmol/l or if it is 300 mosmol/l. Although urinary concentrating ability may be limited to approximately 700 mosmol/l in the immediate newborn period (Hansen and Smith, 1953), most normal infants older than two weeks of age can concentrate the urine to 1000 mosmol/l (Pratt et al., 1948; Poláček et al. 1965). Infants with severe renal disease may not be able to concentrate the urine above 300 mosmol/l, and infants with diabetes insipidus may have even greater impairment of concentrating ability.

Although renal solute load is of primary importance in management of the infant with severe impairment of renal concentrating ability, the normal infant fed ad libitum will usually ingest an amount of water well in excess of requirements and this excess must be excreted by the kidneys. With an abundant supply of water available for renal excretion, it matters little whether the normal infant uses a greater or smaller portion of this water for excretion of solutes. Thus, the fact that human milk presents a renal solute load only about one-third that presented by whole cow milk is usually not of great medical or nutritional significance.

As may be appreciated from the calculations presented in Table 9–10, difficulties arising from excessive renal solute load will rarely occur unless (1) total fluid intake is exceptionally low, (2) extrarenal losses are unusually high, as is true with diarrhea, fever, hyperventilation or elevated environmental temperature, (3) renal concentrating ability is seriously impaired, (4) a gross error in diet has occurred, or (5) a combination of these factors is involved.

(Text continued on page 158.)

Table 9–8. Potential Renal Solute Load from Ingestion of 100 Milliliters of Milk or Formula

	Urea (mosmol)	Na (meq)	Cl (meq)	K (meq)	Renal Solute Load (mosmol)	Water for Renal Excretion (ml) Urine Conc. 1000 mosmol/l	Urine Conc. 300 mosmol/l
Milks and Formulas							
Human milk	6.3	.7	1.1	1.3	9.4	9	30
Cow milk							
fresh, fluid	18.9	2.5	2.9	3.5	27.7	28	92
evaporated	21.7	2.8	3.2	3.9	31.6	32	109
Klim	18.9	2.2	2.8	3.5	27.3	27	91
Goat milk							
fresh	18.9	1.8	4.5	4.6	29.7	30	99
Dale's	18.9	1.8	4.5	4.6	29.7	30	99
Half skim							
Alacta	20.6	2.1	2.3	3.9	28.9	29	96
Dryco	22.9	2.7	3.2	3.8	32.5	33	108
Skim-fluid	20.0	2.3	2.9	4.3	29.5	30	98
Skim-powdered	20.0	2.6	3.2	3.4	29.2	29	97
Lactum	15.4	1.6	2.1	2.8	21.9	22	73
Carnalac	13.7	1.6	2.1	2.4	19.8	20	60
Purevap	13.1	1.6	2.1	2.4	19.7	20	66
Bottle Ready							
Infant Formula	8.6	1.1	1.2	1.6	12.5	13	42
Bremil	8.6	1.1	1.3	1.5	12.5	13	42
Enfamil	8.6	1.1	1.3	1.6	12.6	13	42
Formil	9.7	1.1	1.3	1.5	13.6	14	45
Infant Formula	12.6	1.7	1.9	2.3	18.5	19	62

Table 9–8. *Potential Renal Solute Load from Ingestion of 100 Milliliters of Milk or Formula (Continued)*

	Urea (mosmol)	Na (meq)	Cl (meq)	K (meq)	Renal Solute Load (mosmol)	Water for Renal Excretion (ml) Urine Conc. 1000 mosmol/l	Urine Conc. 300 mosmol/l
Modilac	12.6	1.7	1.9	2.3	18.6	19	62
Olac	19.4	2.6	3.0	3.6	28.6	29	95
Similac	9.7	1.1	1.5	1.8	14.1	14	47
Varamel	14.3	1.9	2.2	2.7	21.1	21	70
Similac PM 60/40	8.6	.7	1.2	1.4	11.9	12	39
SMA	8.6	.7	1.2	1.4	11.9	12	40
Lonalac	19.4	.1	1.7	2.7	23.9	24	80
Protein Milk	21.7	2.2	2.8	2.1	28.8	29	97
Probana	22.3	2.6	3.0	3.1	31.0	31	103
Sobee	18.3	1.4	1.4	4.0	25.1	25	83
Mull-Soy							
liquid	17.7	1.6	1.6	4.1	25.0	25	83
powder	17.7	1.6	1.6	4.1	25.0	25	83
Soyalac							
liquid	12.0	.6	?	2.2	>14.8	>15	>49
powder	18.9	2.8	?	2.6	>24.2	>24	>81
Prosobee	14.3	2.0	0.8	2.5	19.6	20	65
Nutramigen	12.6	2.1	2.6	2.9	20.2	20	67
Meat Base Formula*	16.0	1.6	2.6	1.2	18.6	19	62
Lambase	13.7	1.1	.7	.9	16.4	16	55
Lofenalac	12.6	2.1	2.7	3.3	20.7	21	69

*With added carbohydrate as indicated in Table 12–3.

*Table 9-9.   Potential Renal Solute Load from Ingestion of 100 Grams of Strained or Chopped Food**

	Urea (mosmol)	Na (meq)	Cl (meq)	K (meq)	Renal Solute Load (mosmol)	Water for Renal Excretion (ml) Urine Conc. 1000 mosmol/l	Water for Renal Excretion (ml) Urine Conc. 300 mosmol/l
Cereals, precooked†							
barley	27.1	3.9	4.2	3.6	38.8	39	129
high protein	44.7	4.1	4.4	3.1	56.3	56	188
mixed	28.6	4.1	4.4	3.2	40.3	40	134
oatmeal	29.5	4.6	4.9	3.3	42.3	42	141
rice	21.6	4.0	4.3	3.4	33.3	33	111
Desserts							
custard pudding	13.1	6.5	5.2	2.4	27.2	27	91
fruit pudding	6.9	5.6	4.5	1.9	18.9	19	63
Dinners							
beef noodle	16.0	11.7	9.4	4.1	41.2	41	137
cereal, egg yolk and bacon	16.6	13.1	10.5	.9	41.1	41	137
chicken noodle	12.0	12.9	10.3	1.1	36.3	36	121
macaroni, tomatoes, meat and cereal	14.9	16.6	13.3	2.0	46.8	47	156
split peas, vegetables and ham or bacon	22.9	12.8	10.2	2.9	48.8	49	163
vegetables and meat							
bacon	9.7	12.3	9.8	3.3	35.1	35	117
beef	15.4	13.3	10.6	3.7	43.0	43	143
chicken	12.0	13.3	10.6	1.4	37.3	37	124
ham	16.0	15.7	12.6	2.3	46.6	47	155
lamb	12.6	11.7	9.4	3.8	37.5	38	125
liver	17.7	10.3	8.2	4.2	40.4	40	135
liver and bacon	13.7	12.3	9.8	3.4	39.2	39	131
turkey	12.0	13.3	10.6	1.2	37.1	37	124

Table 9-9. *Potential Renal Solute Load from Ingestion of 100 Grams of Strained or Chopped Food* (Continued)*

	Urea (mosmol)	Na (meq)	Cl (meq)	K (meq)	Renal Solute Load (mosmol)	Water for Renal Excretion (ml)	
						Urine Conc. 1000 mosmol/l	Urine Conc. 300 mosmol/l
meat and vegetables							
beef	42.3	13.2	10.6	2.9	69.0	69	230
chicken	42.3	11.5	9.2	1.8	64.8	65	216
turkey	38.3	15.1	12.1	3.1	68.6	69	229
veal	40.6	14.0	11.2	2.4	68.2	68	227
Fruits							
applesauce	1.1	.3	.2	1.6	3.2	3	11
applesauce and apricots	1.7	1.0	0.8	2.7	6.2	6	21
bananas	2.3	1.3	1.0	3.0	7.6	8	25
bananas and pineapple	2.3	2.6	2.1	1.8	8.8	9	29
fruit dessert	1.7	2.3	1.8	1.9	7.7	8	26
peaches	3.4	1.9	1.5	2.1	8.9	9	30
pears	1.7	.2	.2	1.6	3.7	4	12
pears and pineapple	2.3	.1	.1	1.8	4.3	4	14
plums with tapioca	2.3	1.7	1.4	1.1	6.5	7	22
prunes with tapioca	1.7	1.4	1.1	3.1	7.3	7	24
Meats and eggs							
beef strained	84.0	9.9	15.8	4.7	114.4	114	381
beef junior	110.3	12.3	19.7	6.2	148.5	149	495
beef heart	77.1	9.0	14.4	6.2	106.7	107	356
chicken	78.3	11.4	18.2	2.5	110.4	110	368
egg yolk	57.1	11.9	10.7	1.5	81.2	81	271
egg yolk with ham	57.1	13.6	21.8	2.1	94.6	95	315
lamb strained	83.4	10.5	16.8	4.6	115.3	115	384
lamb junior	100.0	12.8	20.5	5.8	139.1	139	464
liver strained	80.6	11.0	17.6	5.2	114.4	114	381

Table 9-9. *Potential Renal Solute Load from Ingestion of 100 Grams of Strained or Chopped Food * (Continued)*

	Urea (mosmol)	Na (meq)	Cl (meq)	K (meq)	Renal Solute Load (mosmol)	Water for Renal Excretion (ml) Urine Conc. 1000 mosmol/l	Urine Conc. 300 mosmol/l
liver and bacon	78.3	13.1	21.0	4.9	117.3	117	391
pork strained	88.0	9.7	15.5	4.6	117.8	118	393
pork junior	106.3	10.3	16.5	5.4	138.5	139	462
veal strained	88.6	9.8	15.7	5.5	119.6	120	399
veal junior	107.4	12.0	19.2	5.3	143.9	144	480
Vegetables							
beans	8.0	9.3	7.4	2.4	27.1	27	90
beets	8.0	9.2	7.4	5.8	30.4	30	101
carrots	4.0	7.3	5.8	4.6	21.7	22	72
mixed vegetables	9.1	11.8	9.4	4.3	34.6	35	115
peas	24.0	8.4	6.7	2.6	41.7	42	139
spinach	13.1	11.8	9.4	3.6	37.9	38	126
squash	4.0	12.7	10.2	3.5	30.4	30	101
sweet potatoes	5.7	8.1	6.5	4.6	24.9	25	83
tomato soup	10.9	12.8	10.2	7.7	41.6	42	139
Campbell soups ‡							
Scotch broth	26.3	43.5	43.5	3.3	116.6	117	389
consomme	26.9	24.0	24.0	3.2	78.1	78	260
cream of chicken	18.3	34.8	34.8	1.7	89.6	90	299

*Calculated as indicated in Table 9–7 from data in Appendix I (p. 280). Since concentrations of chloride are not listed in Appendix I, these have been estimated for strained and "junior" foods on the assumption that the milliosmolar ratio of chloride to sodium is 1.0 for dry cereal and Campbell soups, 1.6 for meats and 0.8 for other foods. These ratios have been calculated on the basis of data supplied by the Beech-Nut Baby Foods Company (1964).

†Cereal composition as fed. Assumes that one part of dry cereal has been mixed with six parts of whole cow milk.

‡Three examples have been chosen from Table 9–10 to represent the highest, the lowest and the median content of sodium.

Table 9-10. Relation Between Fluid Intake, Renal Solute Load and Water Balance (Hypothetic Two-month-old Infant Weighing 5.5 kg)

Type of Feeding	Amount Consumed (ml or gm)	Renal Solute Load (mosmol)	Water Available for Urinary Excretion° (ml)	With Urine Concentration 1000 mosmol/l	
				Water for Renal Excretion (ml)	"Free Water" (ml)
Environmental temperature 22°C (72°F); extrarenal losses assumed to be 215 ml					
Human milk	500	47	285	47	238
Cow milk	500	139	285	139	146
Cow milk	400	111 ⎫ 225	285	225	60
Strained beef	100	114 ⎭			
Environmental temperature 32°C (90°F); extrarenal losses assumed to be 380 ml					
Human milk	500	47	120	47	73
Cow milk	500	139	120	139	-19
Cow milk	700	194	320	194	126
Cow milk	500	139 ⎫ 253	220	253	-33
Strained beef	100	114 ⎭			
Cow milk	500	139 ⎫ 142	220	142	78
Applesauce	100	3 ⎭			

°Difference between total fluid intake and amount of water required for extrarenal excretion. Although solids account for approximately 15 per cent by weight of milk or applesauce and nearly 20 per cent by weight of strained beef, water of oxidation will be nearly equal to the weight of solids.

Low Fluid Intakes

An intake of only 500 ml of human milk or cow milk (Table 9–10) by a two-month-old infant receiving milk as the sole source of calories is below the normal range for infants of this age (Fig. 4–1). Yet, when extrarenal losses are not excessive, the urinary concentrating mechanism will be sufficient to maintain water balance with ease. Even when a strained food presenting a high renal solute load replaces 100 ml of cow milk, the normal infant will maintain water balance. However, when low fluid intakes are combined with high extrarenal losses, as illustrated at an environmental temperature of 32°C (90°F) and fluid intake of 500 ml, choice of feeding becomes important. With an intake of 500 ml of cow milk, water balance will not be maintained. When the intake of cow milk is increased from 500 to 700 ml, losses from skin and lungs and in feces do not increase and, therefore, additional water is available for urinary excretion. There is then no difficulty in maintaining water balance. The manner in which choice of strained foods may influence renal solute load (e.g., choice of beef versus choice of applesauce) is also shown.

The volume of intake that must be considered is the "net" or effective intake — subtracting any amount lost through regurgitation. Low volumes of intake may be encountered temporarily in normal infants at the time they are weaned from breast or bottle to cup. Since cow milk is frequently fed at this age, strained foods should be selected with preference for those providing low renal solute loads. As may be seen from Table 9–9, fruits are particularly valuable in this respect.

Calorically Concentrated Formulas

Infants with various types of cerebral damage, gastrointestinal abnormalities and congenital heart disease may be unable to tolerate amounts of food equal to those commonly ingested by normal infants. In such cases it is frequently desirable to utilize formulas more concentrated than 67 kcal/100 ml (20 kcal/oz). Commercially prepared formulas that provide relatively low renal solute loads are then desirable (Table 9–8).

Treatment of Diarrhea

Particular caution is necessary in management of infants with diarrhea. Misuse of the commercially prepared electrolyte mixture, Lytren, and of improvised mixtures of salts have been responsible for production of hypertonic dehydration in infants mildly ill with diarrhea (Colle et al., 1958; Franz and Segar, 1959; DeYoung and Diamond, 1960). Grave consequences have also resulted from a parent's misunderstanding of instructions for preparation of dilute salt solutions. For this reason it seems preferable to utilize dilute skim milk, dilute whole milk or formula rather than salt solutions. The practice of feeding boiled skim milk to infants with diarrhea is not medically sound since the renal solute load is as great in skim milk as in whole milk and water content is reduced by boiling.

Impaired Renal Concentrating Ability

Infants with impaired renal concentrating ability should receive low renal solute loads. Choice of formula and strained foods should be made with primary attention to this feature. Infants with renal diabetes insipidus should receive renal solute loads as low as can be achieved. With such infants it will frequently be desirable to utilize a formula more dilute than 67 kcal/100 ml or to offer breast or formula at one time and water at another.

Summary

As a general guideline it may be stated that the renal solute load will rarely be of importance in the choice of the feeding for infants unless (1) total volume of intake is less than 100 ml/kg/day, (2) protein supplies are appreciably more than 20 per cent of caloric intake (with the increased intake of salts that usually accompany diets high in protein), (3) extrarenal losses of water are excessive or (4) renal concentrating ability is seriously impaired.

Sodium Chloride and Hypertension

As pointed out by Dahl et al. (1963) and Puyau and Hampton (1966), intake of sodium chloride by infants in the United States is likely to be high. Harmful effects of such diets have not been demonstrated, but this may be primarily because appropriate studies have not yet been carried out. Studies of rats provide some cause for concern.

When rats of a strain bred for their propensity to develop hypertension are fed a diet high in salt, hypertension develops at a relatively early age and is self-sustaining after withdrawal of salt from the diet (Dahl et al., 1963). Ease of production of hypertension by addition of salt to the diet is greater with weanling than with older rats.

Employing a strain of rat prone to develop hypertension, Dahl et al. (1963) found that five of seven weanling rats fed commercially prepared strained foods for infants developed hypertension within four months; hypertension did not develop in any of seven control rats fed a low salt diet.

Strained and "junior" foods commercially prepared for infants are generally selected by mothers with little direction from their physicians. If a food is unpalatable to a mother, she is unlikely to purchase it for her infant; thus, the manufacturer of infant foods has found it profitable to cater to the tastes of adults. Salt is added to nearly all strained and "junior" foods for infants except fruits and fruit juices. Table 9–9 indicates the approximate content of sodium and chloride in various foods commercially prepared for infants in the United States. Because the salt content of canned soups (at least those marketed by the Campbell Soup Company) is high (Table 9–11), the practice of feeding these soups undiluted to infants as a substitute for "junior" foods results in particularly large intakes of sodium chloride.

As may be seen from Figure 9–3, intake of sodium by infants 11 to 13 months of age was found by Puyau and Hampton (1966) to average 60 meq/day—approximately 0.35 gm of sodium chloride per kilogram per day and, assuming that the 11- to 13-month-old infant is 0.45 m², 13.4 gm of sodium chloride per m² of body surface area per day. These intakes per unit of body weight, although perhaps not per unit of surface area, are in the range encountered in populations with high incidence of hypertension (Meneely and Dahl, 1961). Because of considerable variability in salt intake from infant to infant, a few infants undoubtedly receive intakes well in excess of the average figure. Concern about the possibility of development of hypertension in such infants seems justified.

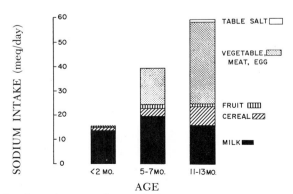

Figure 9–3. Contributions of various dietary components to sodium intake of normal infants at selected ages. (From Puyau, F. A., and Hampton, L. P.: Am. J. Dis. Child. *111*:370, 1966.)

Table 9-11. Proximate, Mineral and Vitamin Composition of Campbell Soup Company Products (Contents of 100 gm)

Variety / Heat Processed Soups	Calories	Protein gm	Fat gm	Carbohydrate gm	Crude Fiber gm	Ash (Salt Free) gm	Solids gm	Calcium mg	Phosphorus mg	Iron mg	Sodium mg	Potassium mg	Vitamin A I.U.	Thiamine mg	Riboflavin mg	Niacin mg
Asparagus, cream of	51	2.0	1.4	7.8	0.6	0.3	14.2	21	31	0.6	820	100	254	0.03	0.07	0.6
Bean with bacon	133	6.8	4.2	17.1	1.3	0.9	32.2	38	98	1.9	750	300	550	0.08	0.05	0.7
Beef	87	8.0	2.0	9.2	0.3	0.1	21.7	3	32	0.9	773	135	1067	0.01	0.06	1.2
Beef broth	22	3.6	0.0	2.1	0.1	0.3	7.8	trace	24	0.2	708	90	trace	trace	0.02	1.0
Beef noodle	58	3.2	1.9	7.2	0.1	0.5	14.5	trace	37	0.8	795	69	52	0.06	0.07	1.2
Black bean	80	4.7	1.4	12.2	0.8	1.4	22.3	24	75	1.9	860	250	258	0.06	0.07	0.4
Celery, cream of	66	1.4	3.9	6.4	0.2	0.2	14.1	34	31	0.8	860	90	173	0.01	0.04	0.8
Cheddar cheese	142	4.8	9.9	8.3	0.2	0.4	25.5	134	106	1.3	780	120	795	0.01	0.12	0.1
Chicken, cream of	93	3.2	5.8	6.9	0.1	0.3	18.3	21	29	0.5	800	68	484	0.01	0.04	0.6
Chicken gumbo	49	2.2	1.1	7.5	0.2	0.3	13.2	14	20	0.6	900	60	179	0.02	0.04	1.4
Chicken noodle	55	3.3	1.6	6.9	0.1	0.1	14.1	5	28	0.4	870	40	47	0.01	0.02	0.7
Chicken vegetable	60	3.4	1.8	7.6	0.3	0.3	15.5	14	34	0.5	820	136	1750	0.02	0.03	0.9
Chicken with rice	43	2.8	1.3	4.9	0.1	0.1	10.9	3	17	0.3	756	82	133	trace	0.02	0.6
Consomme	28	4.7	0.0	2.5	0.1	0.4	8.9	trace	26	0.7	550	125	trace	trace	0.02	0.9
Green pea	116	6.9	1.6	18.5	0.5	0.6	29.9	24	96	1.3	760	130	206	0.01	0.05	1.0
Minestrone	83	4.9	3.0	9.2	0.7	0.5	20.3	27	46	0.7	788	255	1917	0.06	0.05	0.9
Mushroom, cream of	115	1.7	8.7	7.5	0.1	0.2	20.3	22	31	0.4	842	60	79	0.01	0.08	0.6
Onion	52	4.4	2.1	3.9	0.4	0.1	13.1	23	23	0.4	966	86	trace	trace	0.02	0.3
Pepper pot	83	6.1	3.2	7.6	0.3	0.3	20.1	17	34	0.8	1000	124	478	0.02	0.02	0.9
Potato, cream of	59	1.4	1.9	9.0	0.2	0.2	14.8	29	37	0.7	914	109	trace	0.06	0.05	0.5
Scotch broth	74	4.6	2.4	8.6	0.4	0.3	18.4	10	45	0.8	1000	130	2623	0.01	0.03	1.4
Split pea with ham	130	8.1	2.4	19.1	0.4	0.8	32.5	16	165	1.6	803	300	480	0.04	0.09	1.0
Tomato	69	1.4	1.6	12.3	0.3	0.4	18.0	10	27	0.9	810	210	946	0.06	0.03	1.2
Tomato rice, old-fashioned	82	1.6	1.9	14.7	0.3	0.3	20.4	16	26	0.8	662	260	917	0.07	0.04	0.9
Turkey noodle	63	3.3	2.6	6.6	0.1	0.2	14.7	8	38	0.6	760	60	120	0.06	0.06	1.1
Turkey vegetable	58	2.8	2.3	6.6	0.3	0.2	14.0	12	33	0.7	710	143	2780	0.07	0.04	0.7
Vegetable	62	2.8	1.6	9.1	0.4	0.3	15.9	14	34	0.9	730	170	2345	0.03	0.02	1.0
Vegetable, cream of	89	2.0	5.3	8.4	0.2	0.3	18.3	42	44	0.4	888	168	967	0.03	0.07	0.3
Vegetable bean	81	4.4	1.8	11.7	0.7	0.6	21.3	20	36	0.8	938	240	2846	0.08	0.06	1.2
Vegetable beef	61	5.9	1.6	5.9	0.5	0.3	16.4	4	35	0.5	788	131	2250	0.03	0.04	0.8
Vegetarian vegetable	62	1.8	1.5	10.4	0.5	0.5	16.2	15	30	0.8	594	200	2318	0.03	0.03	0.7

161

APPENDIX
Calculations of Requirements of Minerals
For Incorporation into Newly Formed Tissues

The requirement for growth can be estimated on the basis of rate of growth of fat-free body tissue and an assumed concentration of the mineral in question per unit of gain in fat-free tissue. As may be seen from Figure 2–8, the "male reference infant" is calculated to gain 3.50 kg between birth and four months of age, of which 56.4 per cent (or 1.97 kg) is fat-free tissue. Assuming, as discussed in Chapter Five, that 115 days are available for tissue synthesis, gain in fat-free tissue must average 17.2 gm/day. Similarly, between four and 12 months of age, this hypothetic infant gains 3.50 kg of which 83.0 per cent (or 2.90 kg) is fat-free tissue. Assuming 235 days available for synthesis of this tissue, gain in fat-free tissue between four and 12 months of age must average 12.3 gm/day. Because requirements of sodium, chloride and potassium for growth are appreciably greater between birth and four months of age than between four and 12 months of age, separate calculations are presented. For calcium, phosphorus and magnesium, requirements are probably more uniform throughout the first year and one value for the daily requirement seems adequate.

Sodium

Concentration of sodium per kilogram of fat-free body mass is approximately 85 meq/kg both in the normal newborn and in the adult (Forbes, 1962). Assuming a similar concentration in the fat-free tissue gained between birth and four months and between four and 12 months of age, the amounts of sodium required for growth during these intervals are 157 and 247 meq, respectively.

Because the infant may lose weight immediately after birth and may fail to gain during periods of illness, 115 days are estimated to be available for tissue synthesis during the first four months of life and 235 days for tissue synthesis between four and 12 months of age. Therefore, the requirements of sodium for growth are approximately 1.4 and 1.0 meq/day, respectively.

Chloride

Since chloride concentration is approximately 57 meq/kg of fat-free body mass in the newborn and 50 meq/kg in the adult (Forbes, 1962), it seems reasonable to assume a concentration in the tissue gained between birth and 12 months of age to be 50 meq/kg. On this basis, the requirements for chloride for growth are calculated to be 93 and 145 meq during the two age intervals or approximately 0.8 and 0.5 meq/day, respectively.

Potassium

Because concentration of sodium is nearly the same per unit of fat-free body mass in the newborn infant and in the adult, one may rather confidently assume that a similar concentration applies per unit of fat-free body mass gained between birth and age one year. For the same reason, the concentration of chloride per unit of gain in fat-free body mass can also be confidently assumed. In the case of potassium, concentration per unit of fat-free body mass differs appreciably between the newborn (52.1 meq/kg) and the adult (68.6 meq/kg) (Forbes, 1962).

The estimation presented here is based on the assumption that concentration of potassium in fat-free tissue gained between birth and one year of age is equal to that of the adult: 68.6 meq/kg. The amount of potassium required for growth is therefore 127 meq between birth and four months of age (68.6 meq/kg $\times$ 1.85 kg) and 199 meq (68.6 meq/kg $\times$ 2.90) between four and 12 months of age. Assuming as previously discussed that synthesis of body tissue occurs during 115 days of the first four months of life and during 235 days of the next eight months, requirements for growth will be approximately 1.1 meq daily during the first four months of life and 0.8 meq daily between four and 12 months of age.

Calcium

Concentration of calcium per unit of fat-free tissue is considerably greater in the adult than in the newborn infant: 21.7 versus 9.5 gm/kg (Forbes, 1962). The data of Dickerson (1962) indicate that the calcium concentration of bone of the newborn is 8.95 gm/100 gm. Therefore, bone must account for 10.7 per cent of fat-free body mass (FFBM) at birth (0.95 gm/100 gm ÷ 0.0895).

Assuming that calcium concentration of bone is similar at birth and age one year and that bone accounts for a similar percentage of fat-free body mass, bone mass will be 860 gm (10.5 kg $\times$ 76.1 per cent FFBM $\times$ 10.7 per cent bone in FFBM) and calcium content of the body will be 81 gm (860 gm $\times$ 9.42 gm/100 gm) at age one year.

Calcium content of the body of the male reference infant, therefore, increases from 29 gm at birth to 81 gm at age one year, and the increase of 52 gm in 350 days amounts to 148 mg/day.

Phosphorus

The ratio of phosphorus to nitrogen (both expressed in grams) in the human body is approximately 0.25 at birth and 0.34 in the adult (Forbes, 1962). The ratio of phosphorus to calcium (expressed in grams) is approximately 0.60 at birth and 0.51 in the adult. The ratio of phosphorus to calcium in the tissue gained between birth and one year of age is probably no greater than the ratio at birth. Therefore, if the tissue increment of calcium is estimated to be 148 mg/day (Table 9–2), the tissue increment of phosphorus will be 89 mg/day.

Magnesium

As is true of phosphorus, magnesium is a component of both hard and soft tissues. The ratio of the amount of magnesium in the body to that of nitrogen changes relatively little between birth and adult life (0.012 to 0.014); the ratio of magnesium to calcium decreases from 0.027 to 0.021 (Forbes, 1962). Assuming that the ratio of magnesium to calcium in tissue formed between birth and one year of age is 0.027, an increase in calcium content of the body of 148 mg/day will be accompanied by an increase in magnesium content of the body of 4 mg/day.

REFERENCES

Bruck, E., and Weintraub, D. H.: Serum calcium and phosphorus in premature and full-term infants. A. M. A. J. Dis. Child. 90:653, 1955.

Colle, E., Ayoub, E., and Raile, R.: Hypertonic dehydration (hypernatremia): The role of feedings high in solutes. Pediatrics 22:5, 1958.

Cooke, R. E., Pratt, E. L., and Darrow, D. C.: The metabolic response of infants to heat stress. Yale J. Biol. Med. 22:227, 1950.

Dahl, L. K., Heine, M., and Tassinari, L.: High salt content of western infant's diet: Possible relationship to hypertension in the adult. Nature 198:1204, 1963.

DeYoung, V. R., and Diamond, E. F.: Possibility of iatrogenic factors responsible for hypernatremia in dehydrated infants. J.A.M.A. 173:1806, 1960.

Dickerson, J. W. T.: Changes in the composition of the human femur during growth. Biochem. J. 82:56, 1962.

Drescher, A. N., Barnett, H. L., and Troupkou, V.: Water balance in infants during water deprivation. The effects of the protein content of the diet on renal water requirements. Am. J. Dis. Child. 104:366, 1962.

Fomon, S. J., Owen, G. M., Jensen, R. L., and Thomas, L. N.: Calcium and phosphorus balance studies with normal full term infants fed pooled human milk or various formulas. Am. J. Clin. Nutr. 12:346, 1963.

Fomon, S. J., Younoszai, M. K., and Thomas, L. N.: Influence of vitamin D on linear growth of normal full-term infants. J. Nutrition 88:345, 1966.

Forbes, G. B.: Methods for determining composition of the human body. With a note on the effect of diet on body composition. (Report of the Committee on Nutrition). Pediatrics 29:477, 1962.

Franz, M. N., and Segar, W. E.: The association of various factors and hypernatremic diarrheal dehydration. A.M.A. Am. J. Dis. Child. 97:298, 1959.

Hansen, J. D. L., and Smith, C. A.: Effects of withholding fluid in the immediate post-natal period. Pediatrics 12:99, 1953.

Meneely, G. R., and Dahl, L. K.: Electrolytes in hypertension: The effects of sodium chloride. M. Clin. North America 45:271, 1961.

Nelson, M. V. K.: Calcium and phosphorus metabolism of infants receiving undiluted milk. Am. J. Dis. Child. 42:1090, 1931.

Owen, G. M., Garry, P., and Fomon, S. J.: Concentrations of calcium and inorganic phosphorus in serum of normal infants receiving various feedings. Pediatrics 31:495, 1963.

Poláček, E., Vocel, J., Neugebauerová, L., Šebková, M., and Věchetová, E.: The osmotic concentrating ability in healthy infants and children. Arch. Dis. Child. 40:291, 1965.

Pratt, E. L., Bienvenu, B., and Whyte, M. M.: Concentration of urine solutes by young infants. Pediatrics 1:181, 1948.

Puyau, F. A., and Hampton, L. P.: Infant feeding practices, 1966. Salt content of the modern diet. Am. J. Dis. Child. 111:370, 1966.

Widdowson, E. M.: Absorption and excretion of fat, nitrogen, and minerals from "filled" milks by babies one week old. Lancet 2:1099, 1965.

Widdowson, E. M., McCance, R. A., Harrison, G. E., and Sutton, A.: Effect of giving phosphate supplements to breast-fed babies on absorption and excretion of calcium, strontium, magnesium, and phosphorus. Lancet 2:1250, 1963.

Chapter Ten

Iron, Fluoride and Trace Minerals

Less than 40 years ago, the only trace elements that could unequivocally be called essential for higher animals were iron and iodine (Underwood, 1962). At present, chromium, cobalt, copper, fluorine, manganese, molybdenum, selenium and zinc must be included. Fluorine, while probably not essential to survival, is certainly highly conducive to dental health. Bromine, barium and strontium are currently classed as probably essential (Underwood, 1962). Many other trace elements, including radioactive materials resulting from the testing of nuclear weapons, are considered to be environmental contaminants.

Iron Deficiency Anemia and Its Prevention

Definition

Disagreements regarding the definition of anemia during infancy have often been a source of confusion in discussion of iron requirements during infancy. For purposes of the present discussion, anemia during infancy is defined as a condition in which concentration of hemoglobin is less than 10 gm/100 ml. Tentatively, at least, such anemia can be attributed to iron deficiency if the erythrocytes demonstrate hypochromia, anisocytosis and poikilocytosis.

166

Decrease in the concentration of serum iron and increase in the serum iron-binding capacity will also be present. Although it may be argued that a relatively late stage of iron deficiency exists by the time the concentration of hemoglobin falls to 10 gm/100 ml, the proposed definition has at least the advantage of simplicity and specificity and is believed adequate for practical purposes.

Hemoglobin concentrations regularly decrease between birth and age two or three months. The bone marrow is relatively inactive for the first month or two of extrauterine life and during this time more erythrocytes are destroyed than are produced, with the result that the total body content of hemoglobin decreases. Iron released from destroyed cells is stored for subsequent use. In addition to the progressively decreasing body content of hemoglobin during the early months of life, increasing total blood volume results in dilution of the erythrocyte mass. To the extent that these changes occur in the face of adequate body stores of iron, they may be considered truly physiologic.

Increase in total body content of hemoglobin generally begins by about two months of age, but whether this increase is reflected in concentrations of hemoglobin in peripheral blood depends largely on the balance between rate of hemoglobin production and rate of expansion of blood volume with growth. Figure 10–1 illustrates the effect of the presence or the absence of exogenous iron on the body content of hemoglobin and on the hemoglobin concentration of two hypothetic infants.

Incidence

If the proposed definition is accepted, iron deficiency during infancy and early childhood is prevalent throughout the world and ranks next to deficiency of fluoride as the most common nutritional deficiency disease in the United States and Canada. However, there is great variability in incidence, generally related to socioeconomic and educational factors. Concentrations of hemoglobin less than 10.0 gm/100 ml are frequently encountered in six- to 24-month-old infants in clinics that provide care for lower socioeconomic groups but are relatively infrequently seen among infants of similar age cared for by private practitioners in certain geographic areas.

Random sampling of children from the three busiest child health stations in New York City demonstrated that 19 of 46 infants (41 per cent) less than one year of age and 31 of 137 children (23 per cent) one to three years of age had concentrations of hemoglobin less than 10.0 gm/100 ml (Haughton, 1963). Andelman and Sered (1966) have reported that 76 per cent of 337 infants followed in the Child Welfare Stations of the Eighth Health District of Chicago

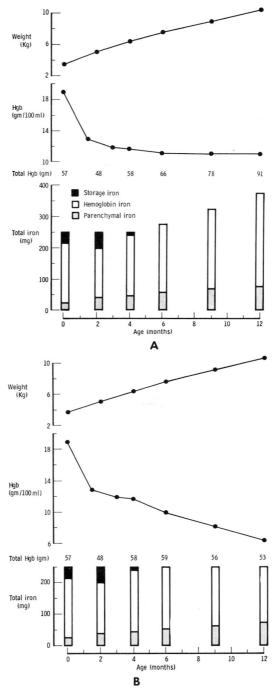

Figure 10-1. Events during the first year of life in a full-term infant with normal concentration of hemoglobin at birth and (A) access to sufficient exogenous supplies of iron to meet requirement during period of active growth or (B) denied access to exogenous supplies of iron. (From Erlandson, M. E.: Pediat. Clin. North America 9:673, 1962.)

became anemic, usually before age one year. Iron-deficiency anemia as defined previously has been reported to be present in about 30 per cent of infants admitted to various hospitals in larger cities in the United States (Holowach and Thurston, 1963; Lahey, 1957; Woodruff, 1958). Schulman (1961) found that 44 per cent of infants between six and 24 months of age admitted to Children's Memorial Hospital in Chicago had hemoglobin concentrations less than 10.5 gm/100 ml. Shaw and Robertson (1964) reported that 24.7 per cent of 775 infants age six to 24 months entering the Columbus Children's Hospital in 1960 had hemoglobin concentrations less than 10.0 gm/ 100 ml. During the same period not a single case of scurvy or of vitamin D deficiency rickets was identified at that hospital.

Although few reports are available to indicate the frequency of iron deficiency anemia among infants from more privileged socio-economic communities, verbal reports from many private practitioners suggest that the incidence is often quite low. Beal et al. (1962) reported that among 60 12-month-old infants cared for by pediatricians in private practice in Denver only two had concentrations of hemoglobin less than 10.0 gm/100 ml. Surveys of the incidence of iron deficiency anemia among infants from rural areas or among socioeconomically and educationally favored urban populations of the United States have not been reported. However, in Norway incidence of iron deficiency anemia in a rural and urban population was found to be less than 1 per cent in infants ranging from six to nine months and from 26 to 34 months of age (Mellander et al., 1959). It must be presumed that the incidence was also low in these infants between the ages of nine and 26 months.

Aims in Prevention

There is still much difference of opinion concerning the hematologic indices that one should attempt to maintain in the infant population. Nearly all pediatricians, nutritionists and hematologists would agree that concentrations of hemoglobin less than 7 gm/ 100 ml are sufficiently hazardous to warrant vigorous therapy, and most would agree that concentrations below 10 gm/100 ml are undesirable. Reports by Sturgeon (1956, 1958), Moe (1963, 1964, 1965) and others demonstrate that generous supplementation of the diet with iron will result in higher mean concentrations of hemoglobin than are to be found with less vigorous iron supplementation. Whether concentration of 12 gm/100 ml at 12 months of age is evidence of a more satisfactory state of health than 10 gm/100 ml is uncertain. Therefore, it seems unreasonable to set as a goal the achievement of maximal concentrations of hemoglobin in the infant population. Future studies may help to clarify this point.

Recommendations concerning advisable intakes of iron by infants vary in relation to the desired goals of management. Recommendations to be presented here are based on the assumption that concentrations of hemoglobin of practically all (i.e., 98 or 99 per cent) of normal infants should be maintained at or above 10 gm/ 100 ml. If one chooses, instead, to set as a goal the attainment of maximal concentrations of hemoglobin in practically all infants, much greater intakes will be necessary.

Although some infants will maintain relatively high concentrations of hemoglobin even when intakes of iron are small, no tests are available to predict which infants will become anemic and which will not. It is therefore preferable to manage the many in such a way as to benefit the few. From this point of view, knowledge of the mean concentration of hemoglobin in a specified population of infants is of less interest than knowledge of the fifth or tenth percentile value—a value that may provide some indication of the incidence of anemia in a relatively small percentage of infants.

Factors Influencing Requirement for Iron

Requirement for dietary iron is related to (1) the amount of iron accumulated by the fetus during gestation, (2) the perinatal and subsequent losses of blood and (3) the rate of growth. The amount of iron accumulated by the fetus during gestation is relatively small in premature infants, mature infants of low birth weight, twins, and infants born to iron-deficient mothers. Perinatal losses may be occasioned by fetal-maternal transfusion through the placenta, by transfusion from one twin to another, by clamping of the umbilical cord before pulsations have ceased or by bleeding during or after circumcision. Subsequent blood loss is, of course, equally important, and recent reports indicate that occult loss of blood from the gastrointestinal tract may be a quite frequent cause or complication of iron deficiency anemia of infancy (Wilson et al., 1962, 1964). Finally, the greater the rate of growth, the greater the extent of dilution of the initial mass of iron available for subsequent hemoglobin production.

Estimation of Requirement

The requirement of an infant for iron during the first year of life is the difference between the amount present at birth and that needed for growth and production of hemoglobin between birth and age one year. Sturgeon (1958) has estimated that one normal full-term infant may have 300 mg of iron in his body at birth while another may have only 129 mg. If each infant weighed 10 kg at age one year, had 100 mg of iron in tissues, a blood volume of 70 ml/kg and a hemoglobin concentration of 10.0 gm/100 ml, the total body content of iron in each infant would be 338 mg. To achieve this body content of iron at age one year, one normal infant might therefore require a net increment of only 38 mg of iron in 12 months while another might require a net increment of 209 mg.

According to the philosophy already presented—that recommendations for intake should be stipulated in terms of the few infants with greatest need—it seems desirable to provide for a net increment in body content of iron during the first year of life of about 200 mg.

Studies with non-radioactive iron and with ^{59}Fe suggest that more than 10 per cent of ingested iron is absorbed by most infants (Schulz and Smith, 1958a and b; Garby and Sjölin, 1959). Thus, a daily intake of 10 times the estimated requirement should result in assimilation of an adequate quantity of iron. Although blood loss and physiologic losses of iron in desquamated epithelium and bile cannot be precisely estimated, such losses are probably not great and have been ignored in the present calculations. Therefore, a cumulative intake of 2000 mg of iron during the first year of life seems reasonable.

Stating the recommendation for intake of iron in terms of a cumulative figure for the first year rather than in terms of mg/kg/day has some practical advantage. Iron is efficiently stored in the body, and the requirement is therefore conveniently stated in terms of total needs during a particular age span.

Although the extent of absorption of dietary and medicinal iron during the early months of life remains uncertain, there can be little doubt that absorption does occur and iron may, in fact, be more actively absorbed at this age than later (Gorten et al., 1963). If one employs a formula fortified with iron to the extent of 8 to 12 mg/liter together with early introduction and daily feeding of an iron-fortified cereal, an infant could ingest 2000 mg of iron during the first five or six months of life. By use of medicinal iron, the same total dose could be given in a much shorter interval. Exactly how short the interval could be and still permit adequate absorption is unknown. The minimum duration of oral administration effective in preventing anemia has not been established, and since we are not certain whether iron deficiency anemia can regularly be prevented by a program of iron administration restricted to the first six months of life, it seems desirable to pay close attention to intakes of iron during the latter months as well as during the early months of the first year of life.

Relatively few studies have been reported that are suitable for testing the hypothesis presented; namely, that cumulative intakes of 2000 mg of iron provided in small daily increments during the first year of life will regularly prevent development of iron deficiency anemia. In a study by Moe (1963), 79 infants received cumulative intakes of iron of approximately 1500 mg during the first year of life. Three of these infants had hemoglobin concentrations of less than 10.0 gm/100 ml (8.6, 9.8 and 9.45 gm/100 ml, respectively). Subsequent follow-up of these infants demonstrated that concentrations of hemoglobin were well maintained between one and three years of age even though supplements of iron were not given after one year of age (Moe, 1964). In the study by Beal et al. (1962), 19 infants received cumulative intakes of iron less than 2000 mg (average 1700 mg) and two of these had hemoglobin concentrations less than 10.0 gm/100 ml (9.7 and 9.8 gm/100 ml with cumulative intakes of 1613 and 1032 mg, respectively).

Foods as Sources of Iron

Iron may be provided for the infant in four main forms: an iron-fortified commercially prepared formula, an iron-fortified precooked cereal, foods naturally rich in iron and medicinal iron.

Amounts of iron provided by various commercially prepared formulas are indicated in the tables in Chapters Eleven and Twelve. Several such formulas provide from 5 to 13 mg of iron per liter and afford a convenient method for administration of iron to small infants. It must be noted, however, that most infants do not receive formula feedings after four or five months of age and very few are still taking formulas after six months of age (Fig. 1–3).

Iron-fortified precooked cereal is a rich source of iron, providing 7 to 12 mg of iron in 100 gm of cereal (about a cupful) as it is ordinarily fed after being mixed with milk to the consistency of a thin gruel (Table 10–1). A volume of such food equal to that provided by one jar of commercially prepared strained food will therefore fulfill the recommended daily intake for iron even if no other source of iron is provided. Cereal is a popular choice of food for infants during the early months of life but is not regularly given to most infants between eight and 24 months of age.

Beal et al. (1962) have reported median intakes of iron by infants studied in Denver (Fig. 10–2). Intake from cereal gradually increased until this source provided 5 or 6 mg daily at about seven months of age. By 12 months of age the median intake of iron from cereal had fallen to between 3 and 4 mg daily because most parents had ceased to offer cereal. By 15 months of age, intake of iron from cereal was less than 2 mg daily. In many parts of the United States it is customary to discontinue feeding of cereal by five or six months of age. Education of parents with respect to the advantages of feeding this iron-fortified food during later infancy could help greatly in reducing the incidence of iron-deficiency anemia.

(Text continued on page 177.)

Table 10–1. *Iron Content of Commercially Prepared Foods*

	Iron (mg per 100 gm of food)
A. STRAINED FOODS FOR INFANTS	
Cereal°	
Heinz	
high protein	12.7
rice	10.1
mixed	9.9
oatmeal	9.0
barley	8.1
Gerber	
rice	11.8
5 other varieties	7.1–8.4
Beech-Nut	
5 varieties	7.1
Meats, egg yolks, dinners, soups, etc.	
Heinz	
liver	4.0
liver and bacon	4.0
beef heart	3.2
egg yolks and bacon	3.0
beef	1.7
lamb	1.6
chicken	1.4
egg yolks	1.4
beef liver soup	1.3
beef with vegetables	1.1
pork	1.0
veal	1.0
chicken with vegetables	1.0
veal with vegetables	1.0
18 other varieties	0.1–0.8
Gerber	
vegetables and liver with bacon	3.1
egg yolks	2.9
beef	1.8
vegetables and lamb	1.7
chicken	1.6
veal	1.5
chicken with potatoes	1.2
chicken with vegetables	1.2
beef with potatoes	1.1
beef with vegetables	1.1
ham with vegetables	1.0
3 other varieties	0.8–0.9

°Iron content of cereal as fed (assumes 6 to 1 dilution with milk).

Table 10–1. *Iron Content of Commercially Prepared Foods (Continued)*

	Iron (mg per 100 gm of food)
A. STRAINED FOODS FOR INFANTS	
Beech-Nut	
egg yolks	3.7
egg yolks and bacon	2.7
chicken	2.3
vegetables and liver	2.0
lamb	1.9
beef	1.8
veal	1.6
pork	1.6
turkey dinner	1.1
veal dinner	1.1
beef dinner	1.0
13 other varieties	0.1–0.8
Swift	
liver and bacon	4.4
beef liver	3.9
beef and beef heart	2.7
lamb	2.3
beef	2.2
chicken	2.1
veal	1.6
pork	1.6
ham	1.5
Fruits	
Heinz	
11 varieties	0.0–0.4
Gerber	
prunes	2.6
plums	2.1
apple raspberry	1.9
bananas with pineapple	1.1
11 other varieties	0.2–0.8
Beech-Nut	
high protein cereal with applesauce and bananas	1.3
3 varieties cereal and fruit	0.5–0.6
cereal, egg yolks and bacon	0.6
pears	1.1
8 other varieties	0.1–0.8

Table 10–1. *Iron Content of Commercially Prepared Foods (Continued)*

	Iron (mg per 100 gm of food)
A. STRAINED FOODS FOR INFANTS	
Fruit juices	
Heinz	
7 varieties	0.1–0.7
Gerber	
5 varieties	0.3–0.7
Beech-Nut	
8 varieties	0.4–0.9
Vegetables	
Heinz	
creamed peas	0.9
8 other varieties	0.1–0.6
Gerber	
peas and carrots	1.9
peas	1.3
green beans	1.2
vegetable soup	1.2
garden vegetables	1.1
4 other varieties	0.6–0.7
Beech-Nut	
creamed spinach	2.2
squash	1.4
garden vegetables	1.0
beets	1.0
peas	0.9
green beans	0.8
3 other varieties	0.3–0.4
Puddings, custards, desserts	
Heinz	
4 varieties	0.0–0.4
Gerber	
banana custard	1.0
7 other varieties	0.3–0.7
Beech-Nut	
6 varieties	0.2–0.5

Table 10–1. *Iron Content of Commercially Prepared Foods (Continued)*

	Iron (mg per 100 gm of food)
B. JUNIOR FOODS FOR INFANTS	
Meats, egg yolks, dinners, soups, etc.	
Heinz	
beef heart	3.5
beef	2.0
lamb	1.6
vegetables and liver	1.2
chicken	1.2
beef with vegetables	1.1
pork	1.1
cereal, eggs and bacon	1.1
veal	1.0
19 other varieties	trace–0.9
Gerber	
beef	4.4
chicken	2.0
vegetables and lamb	1.7
veal	1.4
beef with vegetables	1.3
chicken with potatoes	1.2
beef with potatoes	1.1
ham with vegetables	1.0
15 other varieties	0.4–0.9
Beech-Nut	
beef	2.3
chicken	2.2
lamb	1.8
pork	1.8
vegetables and liver	1.8
veal	1.5
cereal, egg yolks and bacon	1.3
veal	1.1
turkey	1.0
17 other varieties	0.1–0.9
Fruits	
Heinz	
apricots and applesauce	0.8
5 other varieties	0.1–0.4
Gerber	
apple-raspberry	1.9
bananas with applesauce	1.1
mixed fruit	0.9
fruit salad	0.8
plums	0.7
7 other varieties	0.2–0.5

Table 10–1. *Iron Content of Commercially Prepared*
Foods (Concluded)

	Iron (mg per 100 gm of food)
B. JUNIOR FOODS FOR INFANTS	
Beech-Nut	
prunes with tapioca	1.3
pears	0.8
7 other varieties	0.3–0.5
Vegetables	
Heinz	
3 varieties	0.5–0.6
Gerber	
garden vegetables	4.7
peas and carrots	1.9
3 other varieties	0.5–0.6
Beech-Nut	
creamed spinach	1.2
squash	1.0
3 other varieties	0.4–0.8
Puddings and desserts	
Heinz	
6 varieties	0.1–0.6
Gerber	
3 varieties	0.5–0.7
Beech-Nut	
5 varieties	0.1–0.5

A word of caution is needed concerning "wet-packed" cereals, which are combinations of cereal with fruit or of cereal with egg yolks and bacon. These foods are not fortified with iron.

Many misconceptions exist about foods that are naturally rich in iron. Fruits, with the exception of prunes and plums, are generally poor sources of iron, providing less than 1 mg in 100 gm (Table 10–1). Peas, green beans and spinach generally provide 1 to 2 mg of iron in 100 gm but only nine of 27 varieties of strained vegetables are stated by the manufacturers to contain as much as 1 mg of iron in 100 gm of food. Fruit juices, puddings, custards and desserts are

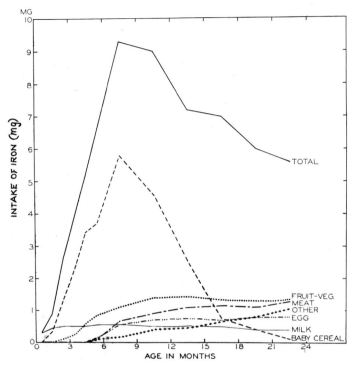

Figure 10-2.   Intake of iron from various dietary sources by infants receiving care from pediatricians in Denver. (From Beal, V. A., Meyers, A. J., and McCammon, R. W.: Pediatrics *30:*518, 1962.)

generally quite poor sources of iron. Many strained meats (Table 10–1) provide 1 to 4 mg of iron in 100 gm but combinations of meat and vegetables and most meat soups and "dinners" provide less than 1 mg in 100 gm. It is clear that an infant who consumes several hundred grams of strained foods daily does not necessarily receive an adequate intake of iron.

Efficacy and Cost of Medicinal Iron

As stated by Lahey (1966): "There are now excellent studies to show that the soluble, dissociated ferrous salts such as the sulfate, succinate, lactate, fumarate, and gluconate are better absorbed and therefore preferable to other ferrous salts . . . and much preferred to the poorly absorbed ferric salts, particularly the chelated iron compounds such as ferric choline citrate . . . and ferric versenate. The evidence that ferrous salts are better absorbed than ferric salts is so overwhelming that it can be concluded that ferric iron has no place in oral iron therapy. Iron salts complexed with large carbohy-

Table 10–2. *Some Preparations of Medicinal Iron for Use with Infants**

Type of Iron	Available Preparations	How Supplied
Ferrocholinate, iron choline citrate† (12% Fe)	Chel-Iron, Ferrolip	Syrup: 20 mg Fe/5 ml 　　　　 50 mg Fe/5 ml Liquid: 50 mg Fe/5 ml Drops (Pediatric): 25 mg Fe/5 ml
Ferroglycine sulfate complex†	Ferronord	Liquid: 40 mg Fe/ml
Ferrous fumarate, U.S.P. (33% Fe)	Feron, Fumiron, Hemoton, Ircon, Toleron	Suspension: 33 mg. Fe/5 ml
Ferrous gluconate, N.F. (12% Fe)	Fergon, Irox, Nionate	Elixir: 37.5 mg Fe/5 ml
Ferrous lactate (36% Fe)	Ferro drops	Drops: 25 mg Fe/ml
Ferrous sulfate, U.S.P. (20% Fe)	Feosol Fer-in-Sol	Syrup (N.F.): 40 mg Fe/5 ml Elixir (Feosol): 40 mg Fe/5 ml Fer-in-Sol: 15 mg Fe/0.6 ml
Polyferose, iron carbohydrate complex† (45% Fe)	Jefron	Elixir: equivalent to 100 mg Fe/5 ml

*Modified from Lahey, 1966.
†Less reliable than ferrous sulfate.

drate molecules . . . appear to be poorly absorbed by some children and therefore cannot be recommended for routine use."

Information about preparations of iron available for oral use with infants is presented in Table 10–2.

Advisable Intake

Every normal full-term infant should receive a cumulative intake of iron amounting to at least 2000 mg during the first year of life, of which at least 1000 mg should be given between age six and 12 months. For simplicity, the daily dose may be prorated over the entire period (e.g., approximately 6 mg of elemental iron daily if begun at age one month and 8 mg daily if begun at age three months). If iron fortification of the diet through use of iron-fortified foods or administration of medicinal iron is emphasized early in the child's life, it will provide an opportunity for educating parents with respect to iron needs during the time when routine well child appointments are most regularly kept.

A program of management aimed at early detection of decreasing hemoglobin concentrations seems less appealing than routine supplementation of the diet from an early age. Clinical acumen cannot be relied upon for detection of mild anemia, and most practitioners find burdensome a program of routine hemoglobin determinations. Furthermore, many parents neglect to seek routine well child care after the first few months of life and, occasionally, an infant will next be seen by a physician at 12 or 18 months of age with a hemoglobin concentration of 3 gm/100 ml.

Those infants with greatest likelihood of developing anemia should, however, be followed with regular laboratory analyses (at least determination of hemoglobin concentration). Included in this group are infants with birth weights below 2800 gm, twins, and infants whose mothers were known to be anemic during pregnancy or who had given birth to several infants in the previous several years. In addition, among infant populations in which anemia is known to be prevalent, concentrations of hemoglobin should be routinely determined even though iron-fortified foods or medicinal iron have been recommended.

The great heterogeneity of premature infants makes any general recommendation difficult. Use of an iron-fortified formula is desirable during the first six months of life. Iron-fortified cereal should be introduced into the diet by three or four months of age, and the importance of giving it regularly should be emphasized to the parents. Medicinal iron (e.g., 10 mg of elemental iron daily as ferrous sulfate) may be utilized instead of an iron-fortified formula or cereal. Concentrations of hemoglobin should be determined at regular intervals and daily iron intake increased if concentrations fall below 10 gm/100 ml.

Fluoride and Dental Caries

To the extent that incidence and severity of dental caries can be reduced by ingestion of fluoride, the condition may be considered a nutritional deficiency disease. In technically advanced countries the magnitude of this problem greatly exceeds that of all other nutritional deficiency diseases, including iron deficiency anemia. In January, 1965, when only 24 communities in Massachusetts were fluoridating their water, a survey of 14-year-old children conducted by the Massachusetts Department of Public Health indicated that almost half of the permanent dentition had already been damaged and that less than half the needed dental restorative treatment had been preformed (Dunning, 1965).

Fluoridation of communal supplies of drinking water has been demonstrated to reduce the incidence of dental caries by about 50 to 60 per cent (Schlesinger, 1963; Dunning, 1965). Reduction in incidence of dental caries can also be brought about by once daily administration of a fluoride supplement (Wrzodek, 1959; Ziemnowicz-Glowacka, 1960; Knychalska-Karwan and Laskowska, 1963; Hennon et al., 1966), although it is not at all certain that such prophylaxis is as effective as ingestion of fluoridated water.

The most pressing practical questions concerning administration of fluoride to the infant seem to be the following: (1) Is it desirable to provide fluoride to the infant prenatally by administration to the pregnant woman? (2) Is it desirable to provide for daily ingestion of fluoride during the first year of life? What are the likely benefits and possible risks? (3) If it is desirable to provide fluoride to the infant, what steps are necessary in communities in which drinking water is fluoridated and what steps are necessary in communities in which drinking water is not fluoridated?

Mechanism of Action

Fluoride is believed to exert its action in prevention of dental caries chiefly by replacement of hydroxyapatite with the less soluble fluorapatite in the crystalline structure of tooth enamel. Possible additional mechanisms are indicated by the fact that fluoride favors the precipitation of calcium phosphate from a saturated solution and that it inhibits some and apparently stimulates other types of enzyme action (Dunning, 1965).

Fluoride in Drinking Water

It is estimated that more than 53 million persons in the United States now live in communities in which drinking water is fluoridated and seven million additional individuals live in communities in which the natural content of fluoride is at the optimum concentration or greater (Dunning, 1965). Although usage of fluoridated water has grown steadily during the past 20 years and may be expected to increase still further, the desirable public health goal of achieving an optimum concentration of fluoride in all communal water supplies may be impossible. In addition, it is estimated that approximately one-third of the population of the United States and Canada does not have access to a communal water supply (Schlesinger,

1963; Nikiforuk and Fraser, 1964). For these individuals another mode of prophylaxis is required.

As will be discussed, the infant represents a special problem in prophylaxis since his intake of fluoride may be little influenced by whether the drinking water of the community is fluoridated.

Prenatal Administration

Because an important effect of fluoridation is considered to relate to formation of tooth structure before teeth erupt into the mouth and because calcification of deciduous teeth begins by the third or fourth month of fetal life (Kraus, 1959), the suggestion that fluoride prophylaxis be initiated prenatally is reasonable. That fluoride does cross the placental barrier has been demonstrated in studies of man and experimental animals (Bawden, 1964; Bawden et al., 1964; Zipkin and Babeaux, 1965).

Studies of the influence of prenatal administration of fluorides on incidence of dental caries have generally suffered from the small number of experimental subjects and from other defects in experimental design (Bawden, 1964; Nikiforuk and Fraser, 1964). As will be discussed subsequently, great variability in fluoride intake may occur between infants living in communities in which water contains optimum amounts of fluoride. It is therefore not surprising that controversy should exist concerning the benefits or lack of benefits of prenatal administration of fluoride (Carlos et al., 1962; Blayney and Hill, 1964; Carlos, 1964).

Tentatively, it is recommended that the pregnant woman receive 1 mg of fluoride daily (in drinking water and food or as a dietary supplement) during the second and third trimesters. Such dosage is almost certainly without hazard and may be of benefit to the fetus. Additional studies are desirable to determine whether the extent of the benefit, if any, warrants continued widespread use of this mode of prophylaxis.

Effect of Fluoride
Administration during Early
Infancy

After eight years of fluoridation in Danvers, Massachusetts, 86.0 per cent reduction in dental caries was found among seven-year-old children and only 49.0 per cent among 10-year-old children. In Athol, Massachusetts, six-year-old children showed 75.0 per cent reduction, while reduction in 11-year-old children was only 53.0 per cent (Dunning, 1965). These differences suggest that fluoride prophylaxis during infancy is desirable. However, review of dental caries incidence in several communities after 10 years of fluoridation has failed to demonstrate similar benefit. For example, in Newburgh, New York, six- to nine-year-old children demonstrated 58.0 per cent reduction in decayed, missing and filled (DMF) permanent teeth, a value almost identical to the reduction in DMF of 10- to 12-year-old children (57.0 per cent). Similarly, in Brantford, Ontario, the percentage reduction in DMF was nearly the same for nine-year-old, 10-year-old and 11- to 13-year-old children (46.0, 41.0, and 44.0 per cent, respectively).

Because an infant lives in a community in which drinking water is fluoridated does not necessarily indicate that he will receive enough of that water to afford significant protection against dental caries. Infants who are breast fed or who receive homogenized milk often consume extremely small amounts of tap water and may be virtually uninfluenced by the fluoride content of such water in their community. Most formulas made with tap water will provide adequate amounts of fluoride: a four-month-old infant receiving 950 ml daily of a commercially prepared liquid formula diluted with an equal volume of water might receive approximately 0.5 mg of fluoride. A formula made from evaporated milk, water and added carbohydrate would provide a slightly greater intake of fluoride, while a commercially prepared powdered formula diluted with water might provide 1 mg of fluoride. Thus, it is apparent that intake of fluoride by an infant living in a community in which the water supply is fluoridated may vary tenfold even when the same volume of milk or formula is consumed. Considerable variability in volume of intake from one infant to another and the presence of appreciable amounts of fluoride in some strained foods commercially prepared for infants will result in even greater variability in fluoride intake. Recommendations regarding fluoride supplementation of the diet must therefore be made in relation to the type of feeding as well as to the fluoride content of the drinking water.

Advisable Intake

From the previous discussion it is apparent that the benefits of providing fluoride during early infancy have not been unequivocally demonstrated. Nevertheless, on theoretic grounds and on the basis of suggestive experimental evidence, benefit seems likely.

The advisable intake is tentatively considered to be 0.5 mg daily, approximately the amount ingested by infants fed evaporated milk formulas or commercially prepared liquid formulas diluted with an equal volume of water in communities in which drinking water contains 1 ppm of fluoride. Recommended supplementation with fluoride in relation to the type of feeding and the fluoride content of the drinking water is indicated in Table 10–3.

Table 10–3. Recommended Fluoride Supplementation During Infancy

Milk or Formula	Fluoride Concentration of Water Supply (ppm)			
	<0.3	0.3–0.7	0.8–1.1	>1.1
Breastfed	0.5	0.5	0.5	0
Cow milk	0.5	0.25	0.25	0
Commercially prepared liquid	0.5	0.25	0	0
Evaporated milk formula	0.5	0.25	0	0
Commercially prepared powder	0.25	0	0	0

Supplementation: With or Without Vitamins?

There seems to be no valid philosophic objection to combining fluoride and vitamins in a single supplement *providing the infant has a need for the vitamins as well as for the fluoride.* A combination of 400 I.U. of vitamin D and 0.5 mg of fluoride in a daily dose of a vitamin preparation (without inclusion of unnecessary additional vitamins) would seem ideal for the breast-fed infant. Such a product is not currently marketed. When use of a vitamin-fluoride supplement would result in administration of amounts of vitamins in excess of the advisable intakes, it is preferable to utilize a fluoride supplement free of vitamins.

Because many parents are firmly convinced of the benefit of administering a daily supplement of vitamins to their infant, it is probably true, as suggested by Hennon et al. (1966), that fluoride will be given more regularly if it is combined with vitamins than if it is given alone. However, the administration of unnecessary supplements of vitamins as a means of assuring a regular dosage of a desirable nutrient is unsound. Parents must be made to understand the importance of daily ingestion of an adequate amount of fluoride just as they must be made to understand that hazards are involved in consumption of excessive amounts of certain vitamins. A vigorous campaign to educate the public in these matters is desirable.

Safety of Fluoride Administration

A great mass of literature documents the safety of fluoride administration (Smith, 1962). The suggestion that mongolism is associated with prenatal administration of fluoride (Rapaport, 1959) appears to be based on inadequate evidence. Berry (1958) has been unable to demonstrate a correlation between the fluoride content of drinking water and the incidence of mongolism.

Chromium

Although chromium has for a number of years been thought to be involved in the activity of certain enzyme systems, more recent studies have suggested other important functions of this element (Underwood, 1962). The suggestion has been made that chromium and other metals may play a role in maintenance of the configuration of the RNA molecule, perhaps linking purine or pyrimidine bases, or both, through covalent bonds. Chromium is also involved in cross-linking of collagen. Beginning with observations made in 1959, it has become increasingly evident that trivalent chromium is essential for normal carbohydrate metabolism (Mertz, 1967).

In rats, deficiency of trivalent chromium results in impairment of glucose tolerance. Oxidation of glucose in vitro by adipose tissue of chromium-deficient rats has been shown to be lower than that of chromium-supplemented rats both in the presence and absence of insulin (Mertz et al., 1965). Glinsmann et al. (1966) have demonstrated that oral supplementation with trivalent chromium was associated with improved glucose tolerance in certain adult patients with diabetes mellitus but that such supplementation did not influence the glucose tolerance of normal individuals. Recently, Hopkins and Majaj (1966) have reported hypoglycemia and impaired glucose tolerance in malnourished infants from the Jerusalem, Jordan, area. Fasting levels of blood sugar rose and glucose tolerance improved promptly after administration of trivalent chromium. It is anticipated that the relation between chromium deficiency, hypoglycemia and glucose tolerance will be extensively investigated during the next few years.

Cobalt

Because cobalt forms a part of the vitamin B_{12} molecule, it must be considered essential. However, cobalt deficiency has not been produced in a nonruminant animal (Underwood, 1962), and the requirements may therefore be assumed to be minute. Possibly its only function is as a component of vitamin B_{12} and, if intakes of this vitamin are adequate, no additional cobalt is required. Whether vitamin B_{12} synthesized by intestinal microorganisms can be absorbed by the human is unknown.

Individuals with anemia of various types have demonstrated an erythropoietic effect after administration of large doses of cobalt (Underwood, 1962; Hawkins, 1964). Such effects are probably pharmacologic rather than nutritional in nature.

Copper

Copper, like iron, is important in cellular respiration as a constituent of the hemocyanins and other oxygen-carrying proteins. It is a constituent of ascorbic acid oxidase, uricase, cytochrome oxidase and several other enzyme systems, is important in formation of bone and in maintenance of myelin in the nervous system, and functions in the utilization of iron in an early stage of hemopoiesis. Copper appears to be involved in development of young erythrocytes, in contrast to iron, which governs the development of normal size and hemoglobin content (Hawkins, 1964).

Manifestations of Deficiency

Manifestations of copper deficiency in various animals include hypocupremia, depletion of tissue copper, anemia, alterations in iron metabolism, skeletal changes, changes in hair and skin, and disorders of neurologic and cardiovascular systems (Cartwright and Wintrobe, 1964). Since other manifestations of copper deficiency are not observed in the absence of hypocupremia, the possibility of copper deficiency can probably be excluded when serum concentration of copper is normal. That hypocupremia does not necessarily indicate copper deficiency is suggested by the low serum copper concentration of the newborn infant in spite of large liver stores of copper (Cartwright and Wintrobe, 1964). Presumably, limited ability of the fetus to synthesize ceruloplasmin, the copper-containing protein of the serum, is responsible for the low serum concentrations at birth.

In the human infant, hypocupremia has been found in association with protein-losing enteropathy, iron-deficiency anemia, cystic fibrosis of the pancreas, celiac disease and kwashiorkor (Cartwright and Wintrobe, 1964). In protein-losing enteropathy and iron-deficiency anemia, abnormal losses of ceruloplasmin from the gastrointestinal tract are probably responsible for low concentrations of copper in serum. Gastrointestinal loss of copper may also be of major importance in other conditions in which hypocupremia is found. The hypocupremia associated with iron deficiency anemia in infants appears to be restricted to those cases in which hypoproteinemia is present (Sturgeon and Brubaker, 1956; Zipursky et al., 1958; Schubert and Lahey, 1959). In some instances, treatment with iron plus copper has been responsible for more complete correction of the anemia than treatment with iron alone (Zipursky et al., 1958; Schubert and Lahey, 1959).

Four infants with severe malnutrition were noted by Cordano et al. (1964) to develop severe anemia, neutropenia, bone changes resembling those of scurvy, and hypocupremia during treatment with a high calorie diet low in content of copper. Two of these infants responded promptly to the administration of copper. Cordano and Graham (1966) have also described a six-and-a-half-year-old child with failure to thrive since early infancy, possibly caused by intestinal lactase deficiency. Hypocupremia, anemia, neutropenia, osteoporosis and pathologic fractures were present. Administration of copper was followed by dramatic improvement in all manifestations.

Requirement and Advisable Intake

Wilson and Lahey (1960) were unsuccessful in producing hypocupremia or other evidences of copper deficiency in premature infants fed milk diets that provided 14 μg of copper per kilogram of body weight daily, suggesting that the requirement is less than this amount. Human milk and cow milk provide approximately 30 μg of copper per liter (Table 11–2), and this amount may tentatively be considered the advisable intake. Strained foods commercially prepared for infants are likely to contribute generous amounts of copper (Table 10–4).

Iodine

Iodine is an essential component of thyroxine and triiodothyronine, which are required for normal thyroid function. No other physiologic function of iodine in man has been identified (Stanbury and Ramalingaswami, 1964). Although iodine has long been recognized as a dietary essential and evidences of deficiency can be

Table 10–4.   *Copper Content of Strained and Junior Foods Commercially Prepared for Infants**

	Concentration of Copper (mg/100 gm)
Cereal, dry†	
high-protein	1.13 - 1.28
rice	0.26 - 0.41
Meats	
beef liver	2.64
other	0.07 - 0.19
High meat dinners	0.07 - 0.19
Egg yolks	0.09
Soups	0.06 - 0.17
Vegetables	0.08 - 0.16
Fruits	0.07 - 0.13
Fruit juices	0.06 - 0.07
Desserts	0.05 - 0.08

*Data of Hughes et al. (1960) concerning foods marketed by Gerber Products Company.

†Values given indicate range found in four widely separated geographic areas. Concentrations in other cereals (oatmeal, barley, mixed) are greater than those in rice cereal and less than those in high protein cereal.

rather readily detected, the combination of difficulties in analytic methods and wide variability in concentration in foodstuffs has made it exceptionally difficult to establish the requirement.

For the adult rat, the requirement for iodine appears to lie between 20 and 40 μg/1000 kcal of food consumed (Levine et al., 1933), and this estimate may be the best basis for arriving at a figure for the human.

As discussed in Chapter Eleven, iodine is unique among the trace elements in the extent to which variations in dietary intake are reflected in concentrations in milk (Underwood, 1962). The infrequency of iodine deficiency in infants in those portions of the United States in which the iodine content of the soil is low may be explained by dairy practices which result in adequate iodine content of cow milk and/or early introduction of strained foods to which iodized salt has been added.

The advisability of adding iodine to soy formulas to counteract the goitrogenic properties of such feedings has been discussed in Chapter Twelve.

Manganese

Because manganese deficiency has been demonstrated convincingly in mice, rats, guinea pigs, rabbits, pigs and poultry, it seems likely that the element is also essential for man (Underwood, 1962). However, deficiency syndromes in the human have not been identified.

Major manifestations of manganese deficiency in experimental animals are impairment of growth, skeletal abnormalities resulting from impaired osteogenesis and probably also impaired chondrogenesis, disturbed reproductive function and ataxia of the newborn. The mechanism of action of manganese is unknown, although several enzyme systems can be activated by this or by other bivalent ions and it appears to be a part of the prosthetic group of arginase.

Since human milk provides only about $7\mu g$ of manganese per liter (Underwood, 1962), it is unlikely that the daily requirement for infants exceeds this amount.

Molybdenum

Molybdenum is a component of xanthine oxidase and of several other metalloenzymes that are probably essential for animals. However, it has been impossible to produce manifestations of deficiency in animals by feeding diets exceedingly low in molybdenum. The addition of tungstate, a known molybdenum antagonist, to diets low in molybdate resulted in increased mortality of chicks; survivors demonstrated a decreased rate of growth, decreased concentrations of molybdenum and of xanthine oxidase in tissues and decreased ability to oxidize xanthine to uric acid (Underwood, 1962).

There is no evidence that molybdenum functions in any manner other than as a constituent for metalloenzymes, and amounts required for this purpose are exceptionally minute. Because it is all but impossible to prepare diets free of molybdenum, clinically significant disorders in the human infant are unlikely to occur as an expression of molybdenum deficiency.

Selenium

Toxicity of selenium for various animals has long been recognized. Much more recent is the appreciation that selenium is an essential element, at least for some animals. The exact nature of the relation between deficiency of vitamin E and that of selenium is unknown, although inhibition of lipid peroxidation in vivo is surely an important property of both.

At least three groups of illnesses have been identified in animals (Underwood, 1962): those caused by vitamin E deficiency alone, such as sterility in rats and encephalomalacia in chicks; those caused by simultaneous lack of vitamin E and selenium, such as liver necrosis in the rat and pig, exudative diathesis in birds and muscular dystrophy in several species; and those caused by lack of selenium alone, for example, lack of growth and muscular wasting in rats receiving adequate intakes of tocopherol.

Selenium deficiency in the human has not yet been identified.

Zinc

Zinc-containing metalloenzymes include carbonic anhydrase, carboxypeptidase, alkaline phosphatase and several pyridine nucleotide dehydrogenases (Prasad, 1967). There can thus be no question about the essential nature of zinc in human nutrition.

The body of the adult human is estimated to contain about 1.6 gm of zinc, i.e., less than half the amount of iron (4.4 gm) and about 16 times the amount of copper (Widdowson and Dickerson, 1964). In the newborn infant, however, concentrations of iron and copper per unit of body weight exceed those of adult animals, while concentrations of zinc are somewhat less in the newborn than in the adult.

As stated by Underwood (1962): "The nature and similarity of the manifestations of zinc deficiency in different species and their prevention by supplemental zinc imply that this element is specifically involved in somatic growth, in the keratinization of skin, hair, and feathers, in osteogenesis and probably in chondrogenesis, and in the development and function of the seminiferous tubules of the male. The precise role of zinc in these processes is unknown."

Important advances in study of zinc metabolism have been reported in a recent publication (Prasad, 1966).

Deficiency in Human Subjects

Although deficiency of any essential nutrient is likely to result in decreased appetite with consequent decrease in food consumption and retardation of growth rate, there is some suggestion that zinc deficiency acts more directly on cell division (Underwood, 1964). Zinc appears to be required for protein and nucleic acid synthesis by certain microorganisms. In animals it may be that zinc deficiency results in diminished production of RNA and, hence, protein and DNA.

Until 1961 zinc deficiency in the human had been described only in patients with advanced cirrhosis of the liver. Since that time several reports by Prasad and co-workers have delineated a syndrome of dwarfism, hypogonadism and decreased plasma concentration of zinc in male subjects in Egypt and Iran (Prasad, 1967). Extensive investigation of the Egyptian patients provided impressive evidence of zinc deficiency: concentrations of zinc in plasma, red cells and hair were decreased; zinc turnover in plasma and the 24-hour exchangeable pool of zinc were decreased. In addition, urinary and fecal excretion of labeled zinc was decreased, and liver function tests and biopsy failed to reveal evidence of cirrhosis.

In the villages in Egypt in which zinc deficiency was recognized, diets of adults were estimated to provide about 1.3 mg of available zinc daily (Prasad, 1967). Under these circumstances, zinc concentrations in human milk would almost certainly be decreased, but evidence is not yet available concerning the presence or absence of zinc deficiency among infants in these areas. Sandstead et al. (1965) have reported low plasma concentration of zinc in Egyptian children with kwashiorkor and have suggested that zinc deficiency in these children may be related to the observed growth failure that antedates the acute illness. It is also possible that zinc deficiency is of importance in the faulty pigmentation of hair in kwashiorkor.

A preliminary report by Strain et al. (1966) suggests that zinc deficiency may be present in a high percentage of infants at the end of the first year of life. These workers reported that the zinc concentration of hair decreased from 138 ppm at birth to 55 ppm or less at age one year. This latter value is similar to that reported in hair of zinc-deficient Egyptian dwarfs. The significance of these low concentrations of zinc in presumably healthy infants cannot be stated at present.

Requirement and Advisable Intake

From the preliminary nature of the reports suggesting a syndrome of zinc deficiency in the human subject, it is clear that a statement of probable requirement cannot be made at present. Under most circumstances the advisable intake is probably no greater than the amount contained in one liter of human milk, i.e., 4 mg. Requirement is greater when calcium content of the diet is high (Hoekstra, 1964). Proteins from soybeans appear to contain zinc in a form which reduces its availability to animals (Luecke, 1965).

REFERENCES

Andelman, M. B., and Sered, B. R.: Utilization of dietary iron by term infants. Am. J. Dis. Child. *111*:45, 1966.
Bawden, J. W.: Prenatal administration of fluorides. J. No. Carolina Dent. Soc. *47*:10, 1964.
Bawden, J. W., Wolkoff, A. S., and Flowers, C. E., Jr.: Placental transfer of F-18 in sheep. J. Dent. Res. *43*:678, 1964.
Beal, V. A., Meyers, A. J., and McCammon, R. W.: Iron intake, hemoglobin, and physical growth during the first two years of life. Pediatrics *30*:518, 1962.
Berry, W. T. C.: A study of the incidence of mongolism in relation to the fluoride content of water. Am. J. Ment. Deficiency *62*:634, 1958.
Blayney, J. R., and Hill, I. N.: Evanston Dental Caries Study XXIV. Prenatal fluorides — value of waterborne fluorides during pregnancy. J. Am. Dent. A. *69*:291, 1964.
Carlos, J. P.: Prenatal fluorides — are they valuable? J. Am. Dent. A. *69*:808, 1964.
Carlos, J. P., Gittelsohn, A. M., and Haddon, W., Jr.: Caries in deciduous teeth in relation to maternal ingestion of fluoride. Pub. Health Rep. *77*:658, 1962.
Cartwright, G. E., and Wintrobe, M. M.: The question of copper deficiency in man. Am. J. Clin. Nutr. *15*:94, 1964.
Cordano, A., Baertl, J. M., and Graham, G. G.: Copper deficiency in infancy. Pediatrics *34*:324, 1964.
Cordano, A., and Graham, G. G.: Copper deficiency complicating severe intestinal malabsorption. Pediatrics *38*:596, 1966.
Dunning, J. M.: Current status of fluoridation. New England J. Med. *272*:30, 1965.
Erlandson, M. E.: Iron metabolism and iron deficiency anemia. Pediat. Clin. North America *9*:673, 1962.
Garby, L., and Sjölin, S.: Absorption of labelled iron in infants less than three months old. Acta Paediat. Suppl. 117, 1959.
Glinsmann, W. H., Feldman, F. J., and Mertz, W.: Plasma chromium after glucose administration. Science *152*:1243, 1966.
Gorten, M. K., Hepner, R., and Workman, J. B.: Iron metabolism in premature infants. I. Absorption and utilization of iron as measured by isotope studies. J. Pediat. *63*:1063, 1963.
Haughton, J. G.: Nutritional anemia of infancy and childhood. Am. J. Pub. Health *53*:1121, 1963.
Hawkins, W. W.: Iron, copper, and cobalt. *In* Beaton, G. H., and McHenry, E. W. (eds.): Nutrition, A Comprehensive Treatise, Vol. 1. New York, Academic Press, Inc., 1964, p. 309.
Hennon, D. K., Stookey, G. K., and Muhler, J. C.: The clinical anticariogenic effectiveness of supplementary fluoride-vitamin preparations. Results at the end of three years. J. Dent. Child. *33*:3, 1966.
Hoekstra, W. G.: Recent observations on mineral interrelationships. Fed. Proc. *23*: 1068, 1964.
Holowach, J., and Thurston, D. L.: Breath-holding spells and anemia. New England J. Med. *268*:21, 1963.
Hopkins, L. L., Jr., and Majaj, A. S.: Normalization of impaired glucose utilization and hypoglycemia by Cr (III) in malnourished infants. (Abstract.) Fed. Proc. *25*:303, 1966.
Hughes, G., Kelly, V. J., and Stewart, R. A.: The copper content of infant foods. Pediatrics *25*:477, 1960.

Knychalska-Karwan, Z., and Laskowska, L.: Fluorowanie tabletkowe dzieci szkól podstawowych rzeszowa. Czas. stomat. *16*:201, 1963. [Use of fluoride tablets in Polish children. D. Abst. *9*:53, 1964.]

Kraus, B. S.: Calcification of the human deciduous teeth. J. Am. Dent. A. *59*:1128, 1959.

Lahey, M. E.: Iron-deficiency anemia. Pediat. Clin. North America *4*:481, 1957.

Lahey, M. E.: Anemia due to inadequate erythrocyte or hemoglobin production. *In* Shirkey, H. C.: Pediatric Therapy. 2nd ed. St. Louis, The C. V. Mosby Co., 1966, p. 623.

Levine, H., Remington, R. E., and Kolnitz, von H.: Studies on the relation of diet to goiter. II. The iodine requirement of the rat. J. Nutr. *6*:347, 1933.

Luecke, R. W.: The significance of zinc in nutrition. Borden's Rev. Nutr. Res. *26*:45, 1965.

Mellander, O., Vahlquist, B., and Mellbin, T.: Breast feeding and artificial feeding: a clinical, serological, and biochemical study of 402 infants, with a survey of the literature. The Norbotten study. Acta Paediat. Suppl. 116, 1959.

Mertz, W.: Biological role of chromium. Fed. Proc. *26*:186, 1967.

Mertz, W., Roginski, E. E., and Schroeder, H. A.: Some aspects of glucose metabolism of chromium-deficient rats raised in a strictly controlled environment. J. Nutr. *86*:107, 1965.

Moe, P. J.: Iron requirements in infancy. Longitudinal studies of iron requirements during the first year of life. Acta Paediat. Scandinav. Suppl. 150, 1963.

Moe, P. J.: Iron requirements in infancy. II. The influence of iron-fortified cereals given during the first year of life, on red blood picture at 1 1/2–3 years of age. Acta Paediat. Scandinav. *53*:423, 1964.

Moe, P. J.: Normal red blood picture during the first three years of life. Acta. Paediat. Scandinav. *54*:69, 1965.

Nikiforuk, G., and Fraser, D.: Fluoride supplements for prophylaxis of dental caries. Am. J. Dis. Child. *107*:111, 1964.

Prasad, A. S. (ed.): Zinc Metabolism. Springfield, Illinois, Charles C Thomas, 1966.

Prasad, A. S.: Nutritional metabolic role of zinc. Fed. Proc. *26*:172, 1967.

Rapaport, I.: Nouvelles recherches sur le mongolisme: A propos du rôle pathogénique du fluor. Bull. Acad. Nat. Méd. (Paris) *143*:367, 1959.

Sandstead, H. H., Shurky, A. S., Prasad, A. S., Gabr, M. K., Hifney, A. E., Mokhtar, N., and Darby, W. J.: Kwashiorkor in Egypt. Am. J. Clin. Nutr. *17*:15, 1965.

Schlesinger, E. R.: Dental caries and the pediatrician. Am. J. Dis. Child. *105*:1, 1963.

Schubert, W. K., and Lahey, M. E.: Copper and protein depletion complicating hypoferric anemia of infancy. Pediatrics *24*:710, 1959.

Schulman, I.: Iron requirements in infancy. J.A.M.A. *175*:118, 1961.

Schulz, J., and Smith, N. J.: A quantitative study of the absorption of food iron in infants and children. Am. J. Dis. Child. *95*:109, 1958a.

Schulz, J., and Smith, N. J.: Quantitative study of the absorption of iron salts in infants and children. Am. J. Dis. Child. *95*:120, 1958b.

Shaw, R., and Robertson, W. O.: Anemia among hospitalized infants. Ohio State Med. J. *60*:45, 1964.

Smith, F. A.: Safety of water fluoridation. J. Am. Dent. A. *65*:598, 1962.

Stanbury, J. B., and Ramalingaswami, V.: Iodine. *In* Beaton, G. H., and McHenry, E. W. (eds.): Nutrition, A Comprehensive Treatise. Vol. 1. New York, Academic Press, Inc., 1964, p. 373.

Strain, W. H., Lascari, A. D., and Pories, W.: Zinc deficiency in babies. Abstracts of papers. Seventh International Congress of Nutrition, Hamburg, Germany. Pergamos-Druck, 1966.

Sturgeon, P.: Iron metabolism. A review with special consideration of iron requirements during normal infancy. Pediatrics *18*:267, 1956.

Sturgeon, P.: Studies of iron requirements in infants and children. *In* Wallerstein, R. O., and Mettier, S. R. (eds.): Iron in Clinical Medicine. Berkeley, University of California Press, 1958, p. 183.

Sturgeon, P., and Brubaker, C.: Copper deficiency in infants. A syndrome characterized by hypocupremia, iron deficiency anemia, and hypoproteinemia. Am. J. Dis. Child. *92*:254, 1956.

Underwood, E. J.: Trace Elements in Human and Animal Nutrition. 2nd ed. New York, Academic Press, Inc., 1962.

Underwood, E. J.: Clinical and physiological aspects of the trace elements. *In* Cuthbertson, D. P., Mills, C. F., and Passmore, R. (eds.): Proceedings of the Sixth International Congress of Nutrition. Edinburgh, E. & S. Livingstone, Ltd., 1964, p. 289.

Widdowson, E. M., and Dickerson, J. W. T.: Chemical composition of the body. *In* Comar, C. L., and Bronner, F. (eds.): Mineral Metabolism. Vol. II. New York, Academic Press, Inc., 1964, p. 1.

Wilson, J. F., Heiner, D. C., and Lahey, M. E.: Studies on iron metabolism. I. Evidence of gastrointestinal dysfunction in infants with iron deficiency anemia. J. Pediat. 60:787, 1962.

Wilson, J. F., Heiner, D. C., and Lahey, M. E.: Milk-induced gastrointestinal bleeding in infants with hypochromic microcytic anemia. J.A.M.A. 189:568, 1964.

Wilson, J. F., and Lahey, M. E.: Failure to induce dietary deficiency of copper in premature infants. Pediatrics 25:40, 1960.

Woodruff, C. W.: Multiple causes of iron deficiency in infants. J.A.M.A. 167:715, 1958.

Wrzodek, G.: Ist eine Kariesprophylaxe mit Fluor-Dragées erfolgversprechend? Zahnärztl. Mitt. 7:258, 1959.

Ziemnowicz-Glowacka, W.: Zapobieganie próchnicy zebów tabletkami „fluodar." Czas. stomat. 13:719, 1960. [Effect of sodium fluoride tablets on teeth of children in Poland. D. Abst. 6:397, 1961.]

Zipkin, I., and Babeaux, W. L.: Maternal transfer of fluoride. J. Oral Ther. & Pharm. 1:652, 1965.

Zipursky, A., Dempsey, H., Markowitz, H., Cartwright, G., Wintrobe, M. M.: Studies on copper metabolism. XXIV. Hypocupremia in infancy. Am. J. Dis. Child. 96:148, 1958.

Chapter Eleven

Milks and
Milk-based Formulas

Most infants are dependent on milk or formula for nearly all of their nutritional needs during the early weeks or months of life. Even after the introduction of other foods into the diet, milk continues to supply a large percentage of caloric intake and is the major source of most of the essential nutrients. Knowledge of the composition of human milk, other milks and various formulas is therefore essential to adequate management in infant feeding.

As pointed out by Kon (1959) "It stands to reason that milk, which only for a limited time and with certain reservations is the ideal food for the young of any one species, is further restricted in value when used by another species, and the limitations of milks of domesticated animals in human nutrition must be frankly accepted and understood." In this respect it is worth noting that growth rates of the human infant and the calf are quite different, the human infant requiring nearly twice as long as the calf to double his birth weight (100 versus 50 days). Thus, the ratio of nutrient requirement for growth to that for maintenance will be greater for the calf than for the human infant. Furthermore, protein and minerals account for smaller percentages of weight gain in the human infant than in the calf. It is, therefore, not surprising that cow milk is richer in protein and minerals than is human milk.

*Table 11–1.   Composition of 24-Hour Samples of Human Milk**

	−1 S.D.†	Mean (gm/100 ml)	+1 S.D.
Protein	0.95	1.21	1.47
Fat	2.76	3.33	3.90
Lactose	6.56	7.23	7.90

*Data of Morrison, 1952.
†Standard deviation.

Human Milk

The extent of variability in composition of milk secreted by different women is not generally appreciated. As may be seen from Table 11–1, milk secreted by two women in the same country and with generally similar diets may vary considerably in caloric concentration and percentage composition of protein, fat and carbohydrate (Morrison, 1952). One-sixth of United States women may be expected to secrete milk with protein content of 0.95 gm/100 ml or less (i.e., mean concentration minus 1 standard deviation) while another one-sixth secrete milk containing 1.47 gm/100 ml or more. Although milk secreted by two cows (or goats) in the same herd also differs considerably in composition, such difference is of less practical importance with respect to infant nutrition since the human infant in our culture will rarely receive human milk except from his mother while the bottle-fed infant will ordinarily receive milk from a pool to which an entire herd of cows have contributed. In the case of evaporated milk or commercially prepared formulas for infants, the milk will usually reflect composition of a pool from many herds. Tabular data on mean composition of cow milk are, therefore, much more meaningful than similar data on human milk.

Composition of Human Colostrum and Transitional Milk

Human milk has a lower mean energy value during the first five days after parturition (67 kcal/100 ml) than does mature milk (75 kcal/100 ml) (Macy and Kelly, 1961).

Ash content of human colostrum is relatively high. Concentrations of sodium, potassium and chloride are greater in colostrum than in mature human milk. Major changes in composition of human milk in transition from colostrum to mature milk are completed by the tenth day (Committee on Nutrition, 1960).

Hytten (1954a) showed that the best prediction of later success in breast feeding is based upon the total fat output on the seventh day. Ninety per cent of the women whose milk contained at least 20 gm of fat on the seventh day were still able to nurse three months later, but only 20 per cent of the women who secreted from 4.9 to 10 gm of fat on the seventh day were still nursing three months later.

A substance present in human milk secreted by some women appears to be responsible for persistent elevation of indirect reacting bilirubin (Arias et al., 1963; Newman and Gross, 1963). This substance, believed to be pregnane-3 alpa, 20 beta-diol, presumably inhibits glucuronide formation (Gartner and Arias, 1964; Stiehm and Ryan, 1965; Gartner and Arias, 1966). Interruption of breast feeding for 24 to 48 hours is generally sufficient to permit concentration of bilirubin to fall below 10 mg/100 ml, and subsequent resumption of breast feeding is not associated with increases in bilirubinemia.

Composition of Mature Human Milk

Average values for composition of mature human milk are presented in Table 11–2.* It must be emphasized again that wide variability occurs from woman to woman and in the same woman from one time of day to another and from one breast to the other. Hytten (1954b) showed that during a single feeding or emptying by pump, the milk from the two breasts might differ in fat content by 1 to 2 gm/100 ml. Furthermore, a diurnal rhythm in total yield and fat content of the milk could be demonstrated. The amount of milk obtainable was greatest at 6 A.M. and least at 10 P.M.

MATERNAL DIET AND COMPOSITION OF MILK. Although differences in diet may affect total volume of milk secreted, moderate changes in dietary intake of protein, fat and calcium do not correlate well with changes in concentrations of these nutrients in human milk (Morrison, 1952). When a woman is poorly nourished, the volume of secreted milk is likely to decrease but the percentage of protein, carbohydrate and fat will be relatively little affected (Committee on Nutrition, 1960). On the other hand, vitamin content generally does reflect maternal intake.

ENZYMES IN MILK. A large number of enzymes are known to be present in human milk and cow milk (Heyndrickx, 1962 and 1963). However, it seems probable that these enzymes are nearly all destroyed in passage through the stomach and are not of great nutritional significance.

---

*The more selective data of Macy and Kelly (1961) are included in Table 11–2 rather than the commonly cited summary values from the compilation of Macy, Kelly and Sloan (1953).

Table 11–2.   *Composition of Mature Human Milk and Cow Milk**

Composition	Human Milk	Cow Milk
Water (100 ml)	87.1	87.3
Energy (kcal/100 ml)	75	69
Total solids (gm/100 ml)	12.9	12.7
Protein	1.1	3.3
Fat	4.5	3.7
Lactose	6.8	4.8
Ash	0.21	0.72
Proteins (% of total protein)		
Casein	40	82
Whey proteins	60	18
Non-protein nitrogen (gm/100 ml)	39	31
(% of total nitrogen)	17	6
Amino acids (mg/liter)		
Essential		
Histidine	23	80
Isoleucine	86	212
Leucine	161	356
Lysine	79	257
Methionine	23	87
Phenylalanine	64	173
Threonine	62	152
Tryptophan	22	50
Valine	90	228
Nonessential		
Arginine	51	124
Alanine	35	75
Aspartic acid	116	166
Cystine	29	29
Glutamic acid	230	680
Glycine	0	11
Proline	80	250
Serine	69	160
Tyrosine	62	190
Fatty acids† (% of total fatty acids)		
Essential		
Linoleic	10.6	2.1
Nonessential, unsaturated		
Oleic	37.4	17.7
Palmitoleic	3.4	3.2
Linolenic	trace	
Nonessential, saturated		
Palmitic	26.7	36.6
Stearic	8.3	8.1
Myristic	7.9	11.8
Lauric	4.7	3.6
Capric	0.8	3.2
Caprylic	0.1	1.2
Caproic	0.1	2.0
Butyric	0.26	2.7

Table 11–2. *Composition of Mature Human Milk and Cow Milk*
(Continued)

Composition	Human Milk	Cow Milk
Ash, major components per liter		
Calcium (mg)	340	1250
Phosphorus (mg)	140	960
Sodium (meq)	7	25
Potassium (meq)	13	35
Chloride (meq)	11	29
Magnesium (mg)	40	120
Sulfur (mg)	140	300
Copper (μg)	30	30
Iodine# (μg)	30	47
Iron (mg)	0.3	1.0
Zinc (mg)	1.2	3.8
Vitamins per liter‡		
Vitamin A (I.U.)	1898	1025§
Thiamine (μg)	160	440
Riboflavin (μg)	360	1750
Niacin (μg)	1470	940
Pyridoxine (μg)	100	640
Pantothenate (μg)	1840	3460
Folic acid (μg)	2	3
B_{12} (ug)	0.3	4
Vitamin C (mg)	43	11
Vitamin D (I.U.)	21	13¶
Vitamin E (mg)	6.6	1.0
Vitamin K (μg)	15	60

*Data of Macy and Kelly, 1961, except as noted.
†Committee on Nutrition, 1960.
‡Hartman and Dryden, 1965, except values for vitamin K which are from Dam et al., 1942.
§Average value summer, 1690; winter, 1425 I.U./l.
‖Average winter value; average summer value 1690 I.U./l.
¶Average winter value; average value summer, 31 I.U./l.
#Chilean Iodine Educational Bureau, 1952.

VITAMIN AND MINERAL CONTENT. Human milk from a well nourished woman if taken in adequate quantity by the infant may be expected to satisfy requirements for vitamin A, thiamine, riboflavin, niacin, pyridoxine, vitamin B_{12}, folic acid, ascorbic acid and vitamin E. Although human milk is not a particularly rich source of niacin, it is a good source of tryptophan so that intake of niacin equivalents is more than adequate (see Chapter Eight). Human milk provides little vitamin D; supplementation of the infant's diet with this vitamin in a dosage of 400 I.U. daily is therefore advisable.

Neither iron nor fluoride is present in human milk in sufficient concentration to provide the advisable dietary intake of these minerals, and supplementation of the diet is recommended as discussed in Chapters Ten and Thirteen.

ANTIBODIES IN HUMAN MILK.   It has been known for some time that bacterial and viral antibodies are present in human milk and that substances in human milk inhibit the growth of the viruses of mumps, Japanese B encephalitis, vaccinia, influenza and poliomyelitis (Vahlquist, 1958). Because little absorption of these antibodies occurs when they are fed to the human infant (Nordbring, 1957), it has been assumed until recently that they were of little importance. However, it has now been shown that infants breast fed by women with high serum titers of antibodies to poliomyelitis are relatively resistant to infection with orally administered poliovaccine (Lepow et al., 1961; Warren et al., 1964). Similar protection is afforded by cow milk containing poliovirus antibody (Gonzaga et al., 1963). Furthermore, stools of newborn and older breast-fed infants contain significant amounts of hemagglutinating antibody to enteropathogenic strains of *Escherichia coli* (Kenny et al., 1967).

Results of animal studies also suggest that ingested antibodies may exert a protective effect. Freter (1956) and Burrows and Ware (1953) have demonstrated that orally administered antibodies can prevent certain bacterial infections and can permit survival of the animals when they are challenged with ordinarily fatal cholera infections. As has been concluded by others (Athreya et al., 1964; Kenny et al., 1967), it therefore appears likely that milk antibody provides some protection to the breast-fed infant. Such antibody probably exerts its influence through production of local immunity in the gastrointestinal tract and cannot be expected to influence frequency or severity of infections due to organisms that enter the body through other portals.

Cow Milk

Protein, Fat and Carbohydrate

As previously mentioned, differences in composition of milk from one cow to another is of relatively little significance in infant nutrition since most infants receive milk taken from a pool to which many cows have contributed. However, composition of milk from various dairy breeds may differ significantly, as indicated in Table 11–3 (Reinart and Nesbitt, cited by Ling et al., 1961). Milk of Guernsey and Jersey breeds is more concentrated in fat and in nonfat solids than is milk of other cows commonly bred in North America and Europe.

Data on composition of cow milk are included in Table 11–2.

Major differences are the greater concentrations of protein and minerals and lower concentrations of lactose in cow milk than in human milk. However, the higher ratio of whey proteins (lactalbumin and lactoglobins) to casein in human milk than in cow milk has not been demonstrated to be of nutritional advantage for the human infant (Chapter Five). Both casein and whey proteins are of exceptionally high quality, and since the content of sulfur-containing amino acids in casein appears to be adequate when requirements for protein are met, the fact that whey proteins contain more of these amino acids than does casein is not relevant for the human. However, the high casein content of whole cow milk is responsible for formation of a large and relatively poorly digested mass of curds in the stomach if the milk is not properly treated (e.g., by dilution, acidification or heating) to reduce curd tension.

Although non-protein nitrogen comprises a lower percentage of total nitrogen in cow milk (7 per cent) than in human milk (17 per cent), little significance is attributed to this difference. When a protein of high quality is fed, at least some of the non-protein nitrogen can be utilized by the infant (Snyderman et al., 1962). It seems likely that the nitrogen of human milk and cow milk can be fully utilized by the infant.

Fat of cow milk is high in content of triglycerides containing two or three saturated fatty acids of C-16 and C-18 chain length (Table 6–2) and is less well digested by full-term infants and infants of low birth weight during the early weeks of life than is the fat of human milk.

Table 11–3. *Composition of Milk of Different Breeds of Cows in Manitoba, 1952–1954**
(Mean values)

	Holstein	Jersey	Guernsey
No. of samples	75	72	23
Composition (gm/100 ml)			
Total solids	11.91	14.15	13.69
Protein	3.05	3.66	3.50
Fat	3.56	4.97	4.58
Lactose	4.61	4.70	4.78
Ash	0.73	0.77	0.75
Calcium	0.117	0.143	0.137

*Data of Reinart and Nesbitt, cited by Ling et al. (1961).

Vitamin and Mineral Content

The cow, as is true of all ruminants, has a paunch in which food undergoes extensive fermentation and microbial digestion before it reaches the true stomach. For this reason the nutritional requirements of the cow differ sharply from those of simple-stomached omnivorous animals, such as man. Microorganisms in the paunch break down food proteins and, from this source as well as from simple nitrogenous compounds such as ammonia and urea, synthesize protein. It is to a large extent this bacterially synthesized protein that the ruminant digests and uses, so that the nutritional quality of food proteins matters much less to ruminant than to nonruminant animals. All vitamins of the B group are synthesized in the paunch through microbial activity, and concentrations of these vitamins in milk of ruminants is therefore less influenced by diet than by factors such as breed and stage of lactation.

Although seasonal variation in content of protein, fat and carbohydrate is not great, amounts of vitamins A[*] and D are somewhat greater in summer than in winter (Table 11–2). But winter or summer, cow milk is a rich source of vitamin A and a poor source of vitamin D.

Thiamine, riboflavin, pyridoxine, vitamin B_{12} and folic acid are present in greater amounts in cow milk than in human milk. Cow milk contains less niacin than does human milk, but the content of tryptophan in cow milk is greater and the total niacin equivalents are similar in the two milks.

A major difference in the feeding of human milk and cow milk is that the former is ordinarily consumed directly from the breast and all vitamins originally present in the milk are transferred to the infant; on the other hand, losses of vitamins from cow milk may occur during collection, processing, transportation, delivery and storage. In the case of most of the B vitamins, the initial content in cow milk is sufficiently high that moderate losses are of little nutritional significance. Vitamin C content of cow milk averages 20 mg per liter as it is obtained from the udder and 15 mg immediately after pasteurization, but decreases to 10 mg during 12 hours of storage and to 5 mg during 24 hours of storage (McCance and Widdowson, 1960).

Although the bacterial flora of the gastrointestinal tract consists primarily of lactobacilli in the breast-fed infant and of coliform organisms in the infant fed various formulas of cow milk, the importance of this difference is as yet unknown; no practical advantage of either type of bacterial flora has been demonstrated. As is true of human milk, the amounts of iron and fluoride in cow milk are too low to make it possible to obtain advisable dietary intakes from this source.

---

[*]That is, vitamin A equivalents calculated from content of vitamin A and carotene.

The major minerals are present in cow milk in considerably greater concentrations than in human milk and there is little question that the infant receiving cow milk as a substantial portion of caloric intake also receives adequate intakes of the major minerals.

Available Forms of Cow Milk

The terms, pasteurized, homogenized, whole, skim, evaporated, condensed, roller-dried, spray-dried, and freeze-dried, as applied to milk, are discussed in the chapter Appendix. Composition of evaporated and dried cow milk is indicated in Table 11–4.

Data on composition of half-skim cow milk (i.e., equal parts of whole milk and nonfat milk) and of skim milk are presented in Table 11–5. Infant formulas based on cow milk are discussed subsequently in this chapter.

Renal Solute Load

Because cow milk has higher concentrations of protein and electrolytes than does human milk, the metabolism of cow milk results in a greater load of solutes (electrolytes and urea) for excretion in the urine. Even when cow milk is diluted with water and carbohydrate, as is common in infant feeding, the load of solutes presented for renal excretion is ordinarily considerably greater than that provided by human milk (Committee on Nutrition, 1957). However, the difference between cow milk and human milk with respect to the load of solutes presented to the kidney is of little practical concern except when renal concentrating ability is grossly impaired or when large extrarenal losses of water occur, as in febrile states and during exposure to high environmental temperature.

As a general rule, it is reasonable to consider that milk or formula providing no more than 20 per cent of calories as protein and fed at a concentration no greater than 67 kcal/100 ml will provide adequate water per unit of renal solute load if taken in amounts sufficient to satisfy caloric requirements. However, if Alacta or Dryco (Table 11–5, 31 per cent of calories from protein) is combined with water (without additional carbohydrate) to a caloric density of 67 kcal/100 ml, the renal solute load will be high in relation to available water, and negative water balance with eventual dehydration may occur.

The practice of prescribing boiled skim milk in treatment of diarrhea is also hazardous. Skim milk has the same renal solute load as does whole milk even though providing only one half as many calories per unit of volume. When skim milk is fed to an infant

Table 11–4. *Composition of Evaporated and Dried Cow Milk and Various Forms of Goat Milk*

Composition	Cow Milk*		Goat Milk	
	Evaporated (Many brands)	Klim (Borden)	Fresh (Market average)	Dale's (Cutter)
Normal dilution				
Ratio				
liquid	1:1			1:1
powder		1:7	undiluted	1:8
kcal/100 ml	74	64	76	76
Major constituents (gm/100 ml)				
Protein	3.8	3.3	3.3	3.3
Fat	4.0	3.5	4.1	4.1
Carbohydrate	5.4	4.7	4.7	4.7
Minerals	0.8	0.7	0.8	0.8
Caloric distribution (% of calories)				
Protein	20	20	19	19
Fat	50	50	59	59
Carbohydrate	30	30	27	27
Content of minerals per liter				
Calcium (mg)	1380	1160	1300	1300
Phosphorus (mg)	960	900	1060	1060
Sodium (meq)	28	22	18	18
Potassium (meq)	39	35	46	46
Chloride (meq)	32	28	45	45
Magnesium (mg)	132	120	160	160
Sulfur (mg)	330	300	160	160
Iron (mg)	1	1	0.5	0.5
Content of vitamins per liter				
Vitamin A (I.U.)	1850	1850	2074	—
Thiamine (μg)	280	380	400	480
Riboflavin (μg)	1900	1900	1840	1140
Niacin (mg)	1.0	1.3	1.9	2.7
Pyridoxine (μg)	370	—	70	70
Pantothenate (mg)	3.5	—	3.4	2.9
Folic acid (μg)	7.0	—	2.4	0.3
B_{12} (μg)	0.7	—	0.6	0.2
Ascorbic acid (mg)	5.5	1.9	15	14
Vitamin D (I.U.)	420	420	24	—
Vitamin E (I.U.)	1.3	—	—	—

*For composition of fresh milk see Table 11–2.

Table 11–5. Composition of Half-Skim and Skim Cow Milk

Composition	Half-Skim°		Skim†	
	Alacta (Mead)	Dryco (Borden)	Fluid (Market average)	Powdered (Many brands)
Normal dilution				
Ratio	1:7	1:8	undiluted	1:10
kcal/100 ml	48	53	35	33
Major constituents				
Protein	4.2	4.0	3.5	3.5
Fat	1.5	1.5	0.2	0.3
Carbohydrate	5.9	5.7	5.1	4.9
Minerals	0.9	0.9	0.7	0.7
Caloric distribution (% of calories)				
Protein	31	31	39	39
Fat	25	25	5	7
Carbohydrate	44	44	56	54
Content of minerals per liter				
Calcium (mg)	1550	1300	1240	1270
Phosphorus (mg)	1180	1000	980	1050
Sodium (meq)	26	27	23	26
Potassium (meq)	75	38	43	34
Chloride (meq)	36	32	29	32
Magnesium (mg)	105	—	—	—
Iron (mg)	1.2	1.0	0.8	0.5
Content of vitamins per liter				
Vitamin A (I.U.)	—	2640	—	—
Thiamine (μg)	—	500	400	360
Riboflavin (μg)	—	230	1700	1890
Niacin (μg)	—	220	860	1060
Pyridoxine (μg)	—	—	450	450
Pantothenate (mg)	—	—	3600	3880
Folic acid (μg)	—	—	12.0	4.4
B_{12} (μg)	—	—	3.8‡	3.4
Ascorbic acid (mg)	—	—	19	—
Vitamin D (I.U.)	—	420	—	—
Vitamin E (I.U.)	3.7	—	—	4.8

°Equal parts of whole milk and nonfat milk; available only as powders. Carbohydrate should be added.

†Data of McCance and Widdowson (1960) except for data on vitamins which are from Hartman and Dryden (1965).

‡Fresh milk; average for market milk about 10 mg per liter.

whose fecal water losses are high or whose insensible fluid losses are high because of fever, renal solute load may be excessive in relation to water available for renal excretion. The situation is aggravated by boiling the milk, which further reduces the ratio of water to renal solute load.

The relation between renal solute load and water requirement has been discussed in Chapter Nine.

Goat Milk

Surprisingly little information has been published concerning nutritional evaluations of goat milk. However, wide clinical experience with this milk as a food for infants and children in many parts of the world suggests that it is nutritionally adequate in most respects. Information about its composition is included in Table 11–4. Its energy value (76 kcal/100 ml) is similar to that of human milk. Concentrations of chloride, potassium, phosphorus and magnesium are greater and concentrations of sodium and sulfur are less in goat milk than in cow milk. Goat milk is especially rich in niacin.

Fat of goat milk differs from that of cow milk in that it contains more essential fatty acids (linoleic and arachidonic) than does cow milk (4.1 vs. 2.6 gm per 100 gm of milk fat), and it has a greater percentage of medium and short-chain fatty acids and a somewhat smaller percentage of long-chain, saturated fatty acids (Committee on Nutrition, 1960). These differences suggest that the fat of goat milk may be more readily digested than that of cow milk.

As discussed in Chapter Eight, goat milk is a relatively poor source of folates. Since it is recognized that infants receiving goat milk as a major source of calories are likely to develop megaloblastic anemia as an expression of folate deficiency, it is recommended that a supplement of 20 μg of folic acid be given daily to such infants.

Formulas Based on Cow Milk

Formulas of Cow Milk and Added Carbohydrate

Several commercially available formulas supply approximately two-thirds of the calories from evaporated cow milk and one-third from added carbohydrate, thus providing 14 to 16 per cent of calories from protein, 36 to 38 per cent from fat and 46 to 50 per cent from carbohydrate (Table 11–6). The added carbohydrate in Carnalac is lactose and in the other formulas is corn sugar.

All formulas of this group provide liberal intakes of vitamins A and D as well as various members of the B vitamin group. Only Carnalac is fortified with vitamin C, and none is fortified with iron.

Table 11–6. *Formulas of Cow Milk and Added Carbohydrate*

Composition	Lactum (Mead)	Carnalac (Carnation)	Purevap (Pet)
Components			
Cow milk protein	x	x	x
Butterfat	x	x	x
Carbohydrate			
lactose	x	x	x
corn sugar	x		x
Normal dilution			
Ratio			
ready to feed			x
liquid	1:1	1:1	
powder			
kcal/100 ml	67	67	67
Major constituents			
Protein	2.7	2.4	2.3
Fat	2.8	2.7	2.6
Carbohydrate	7.8	8.2	8.0
Minerals	0.6	0.5	0.5
Caloric distribution (% of calories)			
Protein	16	14	14
Fat	38	37	36
Carbohydrate	46	49	50
Content of minerals per liter			
Calcium (mg)	1000	850	800
Phosphorus (mg)	750	650	600
Sodium (meq)	17	16	16
Potassium (meq)	28	24	23
Chloride (meq)	23	21	18
Magnesium (mg)	100	80	86
Sulfur (mg)	300	—	—
Iron (mg)	trace	trace	trace
Content of vitamins per liter			
A (I.U.)	2643	1095	—[*]
Thiamine (μg)	264	422	—
Riboflavin (μg)	1268	1130	—
Niacin (mg)	0.7	0.6	—
Pyridoxine (μg)	423	221	—
Pantothenate (mg)	2.0	2.0	—
C (mg)	2	84	—
D (I.U.)	423	423	423

[*]Concentrations of vitamins in Purevap probably in same general range as in Lactum and Carnalac.

Wide clinical use of formulas of this type (whether commercially prepared or mixed in a hospital formula room or in the home) provides evidence of the general adequacy of such feedings. As discussed in Chapter Six, fat excretion will generally be somewhat greater when butterfat is fed than when an equal amount of fat is consumed in the form of certain combinations of vegetable oils. The difference in fat absorption will rarely be clinically significant in full-size infants except during the first two weeks of life, but mild to moderate steatorrhea may occur when these formulas are fed to infants of low birth weight. This possibility should be considered when an infant with adequate caloric intake fails to gain weight normally.

Serum concentrations of cholesterol of infants receiving formulas in which the fat is supplied as butterfat are more similar to those of breast-fed infants than is true of infants receiving formulas containing various mixtures of vegetable oils. The physiologic or medical significance of this observation is as yet unknown.

A practical consideration in the use of formulas containing butterfat is the sour odor of the vomitus. This odor arises from butyric acid and is thus absent when butterfat has been replaced by vegetable oils.

Formulas of Nonfat Cow Milk, Vegetable Oils and Carbohydrate

Formulas of this group have in common the combination of nonfat cow milk, vegetable oils (including corn oil) and, with the exception of Varamel, added carbohydrate (Table 11–7). The added carbohydrate is either lactose or corn sugar. Formil contains butterfat in addition to vegetable oils. With the exception of Olac, which is not fortified with ascorbic acid, all formulas in this group provide adequate intakes of vitamins. Some supply rather generous amounts of iron.

Varamel differs rather markedly from the other formulas in this group since it resembles evaporated milk in caloric distribution, being relatively high in content of protein and fat and relatively low in carbohydrate. In practice, carbohydrate is generally added to Varamel before it is fed to the infant. Each of the other feedings listed in Table 11–7 is fed as supplied or after dilution with water.

Protein provides from 9 to 20 per cent of calories. With the exceptions of Modilac and Olac, which are lower in fat content, fat provides from 44 to 50 per cent of calories. Modilac provides 48 per cent of calories as carbohydrate; Varamel, to which carbohydrate is usually added, provides only 32 per cent of calories from this source. The other formulas of the group supply from 41 to 44 per cent of calories from carbohydrate.

With the exception of Olac and Varamel, which provide relatively high renal solute loads, all can be fed at 80 kcal/100 ml (merely by reducing the amount of water used in making up the feeding) without concern about excessive renal solute load. Such calorically concentrated feedings are frequently valuable in management of infants of low birth weight.

Formulas Containing Partially Demineralized Whey Proteins

By combining nonfat cow milk and whey proteins, it is possible to achieve a ratio of whey proteins to casein resembling that of human milk, i.e., approximately 60 per cent of protein from whey and 40 per cent from casein. This differs considerably from cow milk, in which casein accounts for approximately 80 per cent of the protein and whey for only about 20 per cent. Through electrodialysis or ion exchange processes, it is technologically feasible to remove minerals from the protein component of a formula. Minerals can then be added in any amounts desired and it is therefore possible to produce a formula based on cow milk in which concentrations of individual minerals are similar to average concentrations in human milk.

Two formulas in which the protein consists of partially demineralized whey and nonfat cow milk are currently marketed (Table 11–8). SMA S-26 (Wyeth) contains electrodialyzed whey, nonfat cow milk, a mixture of vegetable and oleo oils, lactose, minerals and vitamins. It is available as a ready-to-feed formula (67 kcal/100 ml), as a concentrated liquid (134 kcal/100 ml) or as a powder. Similac PM 60/40 (Ross) contains whey and nonfat cow milk, both of which have been treated by ion exchange to remove minerals. Vegetable oils, additional lactose, minerals and vitamins are added. The product is marketed only as a powder.

As discussed in Chapter Five, it was at one time generally believed that lactalbumin, the predominant protein of human milk, was nutritionally superior to casein for feeding of infants. This belief was based in part on the historically better growth and lower incidence of disease in breast-fed infants than in those fed formulas of cow milk, and in part on the demonstrated nutritional superiority of lactalbumin over casein in studies with various hair-bearing animals. However, it now seems clear that the difficulties once encountered with formula feeding were due at least partially to bacterial contamination and to the relatively high curd tension of

(Text continued on page 213.)

Table 11-7. Composition of Commercial Infant Formulas

Composition	Bottle Ready Infant Formula (Baker)	Bremil (Borden)	Enfamil§‡ (Mead)	Formil°‡ (Pet)	Infant Formula (Baker)	Modilac (Gerber)	Olac (Mead)	Similac°‡ (Ross)	Varamel† (Baker)
Components									
Cow milk protein	x	x	x	x	x	x	x	x	x
Fat									
corn oil	x	x	x	x	x	x	x	x	x
coconut oil	x	x	x	x	x	x	x	x	
peanut oil		x							
oleo oils			x						
soy oil	x								
butterfat				x					
Carbohydrate									
lactose	x	x	x	x	x	x	x	x	
corn sugar	x				x	x	x		x
Normal dilution Ratio									
ready to feed								x	
conc. liquid	–	1:1	1:1	1:1	1:1	1:1	1:1	1:1	1:1
powder	–	1:8	1:6	–	–	–	1:6	1:8	–
kcal/100 ml	45	67	67	67	67	64	67	67	54
Major constituents (gm/100 ml)									
Protein	1.5	1.5	1.5	1.7	2.2	2.2	3.4	1.7	2.5
Fat	2.2	3.5	3.7	3.5	3.3	2.7	2.7	3.4	3.0
Carbohydrate	4.7	7.0	7.0	7.0	7.0	7.8	7.5	6.6	4.3
Minerals	0.4	0.5	0.3	0.4	0.6	0.4	0.7	0.4	0.7
Caloric distribution (% of calories)									
Protein	13	9	9	10	13	14	20	11	15
Fat	45	48	50	48	45	38	36	48	40
Carbohydrate	42	43	41	42	42	48	44	41	45

Table 11-7. *Composition of Commercial Infant Formulas*
(Continued)

Composition	Bottle Ready Infant Formula (Baker)	Bremil (Borden)	Enfamil§‡ (Mead)	Formil°† (Pet)	Infant Formula (Baker)	Modilac (Gerber)	Olac (Mead)	Similac°‡ (Ross)	Varamel† (Baker)
Content of minerals per liter									
Calcium (mg)	588	690	651	615	872	845	1201	670	993
Phosphorus (mg)	438	360	501	492	649	639	901	517	739
Sodium (meq)	11	11	11	11	17	17	22	11	19
Potassium (meq)	16	15	19	15	23	27	41	28	27
Chloride (meq)	12	13	12	13	19	19	29	15	22
Magnesium (mg)	–	56‖	90	68‖	–	48	100	62	–
Sulfur (mg)	–	–	160	–	–	–	300	–	–
Iron (mg)	trace	8.8	8.5	9.2	7.9	10.6	trace	12	7.9
Content of vitamins per liter									
A (I.U.)	1782	2640	1586	2641	2641	1585	2643	2650	2641
Thiamine (µg)	446	440	423	528	661	528	–	710	661
Riboflavin (µg)	743	1100	1000	951	1102	1057	–	1100	1212
Niacin (mg)	7.4	6.6	4.2	6.3	11	5.3	–	4.4	11
Pyridoxine (µg)	297	440	317	264	440	740	–	–	–
Pantothenate (mg)	–	–	2.1	–	–	–	–	–	–
C (mg)	35	55	53	53	53	48	trace	55	53
D (I.U.)	285	423	423	423	423	422	423	440	423

°Also sold as ready-to-feed formula at 43 kcal/100 ml.
†Contains no added carbohydrate.
‡Also available as formula unsupplemented with iron.
§Powdered formula: potassium 36 meq/l; unsupplemented with iron.
‖Author's analysis.

Table 11–8.   *Formulas with Nonfat Cow Milk and Whey Proteins*

Composition	Similac PM 60/40 (Ross)	SMA S-26 (Wyeth)
Components		
Protein		
nonfat cow milk	x	x
partially demineralized whey	x	x
Fat		
corn oil	x	x
coconut oil	x	x
oleo oil		x
soy oil		x
Carbohydrate		
lactose	x	x
Normal dilution		
Ratio		
ready to feed		x
liquid		1:1
powder	1:8	1:8
kcal/100 ml	67	67
Major constituents		
Protein	1.5	1.5
Fat	3.4	3.6
Carbohydrate	7.2	7.2
Minerals	.2	.25
Caloric distribution (% of calories)		
Protein	9	9
Fat	48	48
Carbohydrate	43	43
Content of minerals per liter		
Calcium (mg)	330	420
Phosphorus (mg)	170	330
Sodium (meq)	7	7
Potassium (meq)	14	14
Chloride (meq)	12	12
Magnesium (mg)	40	45
Sulfur (mg)	–	145
Iron (mg)	2	8
Content of vitamins per liter		
A (I.U.)	2750	2650
Thiamine (μg)	710	710
Riboflavin (μg)	1100	1100
Niacin (mg)	3.3	5.3
Pyridoxine (μg)	–	420
Pantothenate (mg)	–	1600
C (mg)	55	53
D (I.U.)	440	420

many of the formulas. The greater requirement of hair-bearing animals than of man for sulfur-containing amino acids is presumably related to the relatively high concentration of cystine in hair. Evidence that whey proteins are nutritionally superior to casein for the human has not been forthcoming (Chapter Five).

Although these formulas have not been demonstrated to be nutritionally superior to other milk-based formulas for the normal infant, they appear to be of high nutritional quality and are likely to be preferable in certain instances. The relatively low renal solute load is an asset in management of the infant with inability to concentrate the urine because of renal disease or diabetes insipidus. It is also an asset in management of children with severe congenital heart disease and other conditions in which difficulty is encountered in achieving an adequate caloric intake. Because renal solute load in relation to caloric concentration is less than that of other formulas, a greater margin of safety is provided when high caloric feedings (i.e., 100 kcal/100 ml or greater) are indicated. In addition, because the sodium content is low but the advisable daily intake of sodium is supplied when caloric requirements are met, these formulas are useful in long-term management of infants with congestive cardiac failure.

Because the naturally occurring minerals in milk are partially removed and the added minerals are free of radionuclide contamination, radionuclide concentrations are low. Comparison of various infant formulas from this point of view is presented in Chapter Twelve.

Special Milk-based Formulas

Special formulas based on cow milk protein or casein are considered in Chapter Twelve.

PROTEIN MILK (MEAD).   In the early 1900's Finkelstein devised a formula for the management of infants with diarrhea. This formula was prepared from whole milk curd (i.e., predominantly the casein component of milk) and skim milk treated with lactic acid. In Finkelstein's time this formulation had several advantages over other formulas available for management of diarrhea: (1) relative freedom from heavy bacterial contamination of the formula by virtue of the lactic acid content; (2) low curd tension; and (3) relatively low content of disaccharide.

At present, nearly all commercially available infant formulas have low curd tension, and clinically important bacterial contamination of formulas is relatively rare. The low disaccharide content of the feeding may be an asset in those instances in which temporary

Table 11-9. Special Formulas*

Composition	Lonalac (Mead)	Protein Milk* (Mead)	Probana (Mead)	Portagen† (Mead)
Components				
Protein				
cow milk	x	x		
casein			x	
casein hydrolysate			x	
Fat				
butterfat		x		
coconut oil	x		x	
Carbohydrate				
lactose	x	x	x	
banana powder			x	
lactic acid		x	x	
Normal dilution				
Ratio‡	1:6	1:10	1:6	1:6
kcal/100 ml	67	46	67	68
Major constituents				
Protein	3.4	3.8	3.9	2.7
Fat	3.5	2.7	2.0	3.2
Carbohydrate	4.8	2.7	7.3	7.7
Minerals	0.6	0.7	0.6	—
Caloric distribution (% of calories)				
Protein	21	30	24	19
Fat	49	48	29	29
Carbohydrate	30	22	47	52

Table 11–9. Special Formulas (Continued)

Composition	Lonalac (Mead)	Protein Milk* (Mead)	Prolana (Mead)	Portagen† (Mead)
Content of minerals per liter				
Calcium (mg)	1163	2000	1200	970
Phosphorus (mg)	1057	1220	900	800
Sodium (meq)	1	30	26	17
Potassium (meq)	27	30	31	33
Chloride (meq)	17	29	28	–
Magnesium (mg)	95	115	120	71
Sulfur (mg)	274	545	400	–
Iron (mg)	2.1	1.3	3.0	11.3
Content of vitamins per liter				
Vitamin A (I.U.)	1015	–	5285	3540
Thiamine (µg)	423	–	–	850
Riboflavin (µg)	1800	–	–	1135
Niacin (mg)	0.9	–	–	11.4
Pyridoxine (µg)	–	–	–	830
Pantothenate (mg)	–	–	–	7.1
Vitamin C (mg)	–	–	–	57
Vitamin D (I.U.)	–	–	1057	284
Vitamin E (I.U.)	–	–	11	7

*Carbohydrate should be added.
†Components: skim milk, sucrose, medium-chain triglycerides, cornstarch, safflower oil, vitamins and minerals.
‡Only powdered formulas are sold.

disaccharidase deficiency interferes with recovery from diarrhea (Chapter Seven).

Some caution is necessary in use of this formula when the state of hydration is inadequate. Renal solute load is high in relation to available water when the formula is fed at 67 kcal/100 ml.

HI-PRO (JACKSON-MITCHELL). Because this is prepared from powdered whole and nonfat cow milk, the percentage of calories provided by protein is exceedingly high (38 per cent), and the renal solute load will frequently be excessive even when it is fed at a caloric concentration considerably less than 67 kcal/100 ml. Composition of the product is not given in Table 11–9 because of limited information available about it.

PROBANA (MEAD). This product is prepared from Protein Milk (Mead), hydrolyzed casein, glucose and banana powder (which contains glucose and sucrose), and is fortified with vitamins A and D but not with other vitamins. It has been recommended for treatment of diarrhea, celiac syndrome and cystic fibrosis of the pancreas.

Two features of this formula may explain its apparently successful use in management of certain infants with steatorrhea or other forms of chronic diarrhea. First, fat contributes only 24 per cent of the calories in Probana (Table 11–9) so that fecal loss of as much as one-third of ingested fat would result in loss of only 8 per cent of the total caloric intake. Second, although carbohydrate contributes 47 per cent of the total calories supplied by the formula, lactose content is relatively low. Thus, the infant with partial lactase deficiency as a cause of persistent diarrhea may be benefited.

Renal solute load in relation to water content of the formula is relatively great. When extrarenal losses of water are high, as in persistent diarrhea, renal solute load may become excessive with development of dehydration.

It is necessary to supplement the formula with ascorbic acid and, in the case of persistent steatorrhea, with vitamins E and K.

LONALAC (MEAD). Lonalac was formulated to provide a feeding low in sodium as an aid in the management of adults and children with congestive cardiac failure. It is prepared from casein, coconut oil, lactose, minerals and vitamins and provides a caloric distribution similar to that of whole milk (Table 11–9). Since it is nearly free of an essential nutrient (sodium), it is clearly not designed for long-term management in the absence of an additional source of sodium.

Infants with severe congenital heart disease will frequently fail to grow normally because they are unwilling to accept a sufficient volume of a formula fed at 67 kcal/100 ml. Increase in caloric concentration should be accomplished by addition of carbohydrate and/or fat rather than by increasing the proportions of powdered formula to water. The renal solute load of Lonalac is somewhat less than that of whole cow milk, but considerable caution must be exercised in view of the limited total volume of feeding likely to be accepted. Vitamins C and D as well as small amounts of sodium (approximately 0.5 meq/kg) should be added when the formula is to be utilized for more than one week.

Lonalac is the only formula marketed in the United States in which fat is derived exclusively from coconut oil. Whether difficulties reported with other formulas containing coconut oil as the sole fat apply to Lonalac is not known.

PORTAGEN (MEAD). Some properties of medium-chain triglycerides (i.e., triglycerides of fatty acids with C-8 or C-10 chain length) have been discussed in Chapter Six. Portagen has been formulated to take advantage of these properties. It is prepared from skim milk, sucrose, medium-chain triglycerides (from coconut oil), cornstarch, safflower oil (to provide essential fatty acids), vitamins and minerals. As mentioned in Chapter Six, medium-chain triglycerides have been demonstrated to be useful in management of patients with chyluria, intestinal lymphangiectasia and various steatorrheas.

Gastrointestinal Passage Time

An interesting difference between human milk and cow milk is the time that elapses between ingestion of carmine and its appearance in the feces. During the first 45 days of life, carmine passage time generally ranges from three to ten hours regardless of diet. After 45 days of age, as may be seen from Figure 11–1, gastrointestinal passage time was less rapid in infants receiving fresh human milk (fed from the breast or by bottle) than in those fed processed human milk (pasteurized, frozen, stored, thawed), cow milk or a formula with protein from cow milk and fat supplied as a mixture of corn and coconut oils. When an infant's diet was changed from fresh to processed or from processed to fresh human milk, gastrointestinal passage time was immediately characteristic of the new feeding, suggesting that alteration in intestinal flora is probably not an important determinant of carmine passage time. The significance of the slower gastrointestinal passage time in the breast-fed infant than in the infant fed cow milk is unknown.

Antigenicity of Milks and Milk-based Formulas

Some general remarks about milk allergy will be included in Chapter Twelve. In this chapter it seems appropriate to comment on

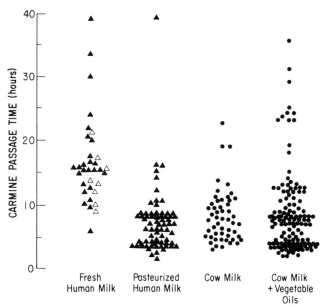

Figure 11–1. Gastrointestinal passage time, as determined by use of a carmine marker, in normal infants between 45 and 180 days of age. Solid triangles refer to observations of infants fed human milk by bottle; open triangles refer to observations of breast-fed infants. (Unpublished data of Fomon, S. J., Younoszai, M. K., and Thomas, L. N.)

the antigenicity of various preparations of cow milk in relation to amounts of heat employed in processing and to refer to data indicating that crossed antigenicity occurs between certain proteins of cow milk and goat milk.

Amounts of casein, beta-lactoglobulin, alpha-lactalbumin and bovine serum albumin present in 100 ml of fluid skim cow milk may

Table 11–10.   *Amount of Casein, Beta-Lactoglobulin, Alpha-Lactalbumin and Serum Albumin in 100 ml of Fluid Skim Cow Milk**

Protein	Amount (mg/100 ml)
Casein	2800
Beta-lactoglobulin	420
Alpha-lactalbumin	70
Bovine serum albumin	20

*From Goldman et al. (1963).

be seen in Table 11–10. Data presented by Goldman et al. (1963) provide some idea of the relative frequency with which these various proteins are responsible for allergic manifestations. Patients who had demonstrated allergic manifestations when challenged with skim milk were given an oral challenge with pure proteins, the amount of protein being equivalent to that present in 100 ml of fluid skim milk. Forty-five such patients were challenged with casein; all but one of these were challenged with bovine serum albumin and most were also challenged with beta-lactoglobulin and alpha-lactalbumin. All developed allergic manifestations to at least one of the proteins and the majority to more than one. As indicated in Table 11–11, evidence of allergenicity was detected with about equal frequency with each of the proteins.

It has long been recognized that casein is quite stable to heat but that bovine serum albumin and, to a lesser extent, bovine gamma globulin are quite heat sensitive. The assumption has frequently been made that the antigenicity of alpha-lactalbumin and beta-lactoglobulin is destroyed by boiling milk, evaporating milk or heat processing canned milk formulas (Fries, 1959; Crawford, 1960; Crawford and Grogan, 1961). Two groups of investigators (Hanson and Månsson, 1961; Saperstein and Anderson, 1962) have demonstrated that alpha-lactalbumin and beta-lactoglobulin persist in antigenically active form after such heat treatment (Table 11–12). Bovine serum albumin and bovine gamma globulin, on the other hand, are quite heat sensitive. Antigenicity of bovine serum albumin or bovine gamma globulin could not be demonstrated in evaporated milk or in commercially prepared liquid formulas, and bovine gamma globulin could not be demonstrated in commercially prepared powdered formulas.

Table 11–11. *Results of Oral Challenges with Isolated Milk Proteins**

Protein	Number of Patients Challenged†	Number Positive	Per Cent Positive
Casein	45	27	60
Bovine serum albumin	44	23	52
Beta-lactoglobulin	37	23	62
Alpha-lactalbumin	34	18	53

*Data of Goldman et al. (1963).
†Each patient had reacted previously to oral challenge with 100 ml of skim milk. Individual challenge doses of purified protein corresponded to the amount of that protein in 100 ml of skim milk.

Table 11–12. Protein Antigenicity of Milk Products Measured
In Vivo by Passive Cutaneous Anaphylaxis in the Guinea Pig*

Milk Product	Antigenicity of Proteins			BSA	BGG
	Casein	Alpha-lactalbumin	Beta-lactoglobulin		
Evaporated milk	+	+	+	–	–
Dried instant skim milk					
(Starlac)	+	+	+	+	+
Pasteurized fluid cow milk	+	+	+	+	+
Prepared infant formulas					
Liquid Similac	+	+	+	–	–
Liquid Baker's	+	+	+	–	–
Liquid Bremil	+	+	+	–	–
Liquid SMA	+	+	+	–	–
Liquid Enfamil	+	+	+	–	–
Liquid Modilac	+	+	+	–	–
Liquid Lactum	+	+	+	–	–
Powdered Similac	+	+	+	+	–
Powdered Bremil	+	+	+	–	–
Powdered SMA	+	+	+	+	–
Powdered Enfamil	+	+	+	+	–
Powdered Lactum	+	+	+	+	–
Powdered Baker's	+	+	+	+	–

*From Saperstein, S., and Anderson, D. W., Jr.: J. Pediat. *61*:196, 1962.

The amount of heat to which milk is subjected during processing will determine whether the product can be tolerated by infants allergic to bovine serum albumin or bovine gamma globulin. In addition, some reduction in amounts of alpha-lactalbumin and beta-lactoglobulin does occur during heating of milk and, in certain instances, evaporated milk or commercially prepared liquid formulas may be tolerated by infants who do not tolerate the larger amounts of these proteins in pasteurized fresh milk.

Since considerable crossed antigenicity exists between alpha-lactalbumin and beta-lactoglobulin of cow milk and goat milk (Saperstein, 1960), infants allergic to one of these proteins will seldom be benefited by substituting goat milk for cow milk.

Pesticides and Radionuclides

Pesticides are needed to achieve maximum production of acceptable foodstuffs, and adequate control of pests is not possible without some of the pesticide remaining on the plant at harvest. Diets of human adults contain relatively small amounts of pesticide residues and amounts of such residues in human milk may be expected to be quite low. Pesticide content of cow milk and of milk-based formulas containing butterfat is greater than that of human milk but is probably not an important public health problem at present. Nevertheless, the United States Department of Agriculture and the Food and Drug Administration continue to monitor milk supplies for pesticide residues. Long-term animal studies of pesticide toxicity are in progress.

Content of various radionuclides in human milk, cow milk, milk-based formulas and milk-free formulas is discussed in Chapter Twelve.

APPENDIX

Pasteurized Milk

Milk is heated to at least 63°C (145°F) and held at or above this temperature continuously for at least 30 minutes, or (as is now more commonly done) heated to at least 72°C (161°F) and held at or above this temperature continuously for at least 15 seconds, then cooled promptly to 50°C (148°F) or lower.

Homogenized Milk

Heated milk is forced under high pressure through small openings to disperse the fat into smaller globules which then remain for days as a fine emulsion throughout the milk.

Evaporated Milk

In older methods, milk was preheated to about 95°C (203°F) for 10 minutes and then concentrated in vacuum pans at a temperature of 50 to 55°C (122 to 131°F). The product was next homogenized and run into cans which were sterilized in a steam autoclave at about 115°C (239°F) for not less than 15 minutes. In modern methods of processing, preheating is done at much higher temperatures for a much shorter time. For example, preheating may be at 120°C (248°F) for 3 minutes, or the concentrated product may be sterilized in a continuous flow and then run aseptically into cans. Such a product has a lower viscosity, whiter color and fresher flavor than the double-heated product. The ratio of fat to nonfatty solids in the original milk is usually standardized so that proportions in the final product remain constant.

Condensed Milk

In the preparation of condensed milk, sugar is added to the milk before the evaporation process is initiated. The added sugar acts as a preservative. Percentages of calories supplied by protein, fat and carbohydrate are approximately 10, 24.5 and 65.5, respectively. The ratio of calories to water is low (321 kcal/100 ml compared to 146 kcal/100 ml in evaporated milk, 67 kcal/100 ml in fresh fluid milk), and therefore mistaken use of condensed instead of evaporated milk in preparation of infant formulas is likely to afford too little water and to lead to dehydration.

Whole Milk

Although the standard of identity from state to state differs, many states define whole milk as milk that contains not less than 3.25 per cent milk fat and not less than 8.25 per cent milk solids-not-fat.

Freeze-Dried Milk

Milk produced by a process in which water is removed by sublimation of the ice crystals from the deep-frozen product at low temperature in a relatively high vacuum.

Roller-Dried Milk

Preheated, and sometimes homogenized, milk is delivered in a thin film on the smooth surface of a single or of twin steam-heated rotating drums; the film of dried milk is scraped off as it forms and is then ground to powder. A refinement of this process includes prior removal of some of the water by enclosing the drums in a vacuum chamber. In its most modern form, the roller process gives a high quality product of relatively good solubility. The process is little used in the United States.

Spray-Dried Milk

Concentrated milk, usually preheated, is "atomized" to a fog-like mist into a current of heated air. The minute milk particles give off their moisture almost instantaneously and drop to the bottom of the drying chamber as small grains of dried milk. Solubility and flavor of the product are good.

REFERENCES

Arias, I. M., Gartner, L. M., Seifter, S., Furman, M.: Neonatal unconjugated hyperbilirubinemia associated with breast-feeding and a factor in milk that inhibits glucuronide formation in vitro. J. Clin. Invest. 42:913, 1963.

Athreya, B. H., Coriell, L. L., and Charney, J.: Poliomyelitis antibodies in human colostrum and milk. J. Pediat. 64:79, 1964.

Burrows, W., and Ware, L. L.: Studies on immunity to Asiatic cholera. VII. Prophylactic immunity to experimental enteric cholera. J. Infect. Dis. 92:164, 1953.

Committee on Nutrition, American Academy of Pediatrics: Water requirement in relation to osmolar load as it applies to infant feeding. Pediatrics 19:339, 1957.

Committee on Nutrition, American Academy of Pediatrics: Composition of milks. Pediatrics 26:1039, 1960.

Crawford, L. V.: Allergenicity of cow's milk proteins. I. Effect of heat treatment on the allergenicity of protein fractions of milk as studied by the dual-ingestion passive transfer test. Pediatrics 25:432, 1960.

Crawford, L. V., and Grogan, F. T.: Allergenicity of cow's milk protein. II. Studies with serum-agar precipitation technique. Pediatrics 28:362, 1960.

Dam, H., Glavind, J., Larsen, E. H., and Plum, P.: Investigations into the cause of the physiological hypoprothrombinemia in new-born children. IV. The vitamin K content of woman's milk and cow's milk. Acta med. Scandinav. 112:210, 1942.

Fomon, S. J., Younoszai, M. K., and Thomas, L. N.: Gastrointestinal passage time in infancy in relation to diet. Unpublished.

Freter, R.: Coproantibody and bacterial antagonism as protective factors in experimental enteric cholera. J. Exp. Med. 104:419, 1956.

Fries, J. H.: Components of milk and their significance to the allergic child. Ann. Allergy 17:1, 1959.

Gartner, L. M., and Arias, I. M.: Production of unconjugated hyperbilirubinaemia in full-term new-born infants following administration of pregnane-3(alpha), 20(beta)-diol. Nature 203:1292, 1964.

Gartner, L. M., and Arias, I. M.: Studies of prolonged neonatal jaundice in the breast-fed infant. J. Pediat. 68:54, 1966.

Goldman, A. S., Anderson, D. W., Jr., Sellers, W. A., Saperstein, S., Kniker, W. T., Halpern, S. R., and collaborators: Milk allergy. I. Oral challenge with milk and isolated milk proteins in allergic children. Pediatrics 32:425, 1963.

Gonzaga, A. J., Warren, R. J., and Robbins, F. C.: Attenuated poliovirus infection in infants fed colostrum from poliomyelitis immune cows. Pediatrics 32:1039, 1963.

Hanson, L. Å., and Månsson, I.: Immune electrophoretic studies of bovine milk and milk products. Acta Paediat. 50:484, 1961.

Hartman, A. M., and Dryden, L. P.: Vitamins in Milk and Milk Products. American Dairy Science Association, 1965.

Heyndrickx, G. V.: Investigations on the enzymes in human milk. Ann. Paediat. 198: 356, 1962.

Heyndrickx, G. V.: Further investigations on the enzymes in human milk. Pediatrics 31:1019, 1963.

Hytten, F. E.: Clinical and chemical studies in human lactation. VII. The effect of differences in yield and composition of milk on the infant's weight gain and the duration of breast-feeding. Brit. M. J. 1:1410, 1954a.

Hytten, F. E.: Clinical and chemical studies in human lactation. II. Variation in major constituents during a feeding. Brit. M. J. 1:176, 1954b.

Kenny, J. F., Boesman, M. I., and Michaels, R. H.: Bacterial and viral coproantibodies in breastfed infants. Pediatrics 39:202, 1967.

Kon, S. K.: Milk and Milk Products in Human Nutrition. FAO Nutritional Studies, #17. Rome, Food and Agriculture Organization of the United Nations, 1959.

Lepow, M. L., Warren, R. J., Guay, N., Ingram, V. G., and Robbins, F. C.: Effect of Sabin Type I poliomyelitis vaccine administered by mouth to newborn infants. New England J. Med. 264:1071, 1961.

Ling, E. R., Kon, S. K., and Porter, J. W. G.: The composition of milk and nutritive value of its components. In Kon, S. K., and Cowie, A. T.: Milk: The Mammary Gland and Its Secretion. New York, Academic Press, Inc., 1961, Vol. II, Chap. 18, p. 195.

Macy, I. G., and Kelly, H. J.: Human milk and cow's milk in infant nutrition, In Kon, S. K., and Cowie, A. T.: Milk: The Mammary Gland and Its Secretion. New York, Academic Press, Inc., 1961, Vol. II, Chap. 18, p. 265.

Macy, I. G., Kelly, H. J., and Sloan, R. E.: The Composition of Milks. A Compilation of the Comparative Composition and Properties of Human, Cow, and Goat Milk, Colostrum, and Transitional Milk. Publication 254. Washington, D.C., National Academy of Sciences–National Research Council, 1953.

McCance, R. A., and Widdowson, E. M.: The Composition of Foods. Med. Res. Coun., Special Report Series #297. London, Her Majesty's Stationery Office, 1960.

Morrison, S. D.: Human Milk: Yield, Proximate Principles and Inorganic Constituents. Commonwealth Agricultural Bureaux, Farnham Royal, Slough Bucks, England, 1952.

Newman, A. J., and Gross, S.: Hyperbilirubinemia in breast-fed infants. Pediatrics 32:995, 1963.

Nordbring, F.: The failure of newborn premature infants to absorb antibodies from heterologous colostrum. Acta Paediat. (Stockholm) 46:569, 1957.

Saperstein, S.: Antigenicity of the whey proteins in evaporated cow's milk and whole goat's milk. Ann. Allergy 18:765, 1960.

Saperstein, S., and Anderson, D. W., Jr.: Antigenicity of milk proteins of prepared formulas measured by precipitin ring test and passive cutaneous anaphylaxis in the guinea pig. J. Pediat. 61:196, 1962.

Snyderman, S. E., Holt, L. E., Jr., Dancis, J., Roitman, E., Boyer, A., and Balis, M. E.: "Unessential" nitrogen: a limiting factor for human growth. J. Nutrition 78:57, 1962.

Stiehm, E. R., and Ryan, J.: Breast-milk jaundice. Am. J. Dis. Child. 109:212, 1965.

Sullivan, L. W., Luhby, A. L., and Streiff, R. R.: Studies of the daily requirement for folic acid in infants and the etiology of folate deficiency in goat's milk megaloblastic anemia. Am. J. Clin. Nutr. 18:311, 1966. (Abstract.)

Vahlquist, B.: The transfer of antibodies from mother to offspring. Advances Pediat. 10:305, 1958.

Warren, R. J., Lepow, M. L., Bartsch, G. E., and Robbins, F. C.: The relationship of maternal antibody, breast feeding, and age to the susceptibility of newborn infants to infection with attenuated polioviruses. Pediatrics 34:4, 1964.

Chapter Twelve

Milk-free Formulas

With Comments
on Milk Allergy

Milk-free diets are utilized most commonly in management of infants who are allergic to milk or are suspected of milk allergy. They have been recommended for management of "the potentially allergic infant" and, as discussed in Chapter Seven, are essential in management of infants with galactosemia and congenital or acquired lactase deficiency. They may also be of value in management of certain infants with inborn errors of amino acid metabolism.

From what has been presented in Chapters Six and Seven, it is clear that the regular occurrence of diarrhea and other manifestations in an infant fed cow milk and the prompt disappearance of these signs when cow milk is withdrawn is not necessarily an evidence of milk allergy. Some otherwise normal infants fed large amounts of butterfat demonstrate considerable steatorrhea which disappears when various mixtures of vegetable oils are given. In addition, lactase deficiency probably occurs with some frequency during diarrhea and may persist for weeks or months. Feeding a milk-free diet will then result in prompt improvement of symptoms, with recurrence of diarrhea if milk or a milk-based formula is fed.

Milk Allergy

Nearly all foods contain some protein and are potentially antigenic. However, dietary proteins are normally converted through digestion and metabolism to amino acids, which are antigenically inactive. The relatively greater frequency of food allergy in the infant than in the adult is believed to be due in part to the incompleteness of normal digestive and metabolic processes. The intestinal epithelium of the newborn of many species is permeable to proteins (Brambell et al., 1958), and in the human infant it is evident that at least certain antibody proteins are absorbed (Leissring et al., 1962).

As pointed out by Taylor (1965), the occurrence and severity of immunologic responses to dietary proteins are dependent on a number of poorly understood relationships. Among these are the amounts and proportions of various proteins in the diet; the extent of denaturation of these proteins (e.g., by heating); rate and completeness of proteolysis; presence or absence of intestinal disease (in the infant, especially diarrhea); the extent and location of such disease; and the intrinsic ability of the individual to respond to the antigenic stimulus.

Food allergy, a more inclusive term than milk allergy, may be defined as the occurrence of abnormal signs or symptoms after ingestion of amounts of a particular food that are innocuous to most individuals. In consideration of the individual patient, use of precise and comprehensive criteria such as those suggested by Pratt (1958) are recommended: "The appearance-disappearance-reappearance of clear-cut clinical abnormalities with the administration-elimination-readministration of a pure, or highly refined substance in much smaller quantities than tolerated by most healthy individuals, during studies conducted in such a manner that the subjective attitudes of the observers and the subjects are properly controlled." Confirmatory evidence from skin testing and various laboratory tests may be helpful, but nearly all investigators report inconsistency of results.

Incidence and Manifestations

The most commonly implicated food allergens during infancy are milk, wheat and egg, and the major allergic manifestations provoked by these substances have traditionally been considered to be diarrhea, vomiting, abdominal pain, wheezing, cough, rhinitis, urticaria, atopic dermatitis and anaphylaxis. Milk allergy probably occurs in no more than 1 per cent of infants (Collins-Williams, 1956, 1962; Bachman and Dees, 1957a and b; Dees, 1959). However, recent evidence has suggested that our previous concept of manifestations of milk allergy may need to be revised. Utilizing agar gel diffusion and immunoelectrophoresis, Heiner et al. (1962; 1964), Wilson et al. (1962;

1964) and Holland et al. (1962) have called attention to a syndrome of chronic iron deficiency anemia, recurrent pneumonia, failure to thrive and presence of serum precipitins to proteins of cow milk. Symptoms subside and titers of precipitins in serum decrease in amount when a milk-free diet is given.

"Potentially Allergic Infants"

On the assumption that immunologic immaturity exists during early infancy and that the infant is therefore more likely to develop milk allergy if milk is introduced into the diet during the first few months of life than if such introduction is deferred until six months or a year of age, Glaser and Johnstone (1953) have recommended that all infants with immediate family histories of major allergies should receive milk-free diets during the early months of life. Several of the criticisms of other authors (Hill, 1953; Lowell and Schiller, 1954a and b) concerning the study on which the recommendation of Glaser and Johnstone was based do not apply to the more recent study reported by Johnstone and Dutton (1966). However, in this study only two of 240 infants demonstrated evidence of milk allergy. It is difficult to interpret the greater incidence of subsequent development of hay fever, asthma and perennial allergic rhinitis in controls than in those fed soy during early infancy. Mueller et al. (1963) studied 299 infants divided almost equally between those with immediate, remote and negative family histories of allergic disease. Two infants, both with negative family history, developed evidence of milk allergy. Twenty-eight infants developed definite or probable evidence of atopy (eczema, wheezing, recurrent rash), but only 15 of these had an immediate family history of allergy.

On the basis of evidence available at present, routine utilization for six months or longer of a milk-free diet for all infants with an immediate family history of allergy does not seem warranted.

Precautions in Use of Milk-free Formulas

The Committee on Nutrition of the American Academy of Pediatrics (1963) has emphasized that "management of the allergic infant often includes extensive dietary restriction in addition to avoidance of milk. A milk-free formula may thus become a major or even sole source of most essential nutrients for many months. Furthermore, the occasional coexistence of anorexia and intercurrent infection in children with allergic manifestations, and losses of protein through the skin of patients with severe eczema, makes adequacy of diet a major concern of the physician caring for such patients."

Published reports of deficiency diseases developing in infants receiving various milk-free formulas indicate the importance of an awareness of the composition and the nutritional properties of these diets.

Deficiencies of vitamin A and thiamine have occurred in infants receiving milk-free diets not fortified with these vitamins, and goiter has occurred in infants receiving soy-based formulas unsupplemented with iodine (Committee on Nutrition, 1963).

Milk-free Formulas

Formulas with Protein from Soy

Formulas of this group contain protein and carbohydrate from soy. As noted in Table 12–1, the fat in Isomil consists of corn and coconut oils while soy oil is the fat in the other formulas. Sobee contains coconut oil as well as soy oil. All formulas in this group contain sucrose and all except Mull-Soy contain corn sugar. Percentage composition of the powdered and liquid products of the same name sometimes differs. Mull-Soy liquid provides a greater percentage of calories from carbohydrate and a smaller percentage from fat than does Mull-Soy powder. Soyalac liquid and powder also differ in percentage of calories provided as protein, fat and carbohydrate. Of greater importance in management, Mull-Soy powder and Soyalac powder are not supplemented with ascorbic acid or vitamins A and D. Soyalac liquid is not fortified with ascorbic acid or vitamin A.

Two published studies have provided quantitative data demonstrating normal growth in length and weight of infants fed a soy-based formula (Mull-Soy) from birth until three months of age (Sternberg and Greenblatt, 1951; Kay et al., 1960). However, only seven infants were included in one study and 14 infants in the other.

One larger study with 102 infants fed a soy-based formula (Sobee) has been reported by Kane (1957), although less detailed information about growth was presented. Sixty-five infants were less than one month of age at the time the soy-based formula was introduced into the diet and 25 were one to two months of age; the remainder were over two months of age. Growth was said to progress normally as measured by Wetzel grids. During the first month that the infants received the diet, the average gain in weight was stated to be 30 ounces and the average increase in length 1⅛ inches.

More extensive testing of two soy-based formulas has been reported by Omans et al. (1963) on the basis of studies of premature

Table 12–1. Formulas with Protein from Soy

Composition	Sobee (Mead)	Mull-Soy Liquid (Borden)	Mull-Soy Powder (Borden)	Soyalac Liquid (Loma Linda)	Soyalac Powder (Loma Linda)	ProSobee (Mead)	Isomil (Ross)
Components							
Soy protein							
from soy flour	x	x	x				
aqueous extract*				x	x	x	x
Fat							
soy oil	x	x	x	x	x	x	x
coconut oil	x						
corn oil	x						x
Carbohydrate							
corn sugar	x			x	x	x	x
sucrose	x	x	x	x	x	x	x
Normal dilution							
Ratio							
ready to feed	x	x				x	x
liquid	1:1	1:1		1:1		1:1	1:1
powder	1:6		1:8		1:7		
kcal/100 ml	67	67	67	67	71	67	67
Major constituents							
(gm/100 ml)							
Protein	3.2	3.1	3.1	2.1	3.3	2.5	2.0
Fat	2.6	3.6	4.0	4.0	3.7	3.4	3.6
Carbohydrate	7.7	5.2	4.5	6.0	6.2	6.8	6.8
Minerals	0.5	0.8	0.7	0.2	0.8	0.5	0.4
Caloric distribution							
(% of calories)							
Protein	19	19	19	12	19	15	12
Fat	35	49	54	36	47	45	48
Carbohydrate	46	32	27	54	34	40	40
Content of minerals							
per liter							
Calcium (mg)	1057	1200	1300	390	810	793	700
Phosphorus (mg)	529	800	1100	340	370	634	500
Sodium (meq)	22	16	16	6 14	28	24	13
Potassium (meq)	33	41	41	22	26	28	18
Chloride (meq)	14	16	16	–	–	7	15
Iodine (µg)	68	158	160	35	34	68	150
Iron (mg)	8.5	5.0	4.0	10	10	8.5	12
Content of vitamins							
per liter							
A (I.U.)	1586	2110	–	–	–	1586	1500
Thiamine (µg)	530	530	80	170	360	530	400
Riboflavin (µg)	1057	845	260	1000	350	1057	600
Niacin (mg)	7.4	9.5	3.5	5.0	1.6	7.4	6.0
Pantothenate (mg)	2.6	1.0	1.0	–	–	2.6	5.0
Pyridoxine (µg)	427	423	235	290	210	427	400
C (mg)	53	42	–	–	–	53	50
D (I.U.)	423	423	–	400	–	423	400
E (I.U.)	5	11	4	–	–	5	5

*Protein of ProSobee and Isomil is the acid precipitated fraction, called soy protein isolate.

infants. As determined by rate of gain in weight and food efficiency ratio (i.e., rate of gain in weight per unit of food consumed), these authors concluded that Sobee and the milk-based control formula (Lactum—see Table 11–6) were nutritionally superior to Soyalac. A significant difference in nutritional quality between Sobee and Lactum was not demonstrated.

PROTEIN.   Although two soy formulas made with soy flour (Mull-Soy and Sobee) have for years been widely used as milk substitutes, the greater whiteness and improved palatability of water-soluble soy isolates makes it likely that in the future such isolates will replace soy flour as the source of protein for most soy formulas. ProSobee and Isomil contain a soy isolate fortified with methionine. As mentioned in Chapter Five, well-processed soy formulas are of high nutritional quality and may be expected to provide adequate protein intake when caloric requirements are fulfilled. Protein efficiency ratios determined with several of these formulas (Sobee, Mull-Soy, Soyalac) are presented in Table 12–2. These results are remarkably similar to the PER values of 2.20 for Sobee, 1.83 for Mull-Soy, 1.39 for Soyalac, and 2.63 for a reference skim milk reported by György et al. (1961).

Two publications have suggested that hypoproteinemia and edema are not rare in chronic atopic eczema, especially when weeping of the skin is present (Wolpe, 1947; Nisenson, 1955). However, information provided in these reports does not warrant the conclusion that feeding of milk substitutes contributed to the development of hypoproteinemia. Concentrations of total protein, albumin and globulin in serum of normal infants fed a soy-based formula (Mull-Soy) have been reported to be normal (Sternberg and Greenblatt, 1951; Kay et al., 1960).

FAT.   Sobee and Soyalac liquid are low in fat. The other formulas provide 45 to 54 per cent of calories from fat. As mentioned in Chapter Six, soy oil is well absorbed by the human infant. Partially hydrogenated soy, which is not well absorbed, is no longer a component of soy formulas, although it was a component of ProSobee when this product was originally marketed.

CARBOHYDRATE.   Amounts of carbohydrate listed in Table 12–1 refer to available carbohydrate since soy-based formulas contain alpha-galactosides (raffinose and stachyose), which are undigestible. However, the amount of these sugars is only about 130 mg per gram of protein and therefore represents only a small percentage of total carbohydrate in the formula (Gitzelmann, 1965; Gitzelmann and Auricchio, 1965). As discussed in Chapter Seven, the fact that stachyose and raffinose contain galactose is not a contraindication to use of these formulas in patients with galactosemia. Soy formulas are also useful in management of infants with lactase deficiency, the most commonly encountered disaccharidase deficiency being seen as a temporary defect in infants recovering from diarrhea.

MINERALS.   All these formulas except Soyalac liquid contain generous amounts of calcium. Soyalac liquid contains as much calcium as does human milk, but whether calcium is as well absorbed from this formula as from human milk has not been studied.

Table 12-2. *Protein Efficiency Ratios of Various Infant Formulas Used as Cow Milk Substitutes**

Diet	Average Initial Weight (gm)	Average Weight Gain (gm) Number of Days						Average Food Consumption (gm)	PER	Adjusted PER
		5	10	14	20	25	28			
1. Casein	64.2	12.2	32.5	38.5	56.7	73.9	94.1	334	2.8	2.5
2. Casein + 10% addidtional fat as Crisco	64.2	8.9	23.9	29.4	44.6	62.8	72.2	260	2.7	2.4
3. Whole milk powder	64.1	12.0	34.1	41.4	58.1	77.3	91.4	363	2.5	2.2
4. Evaporated goat milk, lyophilized	64.2	9.7	31.2	38.8	57.3	72.2	84.3	332	2.5	2.2
5. Infant casein hydrolysate formula, powder	64.1	11.8	35.1	39.3	56.1	73.3	95.4	346	2.7	2.4
6. Infant meat base formula, lyophilized	64.2	11.2	30.5	38.1	54.0	67.6	80.5	360	2.2	2.0
7. Infant soya bean formula 1, lyophilized	64.2	7.6	25.5	31.7	51.8	61.6	75.3	334	2.3	2.0
8. Infant soya bean formula 1, powder	64.1	7.4	23.5	30.4	45.1	57.3	69.0	321	2.1	1.9
9. Infant soya bean formula 2, lyophilized	64.2	6.1	20.6	23.7	37.1	45.1	56.0	297	1.9	1.7
10. Infant soya bean formula 2, powder	64.1	7.8	27.2	34.4	50.0	64.7	80.0	352	2.3	2.0
11. Infant soya bean formula 3, lyophilized	64.2	2.0	10.1	11.9	20.6	28.3	33.2	226	1.5	1.3
12. Infant soya bean formula 3, powder	64.2	3.8	17.2	20.3	32.1	41.7	52.6	289	1.8	1.6
13. Casein	64.1	10.5	32.3	37.2	54.6	73.7	92.6	323	2.8	2.5

*From Committee on Nutrition, American Academy of Pediatrics: Pediatrics 31:329, 1963. Used by permission.

Enlargement of the thyroid gland develops when young rats are fed a diet of raw soybeans or soy flour without additional intake of iodine. The goitrogenic effects of soy flour in rats can be diminished by treatment with organic solvents (presumably extracting some goitrogenic agent) or by heating, and rats are protected against the goitrogenic effects by supplementation of the diet with iodine (Committee on Nutrition, 1963). Several investigators reported development of goiter in infants fed Mull-Soy before this formula was supplemented with iodine. All the soy formulas listed in Table 12–1 are now fortified with iodine, and studies of weanling rats demonstrate no thyroid enlargement when these formulas are fed.

As may also be noted from Table 12–1, soy formulas are relatively rich sources of iron, providing 4 to 12 mg of iron per liter.

VITAMINS.   When organic solvents are employed for the extraction of fat from soy flour, the fat-soluble vitamins native to the bean are lost (Committee on Nutrition, 1963). Reports of vitamin A deficiency in infants receiving soy formulas not supplemented with vitamin A indicate the need for close attention to the label statement concerning the content of vitamin A in the formula (Committee on Nutrition, 1963). When a formula not supplemented with vitamin A is fed (Mull-Soy powder, Soyalac liquid and powder), the advisable daily intake of 500 I.U. (Chapter Eight) should be provided from another source.

Although rickets has not been reported in infants receiving soy formulas, the advisable daily intake of 400 I.U. of vitamin D should be given when formulas unsupplemented with this vitamin (Mull-Soy powder, Soyalac powder) are fed.

The content of vitamin E in all soy formulas, with the possible exception of Soyalac, is probably adequate. Amounts in Soyalac liquid and powder are unknown.

Vitamins of the B complex may be lost during processing of soy (Committee on Nutrition, 1963). Although currently available soy formulas appear to provide adequate amounts of B vitamins, label claims should be examined as new products are marketed. In the past, thiamine deficiency has developed in infants receiving soy formulas not supplemented with thiamine (Davis and Wolf, 1958; Cochrane et al., 1961).

Mull-Soy powder and Soyalac liquid and powder are not supplemented with ascorbic acid; when these formulas are utilized, the advisable daily intake of 20 mg of ascorbic acid should be provided.

HEAT-LABILE SUBSTANCES.   A number of heat-labile, physiologically active substances, including a trypsin inhibitor, have been isolated from raw soybean meal. Presumably because of the presence of these substances, adverse effects are noted when raw soybeans are employed as food for animals. Rats demonstrate poor growth, low protein efficiency ratios and pancreatic hypertrophy when raw soybean meal serves as the sole source of protein. These heat-labile substances are destroyed in the processing of the commercially available soy-based formulas for infants.

Non-Soy Milk-free Formulas

The compositions of several milk-free formulas not based on soy protein are presented in Table 12–3.

MEAT-BASED FORMULAS. Meat Base Formula (Gerber) and Lambase (Gerber) are prepared from beef heart and lamb heart, respectively, with added fat and carbohydrate. Approximately 50 per cent of fat in each formula is derived from the meat, the remainder from sesame oil in Meat Base Formula and from corn oil in Lambase. Since Meat Base Formula is relatively high in protein and fat, but relatively low in carbohydrate, additional carbohydrate is ordinarily added before feeding.

Several studies of growth and nitrogen balance in infants receiving meat as the sole source of protein have been reported (Committee on Nutrition, 1963), but studies with commercially available products have not been published. The protein efficiency ratio of Meat Base Formula was found to be 80 per cent that of casein (Table 12–2).

Although a trace of galactose is present, presumably arising from a galactoside in heart muscle (Committee on Nutrition, 1963), it seems unlikely that the amounts present would be harmful to patients with galactosemia.

NUTRAMIGEN. This product consists of an enzymatic hydrolysate of casein with added sucrose, arrowroot starch, corn oil, minerals and vitamins. Approximately 65 per cent of the amino acids are present in the free form and the remainder are present as polypeptides. The pattern of essential amino acids is the same as that of casein.

Long-term growth studies of normal infants receiving this formula have not been reported. Hill (1953) reported that growth of 36 infants with atopic eczema receiving Nutramigen was "satisfactory" (but less than "average normal") in 19, unsatisfactory in nine and inconclusive in eight. These infants were studied for intervals of two weeks to three months.

Nitrogen retention of children receiving Nutramigen was reported by Hartmann et al. (1942) to be similar to that of infants receiving milk, meat and eggs, but the conditions of testing were not sufficiently rigorous to provide an adequate evaluation. Nevertheless, PER studies suggest excellent nutritional quality (Table 12–2).

Nutramigen contains a trace of lactose (approximately 16 mg/67 kcal), believed to represent a contaminant of the casein from which

Table 12–3. Non-soy, Milk-free Formulas

Composition	Nutramigen (Mead)	Meat Base Formula (Gerber)	Lambase (Gerber)	Lofenalac* (Mead)
Components				
Protein				
meat		x	x	
casein hydrolysate	x			x
amino acids†				x
Fat				
animal fat		x	x	
corn oil	x		x	x
sesame oil		x		
Carbohydrate				
corn sugar			x	x
sucrose	x	x	x	x
arrowroot starch	x			x
Normal dilution				
Ratio				
liquid		13:19.5	1:1	
powder	1:6			1:6
kcal/100 ml	67	58	67	67
Major constituents (gm/100 ml)				
Protein	2.2	2.7	2.4	2.2
Fat	2.6	3.1	2.4	2.7
Carbohydrate	8.5	4.0	7.9	8.5
Minerals	0.6	0.6	0.3	0.8
Caloric distribution (% of calories)				
Protein	15	20	15	15
Fat	35	51	35	35
Carbohydrate	50	29	50	50
Content of minerals per liter				
Calcium (mg)	1000	1030	734	1000
Phosphorus (mg)	700	686	546	700
Sodium (meq)	17	12	11	26
Potassium (meq)	26	12	11	38
Chloride (meq)	23	17	7	27
Iron (mg)	10	9.7	7.9	1.6
Content of vitamins per liter				
A (I.U.)	1586	1585	1585	1586
Thiamine (μg)	486	420	420	486
Riboflavin (μg)	1903	1370	1050	1903
Niacin (mg)	4.2	10.6	5.3	4.2
Pyridoxine (μg)	529	507	630	529
Pantothenate (mg)	3.4	—	—	3.4
C (mg)	32	42	48	32
D (I.U.)	423	422	422	423
E (I.U.)	5.3	5.3	5.3	5.3

*Casein hydrolysate from which phenylalanine has been removed (see text).
†DL-methionine, L-tryptophan, L-tyrosine.

it is prepared (Committee on Nutrition, 1963). It has been used successfully by Isselbacher (1959) and Donnell et al. (1961) in the management of patients with galactosemia.

LOFENALAC. An enzymatic digest of casein (similar to that employed in Nutramigen) is chemically treated to destroy phenylalanine and then supplemented with DL-methionine, L-tryptophan and L-tyrosine to form the "protein" component of Lofenalac. Corn oil, corn sugar, minerals and vitamins are added. With the exception of iron, which is present in much lesser amounts in Lofenalac than in Nutramigen, vitamin and mineral concentrations are in most instances identical in the two products.

Several investigators have reported normal growth of infants with phenylketonuria who have received Lofenalac as the major source of nutrients. Nutritional adequacy of the formula could be further tested by feeding phenylalanine-supplemented Lofenalac to normal infants, but such studies have not been reported. However, as may be seen from Table 12–4, Lofenalac supplemented with 1.0 per cent DL-phenylalanine appears to be nutritionally equivalent to Nutramigen when fed to growing rats, and it seems probable that Lofenalac is a product of relatively high nutritional quality.

Table 12–4. *Food Intake and Weight Gain of Weanling Rats Fed Nutramigen or Phenylalanine-Supplemented Lofenalac**

	Nutramigen	Lofenalac + 1.0% DL-Phenylalanine
Number of survivors †	9	9
Food intake (gm)	274	268
Water intake (ml)	541	456
Weight gain		
mean	117	120
S.D.‡	18	12
Food efficiency§		
mean	42.4	44.8
S.D.	2.3	2.3

*Unpublished data of A. B. Morrison, kindly provided by Dr. Herbert P. Sarett, Mead Johnson Research Laboratories.
†Each group contained 10 animals initially.
‡Standard deviation.
§Food efficiency: grams of body weight gained per gram of food consumed.

Radioactivity of Infant Foods

"We live in a sea of radiation. As far as is known, man always has and always will live in an environment filled with radiation. There are radioactive materials present naturally in the ground, the sea, and the air. Cosmic rays bombard us from outerspace" (Dunning, 1962). To consider radioactivity of foods in proper perspective it is desirable to compare the estimated radiation doses from natural sources, from man-made radiation and from fallout. As may be seen from Table 12–5, natural radiation contributes an estimated 3.8 rem gonadal dose in 30 years, compared with 3.5 rem from man-made radiation and between 0.05 and 0.4 rem from fallout. Gonadal radiation from diagnostic x-ray is likely to be more than ten times that from fallout. Comparison of estimated radiation from natural sources with that from

Table 12–5. *Comparison of Estimated Radiation Doses from Natural Sources, Man-Made Radiation and Fallout**

Sources of Radiation		30 Yr Gonadal Dose (rem)	70 Yr Bone Dose (rem)
Natural sources:			
External:	cosmic rays	0.9	2.1
	terrestrial radiation	2.1	4.9
	atmospheric radiation	0.06	0.1
Internal:	potassium-40	0.6	0.7
	carbon-14	0.06	0.1
	radium-thorium families	0.06	2.9
Subtotal:		3.8	11
Man-made radiation:			
Diagnostic x-ray		3	3.3
Therapeutic x-ray		0.4	†
Internal isotopes		<0.03	†
Atomic energy and medical workers		0.03	0.003+
Luminous dials		0.03	†
Television		<0.03	<0.03
Subtotal		3.5	3.3
Approximate total		7–8	12–16
Fallout contribution:			
Tests cease in 1958		0.05	0.2–0.4
Tests continue indefinitely (steady state 40 years hence)		0.4	1.6–3.8

*From Forbes, G. B.: Pediat. Clin. North America 9:1009, 1962.
†No estimate.

fallout is shown in Table 12–6 for whole body, reproductive cells, bone and bone marrow. Although at age one year the relative contribution from fallout is fairly high, lifetime dosage from fallout is a small percentage of that from the natural background. Not only is the contribution of fallout to total radiation dose relatively small, but a portion of the fallout radiation is of an external nature, being contributed by radioactive materials that do not become associated with foods or water or that are not absorbed by the body. It is highly probable that radioactive contamination of foods constitutes some hazard for the infant, but these hazards are almost certainly small, even in comparison to the rather slight hazards from natural sources of radiation. Fallout effects are estimated to be less than one-tenth the effects of natural radiation (Jones, 1963).

Since the advent of nuclear weapons testing, radioactive fallout has been attributable in large measure to such testing. In the absence of further atmospheric testing, peacetime operations may be expected to be increasingly important as sources of radioactive contamination of the environment. Reactor installations in power plants, submarines, ships and aircraft will contribute radioactivity to the environment both through normal operation and through accidents, and radioisotope application in medicine, industry and agriculture will also be a source of contamination. We must learn to live with radiation and other hazards in such a way that the hazard is kept within reason and exposure expanded only for greater gain (Jones, 1963).

Some 230 radioisotopes are manufactured in the explosion of an

Table 12–6. *Estimated Radiation Doses in the United States from Detonation of Nuclear Weapons and from Natural Sources**

Tissue or Organ	All Tests Through 1961	Natural Background
Whole body		
1 year	10–25	100
70 years	70–150	7000
Reproductive cells		
1 year	10–15	100
70 years	70–150	7000
Bone		
1 year	30–80	130
70 years	400–900	9100
Bone marrow		
1 year	20–40	100
70 years	150–350 ·	7000

*Data of Federal Radiation Council, 1962.

atomic bomb, and additional isotopes are formed by neutron activation of air, soil and bomb components (Forbes, 1962). The half-lives of many of these fission products are so short that they cannot participate in distant fallout. Many other fission products are produced in such small quantities that their contribution to environmental contamination may be disregarded. In addition to physical half-life and the amount of the fission products released into the environment, the relative hazard from a specified radioactive material is governed by the efficiency of transfer through the food chain to the human diet, the degree of absorption by the body, and the length of time retained in the body. By these criteria, the radioisotopes of greatest concern are iodine-131, barium-140, strontium-89, strontium-90 and cesium-137. The first three of these are relatively short-lived and are of biologic significance only for several months after a bomb is exploded. Strontium-90 and cesium-137 are long-lived isotopes and thus constitute the major contaminants of food from fallout during peacetime and in the absence of atomic testing.

Iodine-131, Barium-140 and Strontium-89

Iodine-131, with a half-life of approximately eight days, is present in the infant's diet primarily in cow milk since fallout of this isotope on grass results in a relatively high intake by the cow. As may be seen from Figure 12–1, concentrations of iodine-131 in cow milk are

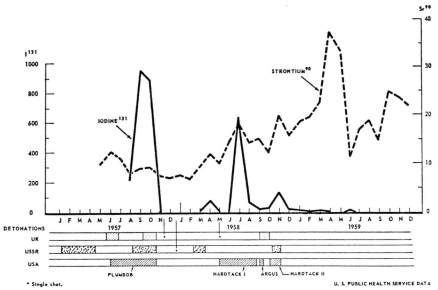

Figure 12–1. Concentrations of iodine-131 and strontium-90 in cow milk in St. Louis, Missouri, from 1957 through 1959. (From Dunning, G. M.: Borden's Rev. Nutr. Res. 23:1, 1962.)

greatest during the summer months that follow detonation of a nuclear device. The concentration of iodine-131 in human milk is only about one-tenth that in cow milk. Iodine-131 is concentrated in the thyroid gland and, because of the relatively large intake of milk by the infant and the relatively small size of the thyroid gland, resulting thyroid radiation will be greater for the infant than for the adult. Because of the short half-life, storing the milk or milk product for a time before it is consumed will result in loss of the isotope. In the case of iodine-131, storage for one month will reduce the concentration to 7 per cent of its original value (Forbes, 1962). After two months, only 0.6 per cent of the original amount remains. Thus, any powdered or evaporated milk product will be nearly free of iodine-131. In addition, it is possible to block uptake of iodine-131 to some extent by daily intake of a few milligrams of stable iodine in the form of potassium iodide (Forbes, 1962).

Barium-140, with a half-life of 13 days, and strontium-89, with a half-life of 53 days, are relatively short-lived radioisotopes whose metabolism is somewhat similar to that of calcium. These materials are deposited primarily in bone, as is true of strontium-90. Because of the short half-lives of these radionuclides, they will continue to be present in the diet for only a limited time after explosion of a bomb and are therefore of less biologic significance than strontium-90.

Strontium-90

Strontium-90, with a half-life of 20 years, is a major radionuclide of fallout responsible for radiation of bone. Because it is handled by the body in much the same fashion as calcium, the ratio of strontium-90 to calcium in food is of more medical significance than the absolute amount of strontium-90 in the diet. Intake of strontium-90 is therefore frequently considered in terms of the "strontium unit," defined as one picocurie (2.2 disintegrations per minute) of strontium-90 per gram of calcium. Proportionately more calcium than strontium is absorbed by the intestine, passed from mother to fetus across the placenta, and secreted in milk. Proportionately more strontium than calcium is excreted in urine. Human milk contains only about one-tenth as much strontium-90 per gram of calcium as the woman's diet (Lough et al., 1960).

Commercially prepared liquid and powdered formulas based on cow milk contain approximately the same ratio of strontium-90 to calcium as does cow milk (Table 12–7). Soy-based formulas, Nutramigen, SMA S-26 and Similac PM 60/40 contain predominantly calcium that has been added from sources uncontaminated with strontium-90 and therefore the strontium to calcium ratio in these products is low.

Table 12-7. Strontium-90 Content of Milks and Formulas

Specimen	Content of Strontium-90 (pCi/gm Ca)		Investigators
	Mean	Range	
Human milk			
Denver, 1959	3.1	0.9–9.5	Straub & Murthy (1965)
Chicago, 1959	3.2	1.1–7.4	Straub & Murthy (1965)
Boston, 1959	1.3		Lough et al. (1960)
Toronto, 1960–61	3.2	1.1–5.6	Brown & Jarvis (1961)
Cow milk			
Chicago, 1959	6.1	4.1–8.9	Straub & Murthy (1965)
Toronto, 1960–61	5.2	4.0–6.8	Brown & Jarvis (1961)
Milk-based formulas			
Commercially prepared			
Formula A	7.1	5.8–8.9	Jarvis & Brown (1962)
Formula B	5.9	5.4–6.7	Jarvis & Brown (1962)
4 Formulas		4.1–9.3	Sarett (1963)
Soy-based formulas			
Formula C	1.6	1.0–1.8	Jarvis & Brown (1962)
2 Formulas		1.0–2.1	Sarett (1963)
Nutramigen		0.7	Sarett (1963)

Figure 12–2 indicates the strontium-90 concentration of pasteurized milk in various cities of the United States from 1961 through September, 1966 (Division of Radiological Health, 1967). It may be seen that appreciable increases in concentration occurred in most cities in 1963 and 1964, reflecting atomic weapons testing in 1961.

The influence of diet on concentration of strontium-90 in relation to calcium content of deciduous teeth is indicated in Table 12–8 for infants in the St. Louis area born in 1957. The protective effect of breast feeding is evident. Peak concentration of strontium-90 in cow milk in the St. Louis area was reached in June, 1963 (Fig. 12–2); Rosenthal et al. (1964) have predicted that deciduous teeth of infants born in 1963 and fed formulas based on cow milk will contain approximately 12.4 pCi of strontium-90 per gram of calcium.

Cesium-137

Cesium-137, with a half-life of 30 years, is distributed through the fat-free body tissues in a manner similar to potassium. The body burden of cesium-137 is contributed primarily by milk, meat and

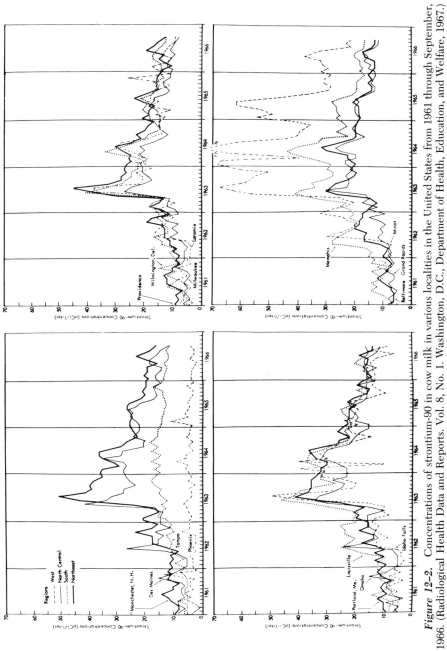

Figure 12–2. Concentrations of strontium-90 in cow milk in various localities in the United States from 1961 through September, 1966. (Radiological Health Data and Reports. Vol. 8, No. 1. Washington, D.C., Department of Health, Education, and Welfare, 1967.)

Table 12–8.   Strontium-90 Content of Deciduous Incisors of St. Louis Children Born in 1957*

Mode of Feeding	Samples	Concentration Strontium-90 (pCi/gm Ca)
Breast fed > 6 months	8	1.73 (0.33)†
Breast fed 6 weeks to 6 months	12	2.19 (0.35)
Breast fed < 6 weeks	21	2.79 (0.08)

*Data of Rosenthal et al. (1964).
†Values in parentheses are standard errors of mean.

Table 12–9.   Cesium-137 Content in Relation to Potassium Content of Infant Formulas*

Infant Formulas	Content of Cesium-137 (pCi/gm K)
Protein from cow milk	
Similac	18
SMA S-26	15 (electrodialysis)
SMA S-26	10
Similac PM 60/40	3 (ion exchange)
Similac PM 60/40	0
Lonalac	3 (ion exchange)
Nutramigen	6 (hydrolysate)
Protein from soy	
Mull-Soy	18
Sobee	13
Soyalac	10
X8711 (Borden)†	17
Protein from soy isolate (Edipro)	
ProSobee	4
Isomil	2
D8815 (Borden)†	3
Protein from meat	
Meat Base	88
Lambase	114

*Data of Filer, Peterson and Fomon (1966).
†Experimental products, not commercially available.

grain. The body does not discriminate against cesium-137 in favor of potassium and the ratio of cesium-137 to potassium in the body eventually becomes about threefold greater than that in the diet. Although the physical half-life is long, the biologic half-life is short, the average value being considered about 75 days for all ages. For the infant, biologic half-life may be as short as 20 days. The content of cesium-137 per gram of potassium in various infant formulas is presented in Table 12–9.

REFERENCES

Bachman, K. D., and Dees, S. C.: Milk allergy. I. Observations on incidence and symptoms in "well" babies. Pediatrics 20:393, 1957a.

Bachman, K. D., and Dees, S. C.: Milk allergy. II. Observations on incidence and symptoms of allergy to milk in allergic infants. Pediatrics 20:400, 1957b.

Brambell, F. W. R., Halliday, R., and Morris, I. G.: Proc. Roy. Soc. London Ser. B. 149:1, 1958.

Brown, J. R., and Jarvis, A. A.: Strontium-90 levels in human milk. A nine-month survey in Toronto. Canad. J. Pub. Health. 52:463, 1961.

Cochrane, W. A., Collins-Williams, C., and Donohue, W. L.: Superior hemorrhagic polioencephalitis (Wernicke's disease) occurring in an infant—probably due to thiamine deficiency from use of a soya bean product. Pediatrics 28:771, 1961.

Collins-Williams, C.: The incidence of milk allergy in pediatric practice. J. Pediat. 48:39, 1956.

Collins-Williams, C.: Cow's milk allergy in infants and children. Int. Arch. Allerg. 20:38, 1962.

Committee on Nutrition, American Academy of Pediatrics: Appraisal of nutritional adequacy of infant formulas used as cow milk substitutes. Pediatrics 31:329, 1963.

Davis, R. A., and Wolf, A.: Infantile beriberi associated with Wernicke's encephalopathy. Pediatrics 21:409, 1958.

Dees, S. C.: Allergy to cow's milk. Pediat. Clin. N. Amer. 6:881, 1959.

Division of Radiological Health: Radiological Health Data and Reports. Washington, D.C., U. S. Department of Health, Education, and Welfare. Vol. 8, No. 1, January, 1967.

Donnell, G. N., Collado, M., and Koch, R.: Growth and development of children with galactosemia. J. Pediat. 58:836, 1961.

Dunning, G. M.: Foods and fallout. Borden's Rev. Nutr. Res. 23:1, 1962.

Federal Radiation Council: Health Implications of Fallout from Nuclear Weapons Testing through 1961. Report No. 3 of the Federal Radiation Council. Washington, D. C., U. S. Gov't. Printing Office, 1962, p. 1.

Filer, L. J., Jr., Peterson, R. E., and Fomon, S. J.: Cesium-137 content of infant formulas. Unpublished, 1966.

Forbes, G. B.: Nutrition in relation to problems of radioactivity. Pediat. Clin. N. Amer. 9:1009, 1962.

Gitzelmann, R.: (Letter to Editor.) Soya alpha-galactosides (continued). Pediatrics 36:806, 1965.

Gitzelmann, R., and Auricchio, S.: The handling of soya alpha-galactosides by a normal and galactosemic child. Pediatrics 36:231, 1965.

Glaser, J., and Johnstone, D. E.: Prophylaxis of allergic disease in the newborn. J.A.M.A. 153:620, 1953.

György, P., Omans, W. B., and Hau, E. W-S.: Feeding value of soy milks for premature infants. Proceedings of Conference on Soybean Products for Protein in Human Foods, September 13–15, 1961. Washington, D. C., U. S. Department of Agriculture, Agricultural Research Service, p. 179.

Hartmann, A. F., Meeker, C. S., Perley, A. M., and McGinnis, H. G.: Studies of amino acid administration: I. Utilization of an enzymatic digest of casein. J. Pediat. 20:308, 1942.

Heiner, D. C., Sears, J. W., and Kniker, W. T.: Multiple precipitins to cow's milk in chronic respiratory disease. Am. J. Dis. Child. 103:634, 1962.

Heiner, D. C., Wilson, J. F., and Lahey, M. E.: Sensitivity to cow's milk. J.A.M.A. 189: 563, 1964.

Hill, L. W.: Soybean as a milk substitute for potentially allergic infants. J. Allergy 24: 474, 1953.

Holland, N. H., Hong, R., Davis, N. C., and West, C. D.: Significance of precipitating antibodies to milk proteins in the serum of infants and children. J. Pediat. 61: 181, 1962.

Isselbacher, K. J.: Galactose metabolism and galactosemia. Am. J. Med. 26:715, 1959.

Jarvis, A. A., and Brown, J. R.: Strontium-90 level in three infant "formula" foods. Canad. M.A.J. 86:73, 1962.

Johnstone, D. E., and Dutton, A. M.: Dietary prophylaxis of allergic disease in children. New England J. Med. 274:715, 1966.

Jones, H. B.: Health hazards from fallout. Fed. Proc. 22:1415, 1963.

Kane, S.: Nutritional management of allergic reactions to cow's milk. Am. Pract. Digest Treat. 8:65, 1957.

Kay, J. L., Daeschner, C. W., and Desmond, M. M.: Evaluation of infants fed soybean and evaporated milk formulae from birth to three months. A comparison of weight, length, hemoglobin, hematocrit, and plasma biochemical values. Am. J. Dis. Child. 100:264, 1960.

Leissring, J. C., Anderson, J. W., and Smith, D. W.: Uptake of antibodies by the intestine of the newborn infant. Am. J. Dis. Child. 103:160, 1962.

Lough, S. A., Hamada, G. H., and Comar, C. L.: Secretion of dietary strontium 90 and calcium in human milk. Proc. Soc. Exper. Biol. & Med. 104:194, 1960.

Lowell, F. C., and Schiller, I. W.: Substitution of soybean milk for cow's milk in allergic infants. J.A.M.A. 154:262, 1954a.

Lowell, F. C., and Schiller, I. W.: It is so — it ain't so. J. Allergy 25:57, 1954b.

Mueller, H. L., Weiss, R. J., O'Leary, D., and Murray, A. B.: The incidence of milk sensitivity and the development of allergy in infants. New England J. Med. 268: 1220, 1963.

Nisenson, A.: Hypoproteinemia and edema in eczema. J. Pediat. 46:544, 1955.

Omans, W. B., Leuterer, W., and György, P.: Feeding value of soy milks for premature infants. J. Pediat. 62:98, 1963.

Pratt, E. L.: Food allergy and food tolerance in relation to the development of good eating habits. Pediatrics 21:642, 1958.

Rosenthal, H. L., Austin, S., O'Neill, S., Takeuchi, K., Bird, J. T., and Gilster, J. E.: Incorporation of fall-out strontium-90 in deciduous incisors and foetal bone. Nature 203:615, 1964.

Sarett, H. P.: Personal communication, 1963.

Sternberg, S. D., and Greenblatt, I. J.: Serum protein values in infants fed soya-bean milk. Ann. Allergy 9:190, 1951.

Straub, C. P., and Murthy, G. K.: A comparison of Sr^{90} component of human and cows' milk. Pediatrics 36:732, 1965.

Taylor, K. B.: Role of immune responses in the gastrointestinal tract. Fed. Proc. 24: 23, 1965.

Wilson, J. F., Heiner, D. C., and Lahey, M. E.: Studies on iron metabolism: I. Evidence of gastrointestinal dysfunction in infants with iron deficiency anemia: A preliminary report. J. Pediat. 60:787, 1962.

Wilson, J. F., Heiner, D. C., and Lahey, M. E.: Milk-induced gastrointestinal bleeding in infants with hypochromic microcytic anemia. J.A.M.A. 189:568, 1964.

Wolpe, L. Z.: Blood protein depletion in infantile eczema. California Med. 67:156, 1947.

Chapter Thirteen

Infant Feeding in Health and Disease

The previous chapters have attempted to review and place in some perspective newer information concerning infant nutrition. It is hoped that this chapter will contribute to practical aspects of putting such information into practice.

Breast Feeding

When hygienic conditions are good and nutritionally sound formulas are readily available and inexpensive, the advantages of breast feeding may be primarily psychologic rather than hygienic or nutritional. Rewards of a psychologic nature seem likely to both mother and infant when a properly motivated woman feeds her infant under favorable circumstances. However, for the woman who considers breast feeding unpleasant or who is constantly harassed by the activity of her other small children while attempting to breast feed, well executed bottle feeding may be preferable.

As discussed in Chapter Eleven, breast feeding may transmit antibacterial and antiviral antibodies that will provide significant protection against organisms which invade the body through the gastrointestinal tract.

It has been remarkably difficult to demonstrate nutritional advantages of human milk over any of several commonly employed formulas. One advantage of breast feeding is that the volume of milk ingested is unknown and, therefore, the tendency of most parents to derive pleasure from feeding large quantities is minimized. However, a problem occasionally arises just because the volume of intake is unknown. When rate of gain in weight has been less than the tenth percentile value during a period of 28 days or longer (Table 2–1), it is wise to weigh the infant before and after a typical feeding to determine the amount ingested. Some infants seem to adapt to relatively small intakes of milk if the supply is limited. Such infants may not cry or fuss excessively so that it is not obvious that they are being underfed.

The widely held belief that complete emptying of the breast is essential to successful lactation appears to rest on folklore rather than fact. In the absence of data clearly demonstrating the advantage of complete emptying of the breast, it seems reasonable to recommend that an infant be fed at both breasts at each feeding, thereby contributing substantially to the comfort of the mother.

In modern society it is frequently not practical for mother and infant to be together at each feeding time. Partly for this reason, many women offer one bottle feeding each day. They then are less prone to worry about the willingness of the infant to accept a bottle feeding when they are to be away from him. When other considerations do not dictate the time at which this bottle feeding is to be given, most women elect to give it at about 6 P.M. Such choice may have some scientific justification since Morrison (1952) has demonstrated that the volume of milk obtained by breast-fed infants gradually decreases from early morning to evening. If a bottle feeding is given at 6 P.M., the supply of milk in the breasts at the time of the next feeding will be particularly abundant and the well-fed infant may sleep for a longer interval than would otherwise be likely.

Vitamin and Mineral Supplementation of the Diets of Full-size Infants

Table 13–1 presents a summary of vitamin and mineral supplementation considered desirable for normal full-size infants. Ascorbic acid may be given in the form of a vitamin concentrate or fruit juice. If fruit juice is used, certain precautions relating to ascorbic acid content of the fruit juice are necessary as discussed in Chapter Eight. Adequate intake of iron may be achieved by daily feeding of iron-fortified cereal or a medicinal iron preparation (Chapter Ten).

Table 13–1. Vitamin and Mineral Supplementation of the Diet of Full-Size Infants

Major Source of Energy	Desirable Supplementation*			
	Vitamin A	Vitamin D	Ascorbic Acid	Iron
Human milk		+		+
Cow milk				
evaporated			+	+
whole, fresh fluid		±	+	+
whole, powdered		±	+	+
skim, fresh fluid	+	+	+	+
skim, powdered	+	+	+	+
Goat milk†				
evaporated		±	+	+
whole, fresh fluid		±	+	+
Commercially prepared formulas based on cow milk				
Lactum			+	+
Purevap			+	+
Olac			+	+
Lonalac		+	+	+
Protein Milk		+	+	+
Probana			+	+
All others				
iron-fortified				
not iron-fortified				+
Soy-based formulas				
Sobee				
Mull-Soy—liquid‡				
—powder‡	+	+	+	
Soyalac —liquid	+		+	
—powder	+	+	+	
ProSobee				
Isomil				
Milk-free, soy-free formulas				
Nutramigen				
Meat Base				
Lambase				
Lofenalac				

*The designation + indicates that supplementation is desirable; the designation ± indicates that supplementation is desirable if the milk or formula has not been fortified with the nutrient in question. Fluoride supplementation is desirable as indicated in Table 10–3.

†Folic acid, 50 μg daily, should be given.

‡Additional iron should be provided if intake of formula is less than 900 ml/day.

Since milks and formulas as supplied to the consumer are uniformly low in content of fluoride, the desirability of supplementing the diet with fluoride will depend on the amount of water, if any, subsequently added to the milk or formula or consumed alone, and the concentration of fluoride in the water (Table 10–3).

When goat milk provides a major source of calories, the diet should be fortified with folic acid.

Infants of Low Birth Weight

Time of First Feeding

History of the controversy regarding time of initiation of feeding in infants of low birth weight has recently been reviewed by Cornblath et al. (1966). It is not yet possible to state with certainty whether feedings should be begun during the first 12 to 24 hours of life or be deferred until 36 to 72 hours of age. From the purely nutritional point of view, it seems probable that the infant of low birth weight is likely to tolerate starvation less well than the full-size infant. However, the advantages of early provision of nutrients must be weighed against such hazards as airway obstruction from an indwelling nasogastric tube, abdominal distention with consequent respiratory difficulty and vomiting.

These hazards appear to be greater for smaller infants. Thus, Wharton and Bower (1965) reported increased mortality in early-fed infants in all weight groups below 2250 gm. Gleiss (1955) and Laurance and Smith (1962) reported decreased mortality in early-fed infants with birth weights above 1250 or 1300 gm, but no difference in mortality among other groups. Other investigators found no difference in mortality in relation to time of first feeding, possibly indicating that the presumed nutritional advantages of early feeding in many cases do not outweigh the consequent hazards (Bauman, 1960; Butterfield et al., 1962; Keitel and Gillen, 1965; Cornblath et al., 1966).

Until more data are available, the following plan of management seems reasonable: Infants of low birth weight are observed during the first 24 hours after birth without feeding. If the Silverman score (Silverman, 1961) is zero at age 24 hours, a nasogastric tube is inserted and a small amount of 10 per cent glucose solution is put into the stomach. If the Silverman score is not zero at age 24 hours the tube is not inserted; if the score increases after insertion of the nasogastric tube, the tube is withdrawn and fluids are given intravenously for 12 to 24 hours. A nasogastric tube is then inserted and if respiratory or other difficulty develops, gastrostomy feedings may be indicated (Silverman, 1961).

Low birth weight infants of diabetic mothers will generally profit from early feedings (begun by 12 hours of age) (Hubbell et al., 1961; Cornblath and Schwartz, 1966) or from intravenous infusions of glucose-containing solutions.

Recent reports suggest that intravenous infusions of solutions containing glucose and sodium chloride or sodium bicarbonate during the first two or three days of life may be associated with decreased mortality in infants of low birth weight (Usher, 1963; Cornblath et al., 1966). Additional studies are needed before a general recommendation is warranted concerning whether intravenous feedings should be employed routinely for infants of low birth weight.

CALORIC CONCENTRATION OF FORMULA

The caloric concentration of the formula chosen for feeding infants of low birth weight will depend to some extent on the objectives of the feeding program. Mortality appears to be unaffected by choice of 67 kcal/100 ml (20 kcal/oz) or 113 kcal/100 ml (34 kcal/oz), and it seems likely that variations in caloric density within this range may be selected on the basis of other considerations. Rate of growth is of obvious importance.

A number of studies have demonstrated that infants of low birth weight gain weight more rapidly when they are fed relatively concentrated formulas (Snyderman and Holt, 1961; Combes and Pratt, 1961; Falkner et al., 1962; Keitel et al., 1965) (Table 4–2). Thus, the physician caring for the infant is able to exert considerable influence over the infant's rate of gain in weight. Unfortunately, we do not yet know what rate of gain in weight is desirable.

In general, it seems reasonable to attempt to achieve a rate of gain in weight equal to that calculated from charts of weight gain in utero (Table 13–2). The following approach is recommended: with infants weighing less than 2000 gm, initial formula feedings are 100 kcal/100 ml (30 kcal/oz) and with infants weighing 2000 gm or more, initial feedings are 80 kcal/100 ml (24 kcal/oz). After about one week, caloric concentration is increased further if it does not appear likely that rate of gain in weight will soon approach the rates indicated in Table 13–2. However, caloric concentration is not permitted to exceed 113 kcal/100 ml (34 kcal/oz). If, at any time, weight gain during one week exceeds by 10 per cent the amounts indicated in Table 13–2, the caloric concentration of the formula is reduced.

Studies of experimental animals have suggested that body com-

Table 13-2.   *Desirable Rates of Gain in Weight by Infants of Low Birth Weight**

Body Weight† (gm)	Gain in Weight (gm/7 days)
840	40
880	75
955	90
1045	105
1150	120
1270	125
1395	145
1540	175
1715	205
1920	280
2200	285
2485	225

*Calculated from data of Lubchenco et al. (1963) as discussed in text. Table applies to infants who are more than one week of age and do not demonstrate respiratory or other difficulty. With larger infants, rates of gain in weight should be evaluated in relation to Table 2-1.

†If body weight at onset of a specified week of observation falls between 840 and 880 gm, desirable rate of gain in weight lies between 40 and 75 gm in seven days.

position varies with caloric concentration of the feeding. Presumably, this may be true of the human infant as well; in addition, body composition may be related to susceptibility to disease. Much further study is necessary before a sound scientific basis can be established for feeding infants of low birth weight.

Congenital Heart Disease

Infants with severe congenital heart disease present rather unique problems in nutritional management. Failure to thrive in such infants is probably explained in most cases by the combination of reduced caloric intake (because the infant readily tires at feedings) and increased energy expenditure as a consequence of increased cardiac work (Pittman and Cohen, 1964; Lees et al., 1965).

It is desirable to manage such infants with formulas of high caloric concentration but without excessive renal solute load (Chapter Nine). In the presence of severe congestive cardiac failure, Lonalac may be a desirable feeding for a brief period. Rarely should administration of Lonalac be continued for more than one week (Chapter Eleven), and caloric concentration should not exceed 67 kcal/100 ml because of the relatively high renal solute load (Table 9–8). Feedings with low renal solute load and fairly low concentrations of sodium are preferable for long-term management: SMA S-26 and Similac PM 60/40 can be concentrated to 100 kcal/100 ml without concern about excessive renal solute load. Feeding by nasogastric tube may be desirable to eliminate the physical exertion associated with bottle feeding.

Management after Bowel Resection

Infants who have had major segments of bowel removed or bypassed often present particularly difficult problems in management. However, a number of reports indicate that survival is possible even when most of the small or large bowel has been removed (Pietz, 1956; Pilling and Cresson, 1957; Lawler and Bernard, 1962; Anderson, 1965). Losses of water, electrolytes and other nutrients in the feces are usually great during the early postoperative period; even when feedings can be initiated orally or through a gastrostomy, it will often be necessary to augment the intake for several days (sometimes for weeks) with fluids given intravenously. Gastrointestinal passage time is rapid, especially after removal or bypassing of the ileocecal valve and right half of the colon (Pilling and Cresson, 1957). Fecal excretion of fat, protein and carbohydrate may account for a relatively large percentage of caloric intake.

During the first few weeks postoperatively, feedings containing medium-chain triglycerides (Chapters Six and Eleven) may be useful. In this early phase of management, major aims should be maintenance of fluid and electrolyte balance and prevention of severe nutritional deficiencies. Parenteral administration of vitamins, minerals and plasma is important at this time. The possibility of development of hypomagnesemia should be considered (Booth et al., 1963). Megaloblastic anemia, presumably because of vitamin B_{12} deficiency, has been reported in adults after resection of the ileum (Kalser et al., 1960), and supplements should be provided. Collection and chemical analysis of stools aids greatly in making a sound decision about therapy.

As soon as fluid and electrolyte balance can be maintained without parenteral administration of supplements, a diet suitable for long-term management should be devised. Feedings should be of low to moderate fat content and include only those fats that are well absorbed. Nutramigen (Table 12–3) and Olac (Table 11–7) are theoretically sound for this purpose, but even such feedings may supply more fat than is desirable for some infants. At times it may be necessary to reduce the percentage of calories provided from long-chain triglycerides in these feedings. This can be accomplished by the addition of carbohydrate and protein and/or medium-chain triglycerides.

Metabolic balance studies are of great value in management because of a need to know the net intake (i.e., intake minus fecal excretion) of water, electrolytes, fat and other nutrients. Regular determinations of solute concentration of the urine is also desirable. When urinary solute concentration consistently exceeds 450 mosmol/l, additional fluid should be supplied either by increasing formula intake, by diluting the formula or by parenteral administration.

Hereditary Metabolic Disease

Comments on management of hypoglycemia, galactosemia and disaccharidase deficiency have been included in Chapter Seven. Idiopathic hypercalcemia, vitamin B_6 dependency and disorders of folic acid metabolism have been discussed in Chapter Eight.

In the present section, discussion will be limited to phenylketonuria, tyrosinemia, gluten-sensitive enteropathy and cystic fibrosis of the pancreas. Table 13–3 lists references to literature concerned with the management of many less common hereditary metabolic disorders.

PHENYLKETONURIA

Because screening tests for phenylketonuria are commonly based on the finding of phenylalaninemia rather than on phenylketonuria, it is important to recognize that there are at least five neonatal conditions associated with phenylalaninemia, some of which do not require dietary restriction of phenylalanine (Committee on Nutrition, 1967). Long-term dietary restriction of phenylalanine has been mistakenly imposed on children subsequently proved not to have phenylketonuria (Allan and Holt, 1965; Rouse, 1966). Berry et al. (1966) have recommended that the following conditions should be met before an unqualified diagnosis of phenylketonuria is made: concentration of phenylalanine in the blood during fasting greater than 15 mg/100 ml, concentration of tyrosine less than 5 mg/100 ml and concentrations of other amino acids normal; urine concentration of phenylalanine greater than 100 μg/ml; and presence of orthohydroxyphenylacetic acid in urine.

In the treatment of phenylketonuria, it is necessary to avoid excessively low as well as excessively high concentrations of phenyl-

(*Text continued on page 257.*)

Table 13–3. *Nutritional Management in Hereditary Metabolic Disease**

Disease	Therapy	Reference
A. Disorders of Amino Acid Metabolism		
i. *Essential amino acids*		
1. Phenylketonuria (classical)	Phenylalanine restriction	Berry et al., 1966 & 1967 Kang et al., 1965 Knox, 1966 Kennedy et al., 1967 Koch et al., 1967
2. Branched-chain keto-aminoaciduria (maple syrup urine disease)	Restriction of leucine, isoleucine and valine	Westall, 1963 Snyderman et al., 1964 Snyderman, 1967 Dancis et al., 1967
3. Hypervalinemia	Valine restriction	Wada et al., 1963
4. Isovalericacidemia ("sweaty-feet" syndrome)	Protein restriction	Tanaka et al., 1966
5. Homocystinuria, with methioninemia	Methionine restriction and cystine supplementation	Perry et al., 1966 Brenton et al., 1966 Komrower, 1967
6. Histidinemia	Early histidine restriction (?)	LaDu, 1966
7. Hyperlysinemia	Protein restriction 1.5 g/kg/day	Woody, 1964 Ghadimi et al., 1965 Colombo et al., 1964
ii. *Nonessential amino acids*		
1. Tyrosinemia		
a. Hereditary form	Tyrosine restriction and phenylalanine adjustment	Halvorsen et al., 1966 Scriver, 1967 Gentz et al., 1967 Halvorsen, 1967
b. Neonatal form	Protein restriction, l-ascorbic acid 75-100 mg/day	Levine, 1946–47 Menkes & Avery, 1963 Avery et al., 1967
2. Diseases of urea cycle		
a. Hyperammonemia	Protein restriction	Efron, 1966 Freeman et al, 1964 Levin & Russell, 1967
b. Citrullinemia		McMurray et al., 1963

Table 13–3. *Nutritional Management in Hereditary Metabolic Disease* (Continued)*

Disease	Therapy	Reference
c. Argininosuccinic-aciduria	Arginine supplementation in early infancy (?)	Westall, 1967 Levin, 1967
3. The hyperglycinemias a. Acetonuric form	Protein restriction	Childs & Nyhan, 1964 Nyhan & Tocci, 1966 Nyhan, 1967
b. Hypo-oxaluric form		Gerritsen et al., 1965
iii. *Disorders of amino acid transport* 1. Hartnup disease	Nicotinic acid supplements; generous protein intake	Scriver, 1965 Jepson, 1966
2. Tryptophanuria	Nicotinic acid	Tada et al., 1963
3. a. Cystinuria	Water; penicillamine	Dent et al., 1965 McDonald & Henneman, 1965
b. ——with protein intolerance	Protein restriction	Fleming et al., 1963 Perheentupa & Visakorpi, 1965
4. Methionine malabsorption	Protein restriction (particularly methionine)	Hooft et al., 1965
5. Tryptophan malabsorption (blue diaper syndrome)	Protein restriction (particularly tryptophan)	Drummond et al., 1964
B. Disorders of Carbohydrate Metabolism		
1. Hyperglycemia (childhood diabetes mellitus)	Dietary control, insulin	O'Brien, 1966 Jackson & Pickens, 1964 Bain & Chute, 1965 Guest & Shirkey, 1966
2. Hypoglycemia a. Toxic: (EDTA, salicylates, sulphonylureas, MOA, inhibitors, etc.)	Remove cause; IV glucose	O'Brien et al., 1966
b. Leucine sensitivity	Protein restriction (steroids); Diazoxide	Roth & Segal, 1964 Drash & Wolff, 1964 Schwartz et al., 1963

Table 13–3. *Nutritional Management in Hereditary Metabolic Disease* (Continued)*

Disease	Therapy	Reference
c. Idiopathic	Steroids	Haworth & Coodin, 1960
d. Ketotic	Frequent feeding	Colle & Ulstrom, 1964
e. Deficient catecholamine response	Ephedrine	Madsen, 1965
f. Hyperinsulinism	Diazoxide; surgery	Drash & Wolff, 1964
3. Glycogen storage diseases (Types I–IX)	Depends on type	Cornblath & Schwartz, 1966
4. Galactosemia (4 types)	Galactose restriction (need may be transient)	Isselbacher, 1966
5. Monosaccharide intolerance	Restriction of the relevant monosaccharides	Dormandy & Porter, 1961 Cornblath, 1966 Cornblath & Schwartz, 1966 Schneider et al., 1966 Burke & Danks, 1966
6. a. True congenital disaccharidase deficiency	Long-term restriction of disaccharide intake	Lifshitz, 1966 Prader & Auricchio, 1965 Auricchio et al., 1965 Dahlqvist, 1966 Burgess et al., 1964
b. Acquired congenital disaccharidase deficiency	Temporary restriction of disaccharides	Sunshine & Kretchmer, 1964 Bowie et al., 1963 and 1965 Dahlqvist, 1966
C. Disorders of Lipid Metabolism†		
1. Idiopathic hyperlipemia (Buerger-Grütz disease		Hsia, 1966
2. Primary hypercholesteremia (xanthelasmatosis)		Hsia, 1966
3. Familial hyperlipoproteinemia (5 types)		Fredrickson, 1966
4. Abetalipoproteinemia		Farquhar & Ways, 1966

Table 13–3. *Nutritional Management in Hereditary Metabolic Disease* (Continued)*

Disease	Therapy	Reference
5. High density lipoprotein deficiency (Tangier disease)		Fredrickson, 1966
D. Miscellaneous Disorders		
1. Vitamin B$_6$ dependency	Pyridoxine HCl 10 mg/day or more	Scriver, 1967
2. Vitamin D dependency	Vitamin D, 25,000 to 100,000 I.U./day	Fraser & Salter, 1958 Fraser, 1966
3. Idiopathic hypercalcemia	Avoid vitamin D; restrict dietary intake of calcium	Fellers, 1966–1967
4. Formimino transferase deficiency	? Histidine restriction	Arakawa et al., 1965
5. Figluuria with mental deficiency, megaloblastic anemia and ataxia	Folic acid	Luhby et al., 1965
6. Cystic fibrosis	Pancreatic enzyme replacement	Shwachman & Khaw, 1966 di Sant'Agnese & Jones, 1962
7. Gluten-sensitive enteropathy	Gluten restriction, with or without milk restriction; decrease in long-chain, saturated fats	di Sant'Agnese & Jones, 1962 Heiner, 1966
8. Wilson's disease	D-Penicillamine	Bearn, 1966
9. Familial hyperuricemia with finger chewing and mental retardation	Probenecid; alkalinization	Lesch & Nyhan, 1964
10. Oroticaciduria	Uridine	Becroft & Phillips, 1965 Smith, 1965.

*This table has been modified from one prepared by the Committee on Nutrition (1967) of the American Academy of Pediatrics. The author gratefully acknowledges the Committee's generosity in permitting its use.

†Dietary restriction of long-chain, saturated fatty acids is generally desirable in disorders of lipid metabolism. In primary hypercholesteremia, dietary cholesterol should also be restricted.

alanine in the blood. Growth retardation, rash, alopecia, bone changes and generalized aminoaciduria occur when phenylalanine deficiency is imposed on normal subjects (Snyderman et al., 1955). Harmful effects of too rigid restriction of phenylalanine, even including death, are well documented (Brimblecombe et al., 1961; Moncrieff and Wilkinson, 1961; Wilson and Clayton, 1962; Medical Research Council, 1963). In general, it is recommended that the concentration of phenylalanine in the blood be maintained between 2 and 6 mg/100 ml. The following guidelines have been recommended by Berry et al. (1966):

There should be indoctrination of the family and family counseling regarding the nature of the illness, the mode of transmission, the need for testing subsequent siblings, the nature of the restrictive diet and the need for long-term clinical, dietary, and biochemical supervision of the treatment. To establish and monitor the dietary treatment there should be regular testing of blood specimens (daily during first week, weekly from second to eighth week, bi-weekly from third month to 1 year, monthly thereafter, except during illness), a regular testing of urine specimens (daily first month, semiweekly during second to sixth month, weekly from seventh month to 1 year, bi-weekly thereafter, except daily during periods of illness), and a regular recording of the amount and type of foods eaten from which calculations of phenylalanine intake may be made. The long-term care and evaluation of the child should include assessment of adequacy of nutrition by height and weight, evaluation of general growth and development, hematologic and roentgenologic examinations to determine nutritional adequacy, assessment of mental development, neurological development, language development, and, later, performance in social situations outside the home environment, including school.

Generally, dietary restriction is considerably simpler in infants than in toddlers or older children. A formula low in concentration of phenylalanine, e.g., Lofenalac (Table 12–3), must be utilized. With an intake of Lofenalac sufficient to provide 120 kcal/kg, intake of phenylalanine will be approximately 15 mg/kg, an amount insufficient to meet requirements for normal growth by most infants with phenylketonuria. It will therefore usually be advisable to include other foods that will provide small amounts of phenylalanine. This may be done conveniently by giving carefully measured amounts of homogenized whole cow milk: 30 ml/kg will provide approximately 5 mg/kg of phenylalanine. After the first few months of life, the diet may be supplemented with strained fruits or other strained foods that are low in content of protein. However, no matter how excellent the dietary record, frequent monitoring of concentrations in the blood is essential for establishing adequate control.

TYROSINEMIA

This disorder exists in at least two forms: one that is transient and benign, occurring in newborn infants, especially those of low birth weight; and another that is hereditary, persistent and serious (Committee on Nutrition, 1967). The benign neonatal form can be corrected by decreasing the intake of protein or by increasing the intake of a reducing agent such as l-ascorbic acid. Intakes of 50 mg of ascorbic acid daily are adequate (Avery et al., 1967).

The hereditary, persistent form of tyrosinemia, characterized by cirrhosis of the liver, renal tubular defects with abnormal tyrosine metabolism and tyrosyluria (Halvorsen et al., 1966), may be at least as frequent as phenylketonuria.

Several recent reports suggest that when a diet low in tyrosine and its precursor phenylalanine is begun in early life, development of hepatic and renal damage will be prevented (Halvorsen and Gjessing, 1964; Halvorsen et al., 1966; Scriver et al., 1967; Gentz et al., 1967).

PROTEIN-LOSING ENTEROPATHY

Excretion of serum proteins into the gastrointestinal tract is part of the normal catabolism of protein (Holman et al., 1959; Wetterfors et al., 1960). The excreted proteins are digested and their amino acids are absorbed and are once again available for synthesis of body proteins. When increased excretion of serum proteins into the gastrointestinal tract occurs, the ability of the body to synthesize sufficient protein to maintain normal body content may be exceeded and hypoproteinemia will result.

Abnormal losses of serum proteins into the gastrointestinal tract occur most commonly in association with morphologic lesions of the intestines but have also been reported in constrictive pericarditis (Holman et al., 1959) and cirrhosis of the liver (Wetterfors et al., 1960). Establishing a specific diagnosis is important since at least half the patients will respond to appropriate therapy (Waldmann, 1965).

The protein-losing enteropathy that is sometimes an expression of gluten intolerance may be relieved by administration of a gluten-free diet. That associated with intestinal lymphangiectasia may be benefited by administration of a diet low in content of long-chain triglycerides. This has been accomplished with diets very low in total content of fat or diets in which the greater part of the fat consists of medium-chain triglycerides (Waldmann, 1965).

CYSTIC FIBROSIS OF THE PANCREAS

For nutritional management of infants with cystic fibrosis of the pancreas, most authorities recommend a diet high in content of protein and carbohydrate and low or moderate in content of fat. Because of greater fecal losses of calories by these patients than by normal individuals, intakes of food will be greater than those listed in Chapter Four. Such fecal losses can be reduced by administration of pancreatic enzymes, but caloric intakes will generally remain toward the upper portion of the normal range.

A reasonable caloric distribution is 20 per cent of the calories from protein, 30 to 40 per cent from fat and the remainder from carbohydrate. The fat should be one that is readily absorbed. Although the formula, Probana, is considered by many physicians to be a particularly suitable formula for management of infants with cystic fibrosis of the pancreas, the author considers Olac a better choice. Fat content of Olac is slightly higher than that of Probana and the fat of Olac is corn oil rather than butterfat and, hence, more readily absorbed. Experience with the formula, Portagen (Table 11–9), is thus far limited.

The practice of administering mineral oil to prevent or alleviate constipation in infants with this disorder is unsound. Use of mineral oil will increase fecal loss of fat-soluble vitamins and, therefore, complicate management. Administration of the surface-wetting agent, dioctyl sodium sulfosuccinate, several times daily will prevent the stools from becoming excessively firm without interfering with absorption of fat-soluble vitamins.

Supplementation of the diet with vitamins A, D, E and K is desirable. Water-miscible preparations should be utilized. Reasonable initial daily doses of vitamins A and D are 5000 and 1000 I.U., respectively.* This dose of vitamin A will almost certainly be adequate and the likelihood of toxicity from it is quite remote. Adjustment of dosage level of vitamin D can be made on the basis of serum concentrations of calcium, phosphorus and alkaline phosphatase, and these should be calculated at intervals of two months or less, and on roentgenograms of the wrist, which should be made at intervals of about four months during infancy.

Reasons for recommending vitamin E supplementation of the diet of infants with cystic fibrosis of the pancreas have been reviewed in Chapter Eight. Ideally, dosage of vitamin E should be regulated to maintain serum concentrations of alpha-tocopherol within the normal range (Chapter Eight). To accomplish this, dosage as high as

---

*For example, 0.125 ml daily of Aquasol A and D (U. S. Vitamin and Pharmaceutical Corporation).

100 mg daily has been recommended (Goldbloom, 1963). Considerably smaller doses may also be adequate, but little information is available.

It is suggested that during the first month of life a water-miscible preparation of vitamin K_1 be given daily by mouth or approximately weekly by injection in a dosage of 1 to 2 mg. After one month of age, 1 mg daily of a water-soluble analogue of menadione should be given daily. One-stage prothrombin should be determined at intervals of one to two months and the dosage adjusted as necessary.

GLUTEN-INDUCED ENTEROPATHY

Gluten is a protein of wheat and rye that constitutes about 10 per cent by weight of flour made from these grains. It contains two fractions which differ on the basis of their solubilities in alcohol—the relatively harmless glutenin and gliadin, which is predominantly responsible for malabsorption in patients with gluten-induced enteropathy. It seems probable that when polypeptides of gliadin are absorbed by susceptible individuals, the manifestations of gluten-induced enteropathy ensue. Gluten that has been subjected to complete enzymic or acid hydrolysis is innocuous (Frazer et al., 1964). Whether absorption of polypeptides of gliadin exert their harmful effects on individuals with gluten-induced enteropathy because the polypeptides are themselves toxic or because they are antigenic is unknown.

Gluten of barley and oats appears to produce in some individuals manifestations similar to those resulting from gluten of wheat and rye. High titers of circulating antibodies against milk proteins as well as against gliadin have been demonstrated in some patients with gluten-induced enteropathy.

References listed in Table 13–3 indicate the steps to be followed in establishing a diagnosis of gluten-induced enteropathy. Only the management will be discussed here.

After correction of any imbalance of fluids and electrolytes, a program of dietary management is undertaken. The recommended diet is free of wheat and rye and, at least initially, is also free of barley, oats and milk. During the initial stages of treatment, intolerance of fat and starch may exist so that a diet relatively low in fat (perhaps 35 per cent of the calories from fat) and free of starch is employed. This diet might consist of a soy-based or other milk-free formula (Tables 12–1 and 12–3), rice cereal and commercially prepared strained fruits and vegetables. After the first few weeks of treatment, the fat-free portion of cow milk will usually be well tolerated, but butterfat is likely to be less well absorbed than vegetable oils. Borgström and

Lindquist (1957), from study of two children in remission (receiving a gluten-free diet), demonstrated that a formula providing 40 per cent of calories from corn oil was well tolerated but that excretion of fat nearly doubled when butterfat was substituted for the corn oil.

Formulas such as Probana and Protein Milk (Table 11–9), commonly employed in treatment of "celiac disease" are not recommended for management of gluten-induced enteropathy since they appear to be unnecessarily low in fat content and contain butterfat rather than the better absorbed vegetable oils. Theoretically, more sound choices are Olac (Table 11–7) or Sobee (Table 12–1), which supply 19 to 20 per cent of calories from protein and 35 to 36 per cent of calories from corn oil or soy oil.

Table 13–4 lists various strained and junior foods likely to be free of gluten. However, it is essential that parents read all labels carefully to be certain that wheat (or rye, barley or oats) has not been included.

Table 13–4. Commercially Prepared Gluten-Free Strained or Junior Foods for Infants

Strained Vegetables

squash	green beans
beets	carrots
garden vegetables	peas
sweet potatoes	

Strained Fruits

applesauce	apricots with applesauce
bananas	plums with tapioca
peaches	pears and pineapple
pears	prunes with tapioca
apricots with tapioca	fruit dessert
bananas with tapioca	

Strained Meats and Egg Yolks

beef	liver and bacon
chicken	beef liver
ham	egg yolks
pork	lamb
egg yolks with ham	veal

Strained Puddings

chocolate-flavored custard	vanilla custard
orange custard	

Table 13–4. *Commercially Prepared Gluten-Free
Strained or Junior Foods for Infants (Continued)*

Miscellaneous Strained Foods

beef with vegetables	vegetables and bacon
creamed cottage cheese with pineapple	vegetables and turkey

Junior Vegetables

carrots	green beans
sweet potatoes	squash

Junior Fruits

plums with tapioca	prunes with tapioca
fruit dessert	pears and pineapple
peaches	applesauce
applesauce and apricots	pears
bananas with pineapple	

Junior Meats and Egg Yolks

beef	chicken
lamb	pork
egg yolks and ham	veal
meat sticks	

Junior Puddings

vanilla custard	chocolate-flavored
banana custard	custard

Miscellaneous Junior Foods

beef with vegetables	vegetables and chicken
ham with vegetables	vegetables and beef
vegetables with liver and bacon	vegetables and ham
creamed cottage cheese with pineapple	split peas with bacon

REFERENCES

Allan, J. D., and Holt, K. S. (eds.): Biochemical Approach to Mental Handicap in Childhood. London, E. & S. Livingstone, Ltd., 1965.

Anderson, C. M.: Long-term survival with six inches of small intestine. Brit. M. J. *1*: 419, 1965.

Arakawa, T., Ohara, K., Takahashi, Y., Ogasawara, J., Hayashi, T., Chiba, R., Wada, Y., Tada, K., Mizuno, T., Okamura, T., and Yoshida, T.: Formiminotransferase-deficiency syndrome: A new inborn error of folic acid metabolism. Ann. Paediat. *205*:1, 1965.

Auricchio, S., Rubino, A., Prader, A., Rey, J., Jos, J., Frézal, J., and Davidson, M.: Intestinal glycosidase activities in congenital malabsorption of disaccharides. J. Pediat. 66:555, 1965.

Avery, M. E., Clow, C. L., Menkes, J. H., Ramos, A., Scriver, C. R., Stern, L., and Wasserman, B. P.: Transient tyrosinemia of the newborn: Dietary and clinical aspects. Pediatrics, 1967. (In press.)

Bain, H. W., and Chute, A. L.: Diabetes in school children. Pediat. Clin. N. America 12:919, 1965.

Bauman, W. A.: Early feeding of dextrose and saline solution to premature infants. Pediatrics 26:756, 1960.

Bearn, A. G.: Wilson's disease. In Stanbury, J. B., Wyngaarden, J. B., and Fredrickson, D. S. (eds.): The Metabolic Basis of Inherited Disease. 2nd ed. New York, McGraw-Hill Book Co., Inc., 1966, p. 761.

Becroft, D. M. O., and Phillips, L. I.: Hereditary orotic aciduria and megaloblastic anaemia: A second case, with response to uridine. Brit. M. J. 1:547, 1965.

Berry, H. K., Sutherland, B. S., and Umbarger, B.: Diagnosis and treatment: Interpretation of results of blood screening studies for detection of phenylketonuria. Pediatrics 37:102, 1966.

Berry, H. K., Sutherland, B. S., Umbarger, B., and O'Grady, D.: Treatment of phenylketonuria. Am. J. Dis. Child. 113:2, 1967.

Booth, C. C., Babouris, N., Hanna, S., and MacIntyre, I.: Incidence of hypomagnesaemia in intestinal malabsorption. Brit. M. J. 2:141, 1963.

Borgström, B., and Lindquist, B.: Favourable effect of liquid formula-feeding high in fat to coeliac children. Acta Paediat. 46:449, 1957.

Bowie, M. D., Brinkman, G. L., and Hansen, J. D. L.: Diarrhoea in protein calorie malnutrition. Lancet 2:550, 1963.

Bowie, M. D., Brinkman, G. L., and Hansen, J. D. L.: Acquired disaccharide intolerance in malnutrition. J. Pediat. 66:1083, 1965.

Brenton, D. P., Cusworth, D. C., Dent, C. E., and Jones, E. E.: Homocystinuria clinical and dietary studies. Quart. J. Med. (NS) 35:325, 1966.

Brimblecombe, F. S. W., Blainey, J. D., Stoneman, M. E. R., and Wood, B. S. B.: Dietary and biochemical control of phenylketonuria. Brit. M. J. 2:793, 1961.

Burgess, E. A., Levin, B., Mahalanabis, D., and Tonge, R. E.: Hereditary sucrose intolerance: Levels of sucrase activity in jejunal mucosa. Arch. Dis. Childhood 39:431, 1964.

Burke, V., and Danks, D. M.: Monosaccharide malabsorption in young infants. Lancet 1:1177, 1966.

Butterfield, J., O'Brien, D., and Lubchenco, L. O.: Respiratory distress syndrome in premature infants. An evaluation of the early feeding of glucose water. Am. J. Dis. Child. 104:230, 1962.

Childs, B., and Nyhan, W. L.: Further observations of a patient with hyperglycinemia. Pediatrics 33:403, 1964.

Colle, E., and Ulstrom, R. A.: Ketotic hypoglycemia. J. Pediat. 64:632, 1964.

Colombo, J. P., Richterich, R., Donath, A., Spahr, A., and Rossi, E.: Congenital lysine inheritance with periodic ammonia intoxication. Lancet 1:1014, 1964.

Combes, M. A., and Pratt, E. L.: Premature infants and concentrated feeding. Am. J. Dis. Child. 102:610, 1961. (Abst. #223.)

Committee on Nutrition. Nutritional management in hereditary metabolic disease. Pediatrics, 1967. (In press.)

Cornblath, M.: Familial carbohydrate intolerance and hypoglycemia. Ann. Rev. Med. 17:161, 1966.

Cornblath, M., Forbes, A. E., Pildes, R. S., Luebben, G., and Greengard, J.: A controlled study of early fluid administration on survival of low birth weight infants. Pediatrics 38:547, 1966.

Cornblath, M., and Schwartz, R.: Disorders of Carbohydrate Metabolism in Infancy. Philadelphia, W. B. Saunders Company, 1966.

Dahlqvist, A.: Disaccharide intolerance. J.A.M.A. 195:225, 1966.

Dancis, J., Hutzler, J., and Rokkones, T.: Intermittent branched-chain ketonuria. Variant of maple-syrup-urine disease. New England J. Med. 276:84, 1967.

Dent, C. E., Friedman, M., Green, H., and Watson, L. C. A.: Treatment of cystinuria. Brit. M. J. 1:403, 1965.

di Sant'Agnese, P. A., and Jones, W. O.: The celiac syndrome (malabsorption) in pediatrics. Classification, differential diagnosis, principles of dietary management. J.A.M.A. *180*:308, 1962.

Dormandy, T. L., and Porter, R. J.: Familial fructose and galactose intolerance. Lancet *1*:1189, 1961.

Drash, A., and Wolff, F.: Drug therapy in leucine-sensitive hypoglycemia. Metabolism *13*:487, 1964.

Drummond, K. N., Michael, A. F., Ulstrom, R. A., and Good, R. A.: The blue diaper syndrome: familial hypercalcemia with nephrocalcinosis and indicanuria. Am. J. Med. 37:928, 1964.

Efron, M. L.: Diseases of the urea cycle. *In* Stanbury, J. B., Wyngaarden, J. B., and Fredrickson, D. S. (eds.): The Metabolic Basis of Inherited Disease. 2nd ed. New York, McGraw-Hill Book Company, 1966, p. 393.

Falkner, F., Steigman, A. J., and Cruise, M. O.: The physical development of the premature infant. I. Some standards and certain relationships to caloric intake. J. Pediat. *60*:895, 1962.

Farquhar, J. W., and Ways, P.: Abetalipoproteinemia. *In* Stanbury, J. B., Wyngaarden, J. B., and Fredrickson, D. S. (eds.): The Metabolic Basis of Inherited Disease. 2nd ed. New York, McGraw-Hill Book Company, Inc., 1966, p. 509.

Fellers, F. X.: Idiopathic hypercalcemia. *In* Gellis, S. S., and Kagan, B. M. (eds.): Current Pediatric Therapy. Philadelphia, W. B. Saunders Company, 1966–1967, p. 414.

Fleming, W. H., Avery, G. B., Morgan, R. I., and Cone, T. E., Jr.: Gastrointestinal malabsorption associated with cystinuria. Report of a case in a negro. Pediatrics 32:358, 1963.

Fraser, D.: Rickets. *In* Conn, H. F., Clohecy, R. J., and Conn, R. B., Jr. (eds.): Current Diagnosis. Philadelphia, W. B. Saunders Company, 1966, p. 391.

Fraser, D., and Salter, R. B.: The diagnosis and management of the various types of rickets. Pediat. Clin. N. America 5:417, 1958.

Frazer, A. C., Schneider, R., Morgan, D. B., Sammons, H. G., and Hayward, M., *In* Munro, H. N. (ed.). The Role of the Gastrointestinal Tract in Protein Metabolism. Oxford, Blackwell Scientific Publications, 1964, p. 349.

Fredrickson, D. S.: Familial high-density lipoprotein deficiency: Tangier disease. *In* Stanbury, J. B. Wyngaarden, J. B., and Fredrickson, D. S. (eds.): The Metabolic Basis of Inherited Disease. 2nd ed. New York, McGraw-Hill Book Company, Inc., 1966, p. 486.

Freeman, J. M., Nicholson, J. F., Masland, W. S., Rowland, L. P., and Carter, S.: Ammonia intoxication due to a congenital defect in urea synthesis. J. Pediat. 65: 1039, 1964.

Gentz, J., Lindblad, B., Lindstedt, S., Levy, L., Shasteen, W., and Zetterstrom, R.: Dietary treatment in tyrosinemia (tyrosinosis) with a note on the possible recognition of the carrier state. Am. J. Dis. Child. *113*:31, 1967.

Gerritsen, T., Kaveggia, E., and Waisman, H. A.: A new type of idiopathic hyperglycinemia with hypo-oxaluria. Pediatrics 36:882, 1965.

Ghadimi, H., Binnington, V. I., and Pecora, P.: Hyperlysinemia associated with retardation. New England J. Med. 273:723, 1965.

Gleiss, J.: Zum Frühgeborenenproblem der Gegenwart. IX. Mitteilung. Ztschr. Kinderh. 76:261, 1955.

Goldbloom, R. B.: Studies of tocopherol requirements in health and disease. Pediatrics 32:36, 1963.

Guest, G. M., and Shirkey, H. C.: Diabetes mellitus. *In* Shirkey, H. C. (ed.): Pediatric Therapy. 2nd ed. St. Louis, The C. V. Mosby Company, 1966, p. 731.

Halvorsen, S.: Dietary treatment of tyrosinosis. Am. J. Dis. Child. *113*:38, 1967.

Halvorsen, S., and Gjessing, L. R.: Studies on tyrosinosis: 1, Effect of low-tyrosine and low-phenylalanine diet. Brit. M. J. *2* :1171, 1964.

Halvorsen, S., Pande, H., Løken, A. C., and Gjessing, L. R.: Tyrosinosis, A study of 6 cases. Arch. Dis. Childhood *41*:238, 1966.

Haworth, J. C., and Coodin, F. J.: Idiopathic spontaneous hypoglycemia in children. Pediatrics 25:748, 1960.

Heiner, D. C.: Celiac syndrome. *In* Shirkey, H. C. (ed.): Pediatric Therapy. 2nd ed. St. Louis, The C. V. Mosby Company, 1966, p. 505.

Holman, H., Nickel, W. F., Jr., and Sleisenger, M. H.: Hypoproteinemia antedating intestinal lesions, and possibly due to excessive serum protein loss into the intestine. Am. J. Med. 27:963, 1959.

Hooft, C., Timmermans, J., Snoeck, J., Antener, I., Oyaert, W., and Van den Hende, C.: Methionine malabsorption syndrome. Ann. Paediat. 205:73, 1965.

Hsia, D. Y.-Y.: Inborn Errors of Metabolism. 2nd ed. Part I. Clinical Aspects. Chicago, Year Book Medical Publishers, Inc., 1966.

Hubbell, J. P., Jr., Drorbaugh, J. E., Rudolph, A. J., Auld, P. A. M., Cherry, R. B., and Smith, C. A.: "Early" versus "late" feeding of infants of diabetic mothers. New England J. Med. 265:835, 1961.

Isselbacher, K. J.: Galactosemia. *In* Stanbury, J. B., Wyngaarden, J. B., and Fredrickson, D. S. (eds.): The Metabolic Basis of Inherited Disease. 2nd ed. New York, McGraw-Hill Book Company, Inc., 1966, p. 178.

Jackson, R. L., and Pickens, J. M.: The child with diabetes. *In* Duncan, G. G. (ed.): Diseases of Metabolism. 5th ed. Philadelphia, W. B. Saunders Company, 1964, p. 1084.

Jepson, J. B.: Hartnup disease. *In* Stanbury, J. B., Wyngaarden, J. B., and Fredrickson, D. S. (eds.): The Metabolic Basis of Inherited Disease. 2nd ed. New York, McGraw-Hill Book Company, 1966, p. 1283.

Kalser, M. H., Roth, J. L. A., Tumen, H., and Johnson, T. A.: Relation of small bowel resection to nutrition in man. Gastroenterology 38:605, 1960.

Kang, E. S., Kennedy, J. L., Jr., Gates, L., Burwash, I., and McKinnon, A.: Clinical observations in phenylketonuria. Pediatrics 35:932, 1965.

Keitel, H. G., and Gillen, A.: Premature infant feeding. IV. The life-death score: a method for evaluating newborn infant survival. Pediat. Clin. N. America 12:357, 1965.

Keitel, H. G., Menduke, H., Smith, T., and Fiorentino, T.: Premature infant feeding. III. The serum bilirubin concentration in premature infants with immediate and delayed feeding of formulas of varying caloric concentration. Pediat. Clin. N. America 12:347, 1965.

Kennedy, J. L., Jr., Wertelecki, W., Gates, L., Sperry, B. P., and Cass, V. M.: The early treatment of phenylketonuria. Am. J. Dis. Child. 113:16, 1967.

Knox, W. E.: Phenylketonuria. *In* Stanbury, J. B., Wyngaarden, J. B., and Fredrickson, D. S. (eds.): The Metabolic Basis of Inherited Disease. 2nd ed. New York, McGraw-Hill Book Company, Inc., 1966, p. 258.

Koch, R., Acosta, P., Fishler, K., Schaeffler, G., and Wohlers, A.: Clinical observations on phenylketonuria. Am. J. Dis. Child. 113:6, 1967.

Komrower, G. M.: Dietary treatment of homocystinuria. Am. J. Dis. Child. 113:98, 1967.

LaDu, B. N.: Histidinemia. *In* Stanbury, J. B., Wyngaarden, J. B., and Fredrickson, D. S. (eds.): The Metabolic Basis of Inherited Disease. 2nd ed. New York, McGraw-Hill Book Company, Inc., 1966, p. 366.

Laurance, B. M., and Smith, B. H.: The premature baby's diet. Lancet 1:589, 1962.

Lawler, W. H., Jr., and Bernard, H. R.: Survival of an infant following massive resection of the small intestine. Ann. Surg. 155:204, 1962.

Lees, M. H., Bristow, J. D., Griswold, H. E., and Olmsted, R. W.: Relative hypermetabolism in infants with congenital heart disease and undernutrition. Pediatrics 36:183, 1965.

Lesch, M., and Nyhan, W. L.: A familial disorder of uric acid metabolism and central nervous system function. Am. J. Med. 36:561, 1964.

Levin, B.: Arginosuccinic aciduria. Am. J. Dis. Child. 113:162, 1967.

Levin, B., and Russell, A.: Treatment of hyperammonemia. Am. J. Dis. Child. 113:142, 1967.

Levine, S. Z.: Tyrosine and phenylalanine metabolism in infants and the role of vitamin C. The Harvey Lectures, Series 42, 303, 1946–1947.

Lifshitz, F.: Congenital lactase deficiency. J. Pediat. 69:229, 1966.

Lubchenco, L. O., Hansman, C., Dressler, M., and Boyd, E.: Intrauterine growth as estimated from liveborn birth-weight data at 24 to 42 weeks of gestation. Pediatrics 32:793, 1963.

Luhby, A. L., Cooperman, J. M., and Pesci-Bourel, A.: A new inborn error of metabolism: Folic acid responsive megaloblastic anemia, ataxia, mental retardation and convulsions. Program and Abstracts, 75th Annual Meeting American Pediatric Society, p. 42, 1965.

Madsen, A.: Spontaneous hypoglycaemia with convulsions and deficient adrenaline reaction. Acta paediat. scandinav. 54:483, 1965.

McDonald, J. E., and Henneman, P. H.: Stone dissolution in vivo and control of cystinuria with D-penicillamine. New England J. Med. 273:578, 1965.

McMurray, W. C., Rathbun, J. C., Mohyuddin, F., and Koegler, S. J.: Citrullinuria. Pediatrics 32:347, 1963.

Medical Research Council: Treatment of phenylketonuria. Brit. M. J. 1:1691, 1963.

Menkes, J. H., and Avery, M. E.: The metabolism of phenylalanine and tyrosine in the premature infant. Bull. Johns Hopkins Hosp. 113:301, 1963.

Moncrieff, A., and Wilkinson, R. H.: Further experiences in the treatment of phenylketonuria. Brit. M. J. 1:763, 1961.

Morrison, S. D.: Human Milk: Yield, Proximate Principles and Inorganic Constituents. Commonwealth Agricultural Bureaux, Farnham Royal, Slough Bucks, England, 1952.

Nyhan, W. L.: Treatment of hyperglycinemia. Am. J. Dis. Child. 113:129, 1967.

Nyhan, W. L., and Tocci, P.: Aminoaciduria. Ann. Rev. Med. 17:133, 1966.

O'Brien, D.: Childhood diabetes. A contemporary re-evaluation. Clin. Pediat. 5:21, 1966.

O'Brien, D., Ibbott, F. A., and Rogerson, D.: Recent advances in clinical biochemistry of diseases of childhood. In Stefanini, M. (ed.): Progress in Clinical Pathology. New York, Grune & Stratton, 1966, p. 512.

Perheentupa, J., and Visakorpi, J. K.: Protein intolerance with deficient transport of basic aminoacids. Lancet 2:813, 1965.

Perry, T. L., Dunn, H. G., Hansen, S., MacDougall, L., and Warrington, P. D.: Early diagnosis and treatment of homocystinuria. Pediatrics 37:502, 1966.

Pietz, D. G.: Nutritional and electrolyte evaluation in massive bowel resection. Gastroenterology 31:56, 1956.

Pilling, G. P., and Cresson, S. L.: Massive resection of the small intestine in the neonatal period. Report of two successful cases and review of the literature. Pediatrics 19:940, 1957.

Pittman, J. G., and Cohen, P.: The pathogenesis of cardiac cachexia. New England J. Med. 271:403, 1964.

Prader, A., and Auricchio, S.: Defects of intestinal disaccharide absorption. Ann. Rev. Med. 16:345, 1965.

Roth, H., and Segal, S.: The dietary management of leucine-sensitive hypoglycemia, with report of a case. Pediatrics 34:831, 1964.

Rouse, B. M.: Phenylalanine deficiency syndrome. J. Pediat. 69:246, 1966.

Schneider, A. J., Kinter, W. B., and Stirling, C. E.: Glucose-galactose malabsorption. New England J. Med. 274:305, 1966.

Schwartz, T. B., Bowyer, A., and Hanashiro, P.: The phenomenon of leucine sensitivity. Med. Clin. N. America 47:219, 1966.

Scriver, C. R.: Hartnup disease. A genetic modification of intestinal and renal transport of certain neutral alpha-amino acids. New England J. Med. 273:530, 1965.

Scriver, C. R.: Vitamin B_6 deficiency and dependency in man. Am. J. Dis. Child. 113:109, 1967.

Scriver, C. R., Larochelle, J., and Silverberg, M.: Hereditary tyrosinemia and the tyrosyluria in a French Canadian geographic isolate. Am. J. Dis. Child. 113:41, 1967.

Shwachman, H., and Khaw, K.-T.: Cystic fibrosis. *In* Shirkey, H. C. (ed.): Pediatric Therapy. 2nd ed. St. Louis, The C. V. Mosby Company, 1966, p. 516.

Silverman, W. A.: Dunham's Premature Infants. 3rd ed. New York, Hoeber Medical Division, Harper and Row, Inc., 1961, p. 186.

Smith, L. H., Jr.: Hereditary orotic aciduria-pyrimidine auxotrophism in man. Am. J. Med. *38*:1, 1965.

Snyderman, S. E.: The therapy of maple syrup urine disease. Am. J. Dis. Child. *113*:68, 1967.

Snyderman, S. E., and Holt, L. E., Jr.: The effect of high caloric feeding on the growth of premature infants. J. Pediat. *58*:237, 1961.

Snyderman, S. E., Norton, P. M., Roitman, E., and Holt, L. E., Jr.: Maple syrup urine disease, with particular reference to dietotherapy. Pediatrics *34*:454, 1964.

Snyderman, S. E., Pratt, E. L., Cheung, M. W., Norton, P., and Holt, L. E., Jr.: The phenylalanine requirement of the normal infant. J. Nutrition *56*:253, 1955.

Sunshine, P., and Kretchmer, N.: Studies of small intestine during development. III. Infantile diarrhea associated with intolerance to disaccharides. Pediatrics *34*:38, 1964.

Tada, K., Ito, H., Wada, Y., and Arakawa, T.: Congenital tryptophanuria with dwarfism ("H" disease-like clinical features without indicanuria and generalized amino-aciduria):—a probably new inborn error of tryptophan metabolism. Tohoku J. Exper. Med. *80*:118, 1963.

Tanaka, K., Budd, M. A., Efron, M. L., and Isselbacher, K. J.: Isovaleric acidemia: a new genetic defect of leucine metabolism. Proc. Nat. Acad. Sci. *56*:236, 1966.

Usher, R.: Reduction of mortality from respiratory distress syndrome of prematurity with early administration of intravenous glucose and sodium bicarbonate. Pediatrics *32*:966, 1963.

Wada, Y., Tada, K., Minagawa, A., Yoshida, T., Morikawa, T., and Okamura, T.: Idiopathic hypervalinemia. Tohoku J. Exper. Med. *81*:46, 1963.

Waldmann, T.: *In* Heiner, D. C. (ed.): Macromolecular Aspects of Protein Absorption and Excretion in the Mammalian Intestine. Report of the Fiftieth Ross Conference of Pediatric Research. Columbus, Ohio, Ross Laboratories, 1965, p. 94.

Westall, R. G.: Treatment in arginosuccinic aciduria. Am. J. Dis. Child. *113*:160, 1967.

Westall, R. G.: Dietary treatment of a child with maple syrup urine disease (branched-chain ketoaciduria). Arch. Dis. Childhood *38*:485, 1963.

Wetterfors, J., Gullberg, R., Liljedahl, S. O., Plantin, L. O., Birke, G., and Olhagen, B.: Role of the stomach and small intestine in albumin breakdown. Acta med. scandinav. *168*:347, 1960.

Wharton, B. A., and Bower, B. D.: Immediate or later feeding for premature babies? Lancet *2*:969, 1965.

Wilson, K. M., and Clayton, B. E.: Importance of choline during growth, with particular reference to synthetic diets in phenylketonuria. Arch. Dis. Childhood *37*:565, 1962.

Woody, N. C.: Hyperlysinemia. Am. J. Dis. Child. *108*:543, 1964.

Chapter Fourteen

The Future of
Infant Nutrition

In the United States and in other countries where gross under-nutrition is no longer widespread, nutritionists have turned their thoughts increasingly toward attempts to define and achieve optimal nutrition. It is quite clear that rapidity of growth or final attainment of a particular size or body composition represents relatively unimportant goals in human nutrition. Longevity is a reasonable goal only if achieved by increasing the duration of a vigorous maturity and not if by mere extension of the duration of senescence. However, the common belief that factors which shorten life spare individuals the consequences of infirmity is to a large extent a misconception (Jones, 1961).

Increase in mortality of rats with advancing age results from the increasing probability of onset of major diseases; it seems likely that in technically advanced countries, the same relation holds for the human.

Diet and Longevity

A number of studies with insects, fish and mammals indicate that longevity can be markedly extended by means of dietary controls

268

Table 14–1. Mortality Ratios* of Rats Maintained on Restricted Intakes of Semisynthetic Diets†

Age	Semisynthetic Diets			
	3.0–6.1‡	3.0–2.0	0.8–8.3	0.8–2.0
First 700 days	48 %	35%	75%	46%
After 700 days	34%	23%	44%	22%

*Mortality ratio is actual deaths as percentage of expected deaths in rats fed commercial diet ad libitum.
†Data of Ross (1961).
‡Diets are expressed as relative amounts of protein and carbohydrate, respectively. Fat content of all diets was the same.

exerted throughout life and that extension of life span by such means results in postponement of the onset of the changes commonly associated with aging (Fomon and Owen, 1964). From the studies of McCay and associates, it has been known for some time that longevity of rats could be increased through severe dietary restriction (McCay et al., 1935, 1943; Saxton, 1945). That less extreme dietary restriction also results in increased longevity has been shown more recently.

It was demonstrated by Berg and Simms (1960) that restriction of food intake by 33 per cent or 48 per cent of that consumed by rats fed ad libitum did not interfere with skeletal growth or sexual maturation. Rats whose food intake was restricted at the 48 per cent level demonstrated an increase in life expectancy of 25 per cent (from 802 to 1005 days) in males and 39 per cent (from 930 to 1294 days) in females. As may be seen from Table 14–1, the data of Ross (1961) are generally similar. Male rats fed restricted amounts of semisynthetic diets from the time of weaning lived considerably longer than those fed a commercially available diet ad libitum. The studies of Ross are of particular interest because even at the same caloric intake some of the restricted diets were more conducive to long life than others.

Diet and Incidence of Disease

McCay and associates found that rats fed ad libitum were more susceptible than underfed rats to chronic lung disease, various tumors and renal disease (McCay et al., 1935, 1943; Saxton, 1945). The frequency of these conditions in the rats fed ad libitum appeared to be sufficient to explain the shortened life span. Findings of other investigators provide general support for the conclusions of McCay et al. (Lane and Dickie, 1958; Ross, 1959; Bras and Ross, 1964; Simms and Berg, 1957, 1962; Berg and Simms, 1965). The relative incidence of lesions of four major diseases in male rats given restricted diets and in those fed ad libitum may be seen from Figure 14–1. Renal disease ("nephrosis") was found by Berg and Simms (1965) to be present in over 90 per cent of 700-day-old rats fed ad libitum but was absent in 700-day-old rats fed restricted amounts of the same diet (Fig. 14–1). Similarly, Bras and Ross (1964) found that the incidence of "progressive glomerulonephrosis" (presumably the same disease) differed remarkably between rats fed ad libitum and those fed the semi-synthetic diets in restricted amounts. Table 14–2 indicates the extent of the difference.

Not only specific diseases but the onset of a variety of changes ordinarily associated with aging can be delayed by dietary restriction. In rats, for example, Ross (1959) found that after one and a half years of ad libitum ingestion of a commercial diet most rats were obese and sluggish, had cataracts, chronic dermatitis of the extremities, coarse, sparse, discolored hair and dry, scaly skin. With restricted diets of various types it was found that even at two and a half years of age the animals were quite active, relatively thin, had thick coats of fine hair, no dermatitis, rarely showed evidence of disease and appeared to be much younger than their actual ages. The extent to which similar age-associated changes in the human may be accelerated or retarded by dietary influences is unknown.

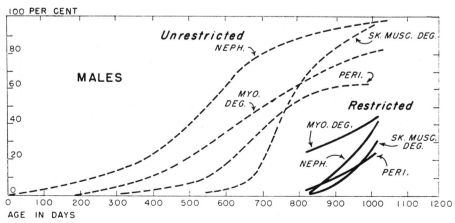

Figure 14–1. Incidence of lesions of four major diseases, namely, "nephrosis" (neph.), periarteritis (peri.), myocardial degeneration (myo. deg.), and skeletal and muscular degeneration (sk. musc. deg.) in male rats fed unrestricted or restricted amounts of the same diet. (From Berg, B. N., and Simms, H. S.: Canadian M.A.J. *93:* 911, 1965. The curves for the restricted rats are reproduced with the permission of the editor from Geriatrics *17:*235, 1962.)

Table 14–2. *Prevalence of "Progressive Glomerulonephrosis"*
in Rats in Relation to Diet

	Commercial Diet Fed Ad Libitum		Semisynthetic Diets Fed in Restricted Amounts							
			High Casein High Sugar		High Casein Low Sugar		Low Casein High Sugar		Low Casein Low Sugar	
Age (days)	Number of Rats	% PGN	Number of Rats	% PGN	Number of Rats	% PGN	Number of Rats	% PGN	Number of Rats	% PGN
600–699	119	3.4	157	0	73	0	161	.6	139	0
700–799	93	20.5	145	1.4	63	0	143	1.4	120	0
800–899	42	33.3	116	4.3	49	2.0	111	0.9	98	0
900–999	15	46.7	89	15.7	39	0	77	5.2	81	0

The possibility that atherosclerosis may have its onset in infancy has been discussed in Chapter Six. It was concluded that major efforts directed at maintenance of relatively low concentrations of lipids in serum throughout infancy is not warranted on the basis of currently available data. Further study is necessary. The possibility that high intakes of sodium chloride during infancy may predispose to subsequent hypertension has also been discussed (Chapter Nine).

Nutritional Imprinting

The animal studies mentioned thus far primarily concern caloric restriction imposed in rats at the time of weaning. Although such studies clearly indicate that consequences of dietary management may have far-reaching implications, they represent experiences of a more mature animal than the human infant. Studies of rats during the preweaning period, therefore, are of particular interest.

Some degree of nutritional imprinting may be produced in animals during early extrauterine life in such a manner as to influence subsequent rate of growth during ad libitum feeding. Undernutrition of calves during early growth results in reduction in size of the mature animal even though an abundant food supply is provided after the period of deprivation (Brookes and Vincett, 1950). Similarly, by reduction in the size of a rat litter with consequent provision of more milk for each individual, more rapid growth is achieved before weaning. As initially shown by Kennedy (1957) (Fig. 14–2) and subsequently confirmed by other investigators (Widdowson & McCance, 1960; Heggeness et al., 1961; McCance and Widdowson, 1962; Winick and

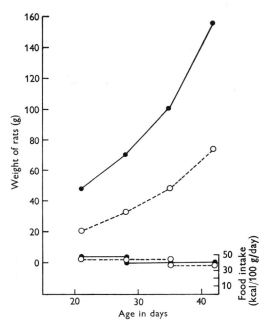

Figure 14-2. Mean growth and caloric intake of rats from small litters (solid dots) and those from large litters (open circles) during the first three weeks after weaning. Rats from small litters were larger at time of weaning (21 days) and remained larger during ad libitum feeding thereafter. (From Kennedy, J. G.: J. Endocrinol. *16*:9, 1957.)

Noble, 1966), rats from small litters not only grow more rapidly before weaning, but continue after weaning in spite of ad libitum feeding to be larger than rats from large litters. McCance and Widdowson (1962) and Winick and Noble (1966, 1967) have demonstrated that these differences in size persist into adult life (Table 14–3). Differences in size of the adult animals reflect differences in cell number in the various organs and tissues. Size of individual cells is little affected (Winick and Noble, 1966, 1967). In both calves and rats the timing of nutritional deprivation is of considerable importance. Prolonged nutritional deprivation during the preweaning period exerts a more profound influence on subsequent growth than does deprivation of shorter duration or deprivation imposed later in life.

When rats are severely restricted in food intake during pregnancy but not during lactation, the offspring are small at birth and remain permanently stunted (Chow and Lee, 1964). Food intake of the offspring after weaning is actually greater than that of normal rats of similar age, but protein metabolism is abnormal (Lee and Chow, 1965).

We do not yet know whether severe and prolonged nutritional deprivation during human infancy will result in reduction in size at maturity when food is permitted ad libitum after infancy. Children recovering from kwashiorkor appear to grow rapidly for several months but, in general, remain smaller than their peers for at least

Table 14–3. *Adult Body Size Attained by Rats Overfed or Underfed During the Preweaning Period and Fed Ad Libitum Thereafter**

	Litter Size	Body Weight (gm)	
		At weaning	Adult
Underfed	18	28.6	297.1
Control	9–12	59.1	376.4
Overfed	3–6	64.2	402.8

*Data of Winick and Noble (1966, 1967).

several years. However, as stated by Dean (1962), it has not yet been possible to conduct a long-continued, well controlled trial with ample diet to reveal the true growth potential of such children.

A point of great importance in nutritional practice in technically highly developed countries is raised by the results of studies with rats that were overfed during the preweaning period.

A concept shared by parents and physicians in highly developed countries depicts the ideally nourished infant as large and strong, with advanced motor skills. This concept probably evolved at a time when undernutrition was prevalent and many infants were small, weak and sickly. In countries in which gross undernutrition is now uncommon, it seems appropriate to ask whether there is a limit to the rate of growth and speed of maturation that we should attempt to achieve during infancy and childhood. Just how large and how well muscled do we wish our infants to be and how rapidly do we wish them to progress in motor skills? It seems possible that maximal rates of growth and maturation during infancy may not be associated with greatest life expectancy and most vigorous maturity. Duration of life in various animals has been shown by several investigators to be closely related to the rate at which the animal approaches its mature weight (Brody, 1945). We must consider the possibility that nutritional (or psychologic) imprinting during early life predisposes to our national problem of obesity in the adult population.

Meal-eating versus Nibbling

Not only the composition of the diet and the quantity consumed, but even the frequency of eating may have significant physiologic consequences. An identical intake of nutrients by rats or by certain other experimental animals produces different results if consumed as spaced meals than if consumed by "nibbling" throughout the day. Consequences of meal-eating as opposed to nibbling in various animals include alteration in activity of enzymes in several tissues, especially liver, alteration in activity of endocrines (thyroid and, possibly, gonads and pancreas), increases in serum lipid concentrations, in lipogenesis and in the development of atherosclerosis (Tepperman and Tepperman, 1958, 1964; Cohn and Joseph, 1960; Fábry et al., 1962; Hollifield and Parson, 1962; Cohn et al., 1962; Cohn, 1963; Stevenson et al., 1964).

From studies of adult human subjects it appears that intake of a small number of large meals tends to promote obesity, hypercholesterolemia and reduced glucose tolerance (Hejda and Fábry, 1964; Fábry et al., 1964; Cohn, 1964; Gwinup et al., 1963a and b).

Recently, children six to 16 years of age in three boarding schools were studied for one year while receiving three, five or seven meals daily (Fábry et al., 1966). Those receiving three meals daily demonstrated greater weight gain per unit gain in height and greater increase in skinfold thickness suggesting that less frequent (and larger) meals contributed to greater fat deposition.

The significance of these observations to infant nutrition is not yet clear. One wonders whether it is indeed reasonable that many parents consider reduction from six to three feedings in 24 hours to be an indication of desirable developmental progress. Whether possible nutritional disadvantages of this practice outweigh the obvious social advantages must await further study.

Consequences of Obesity

Although there can be no doubt that obesity in human adults is associated with decreased longevity and with increased incidence of certain diseases, factors other than diet may be of considerable importance in determining the relation between obesity and incidence of disease. To what extent familial or inherited propensity to obesity may be associated with genetically determined susceptibility to various diseases is unknown.

Marks (1960) has reported on the experience of the Metropolitan Life Insurance Company concerning individuals to whom life insurance policies were issued between 1925 and 1934. Among those charged higher than standard premium rates solely because of overweight, the observed number of deaths in the overweight individuals at the time of the policy anniversary in 1950 was significantly greater than in individuals of standard risk. Among men between 20 and 29 years of age who were overweight when the policies were issued, observed mortality was 180 per cent of the expected; among those between 40 and 49 years of age at the time the policies were issued, observed mortality was 152 per cent of the expected. Deaths from principal cardiovascular-renal diseases, numerically the most important in relation to total mortality, were approximately one and one-half times those of men of standard risk. Among overweight women, the death rate from principal cardiovascular-renal diseases was about one and three-quarters times that of women of standard risk.

An important area for study is the effect of overweight during infancy on subsequent incidence of obesity, on incidence of various diseases and on longevity.

Nutrition, Brain Growth and Mental Development

Questions of extreme importance concern the relation of nutritional status during early development (prenatal or postnatal) to rate of brain growth, rate of mental development and ultimate mental capacity. Unfortunately, it is exceptionally difficult to design studies that will clarify these relationships even in experimental animals, and problems in designing studies with human subjects are even greater.

When littermate rats are caused to differ in size through dietary management in the preweaning period, more rapid rates of physical, motor and sexual development are noted in the larger rats; in addition, during early life the larger rats demonstrate a greater tendency to explore their surroundings, implying a greater degree of maturation of the central nervous system (Lát et al., 1961).

Severe undernutrition of infant pigs has been shown to influence chemical composition of the brain in such a way that concentrations of sodium, chloride and potassium resemble those of considerably younger pigs (Widdowson et al., 1960). Electroencephalograms of malnourished pigs (Platt et al., 1965) resemble in certain respects those of children with kwashiorkor (Nelson and Dean, 1959). Electroencephalograms of young adults living in regions where protein-calorie malnutrition is prevalent demonstrate an abnormality that may conceivably represent residual damage from early malnutrition (Gallais et al., 1951a and b).

In technically underdeveloped countries, motor development in infancy and early childhood has been shown to be significantly correlated with body size (Geber and Dean, 1957; Cravioto, 1963). Among schoolchildren, also, those who are physically advanced in relation to chronologic age score higher in mental tests than those of the same age who are less mature physically (Tanner, 1963).

Infants and children with kwashiorkor perform poorly in motor, adaptive, language and social-personal behavior (Cravioto and Robles, 1965; Cravioto et al., 1966). During recovery from kwashiorkor, rate of progress in behavioral development appears to be related to age. Children 37 to 41 months of age when admitted to the hospital demonstrated relatively rapid behavioral development during recovery; less rapid development was evidenced by those 15 to 29 months of age, and relatively little progress by those three to six months of age. As is true with respect to physical growth of animals after an interval of caloric deprivation, the earlier the period of deprivation, the more serious would seem to be the consequences.

In relation to this latter observation, it may be significant that food restriction from birth to weaning in the rat was shown to be associated with permanent changes in size and chemical composition of the brain (Winick and Noble, 1966), but food restriction for an equal period of time but imposed at weaning resulted in alterations that disappeared during a subsequent period of adequate nutrition. Dobbing and Widdowson (1965) have also demonstrated that the abnormality in myelination of the brain of rats brought about by undernutrition from the time of weaning (age three weeks) to age 11 weeks was corrected during ingestion of a normal diet between ages 11 and 19 weeks.

It seems necessary to consider the possibility that malnutrition during infancy may exert significant adverse effects on later performance even in the absence of permanent mental damage. Adequate achievement in school requires extensive preschool education which must begin during early infancy. Chronic illness during infancy may change a reasonably well-motivated child to one who is apathetic and disinterested in his surroundings. Deficiency of calories or of any essential nutrient is likely to have this effect, and a year or two of interruption in the preschool educational process may yield a child who at six years of age has reached the level of maturity of a normal four to five year old. Such a child may perform poorly in the early school years and then be inadequately prepared to benefit maximally from later schooling.

REFERENCES

Berg, B. N., and Simms, H. S.: Nutrition and longevity in the rat. II. Longevity and onset of disease with different levels of food intake. J. Nutrition 71:255, 1960.
Berg, B. N., and Simms, H. S.: Nutrition, onset of disease, and longevity in the rat. Canad. M. A. J. 93:911, 1965.
Bras, G., and Ross, M. H.: Kidney disease and nutrition in the rat. Tox. & Appl. Pharm. 6:247, 1964.

Brody, S.: Bioenergetics and Growth. New York, Reinhold Publishing Corp., 1945.

Brookes, A. J., and Vincett, L. S.: Beef production experiment at Cambridge. Interim report. J. Roy. Agric. Soc. Engl. V. 111:99, 1950.

Chow, B. F., and Lee, C. J.: Effect of dietary restriction of pregnant rats on body weight gain of the offspring. J. Nutrition 82:10, 1964.

Cohn, C.: Feeding frequency and body composition. Ann. N. Y. Acad. Sci. 110:395, 1963.

Cohn, C.: Feeding patterns and some aspects of cholesterol metabolism. Fed. Proc. 23:76, 1964.

Cohn, C., and Joseph, D.: Role of rate of ingestion of diet on regulation of intermediary metabolism ("meal eating" vs. "nibbling"). Metabolism 9:492, 1960.

Cohn, C., Joseph, D., and Allweiss, M. D.: Nutritional effects of feeding frequency. Am. J. Clin. Nutr. 11:356, 1962.

Cravioto, J.: Application of newer knowledge of nutrition on physical and mental growth and development. Am. J. Pub. Health 53:1803, 1963.

Cravioto, J., DeLicardie, E. R., and Birch, H. G.: Nutrition, growth and neurointegrative development: an experimental and ecologic study. Pediatrics 38:319, 1966.

Cravioto, J., and Robles, B.: Evolution of adaptive and motor behavior during rehabilitation from kwashiorkor. Am. J. Orthopsychiatry 25:449, 1965.

Dean, R. F. A.: Nutrition and growth. In Hottinger, A., and Berger, H.: Modern Problems in Pediatrics, Basel, Karger, 1962, vol. 7, p. 191.

Dobbing, J., and Widdowson, E. M.: The effect of undernutrition and subsequent rehabilitation on myelination of rat brain as measured by its composition. Brain 88:357, 1965.

Fábry, P., Petrásek, R., Braun, T., Bednárek, M., Horáková, E., and Konopásek, E.: Lipogenesis in rats adapted to intermittent starvation or continuous underfeeding. Experientia 18:555, 1962.

Fábry, P., Hejl, Z., Foder, J., Braun, T. and Zvolánková, K.: The frequency of meals. Its relation to overweight, hypercholesterolaemia, and decreased glucose-tolerance. Lancet 2:614, 1964.

Fábry, P., Hejda, S., Černý, K., Ošancová, M. A., Pechar, J., and Zvolánková, K.: Effect of meal frequency in schoolchildren. Changes in weight-height proportion and skinfold thickness. Am. J. Clin. Nutr. 18:358, 1966.

Fomon, S. J., and Owen, G. M.: Influence of age, sex and diet on rate of growth and body composition during early infancy. In Cuthbertson, D. P., Mills, C. F., and Passmore, R. (eds.): Proceedings of the Sixth International Congress of Nutrition. Edinburgh, E. & S. Livingstone, Ltd., 1964, p. 66.

Gallais, P., Bert, J., Corriol, J., and Miletto, G.: Les rythmes EEG des noirs d'Afrique (étude des 100 premiers tracés de sujets normaux). Electroenceph. Clin. Neurophysiol. 3:110, 1951a.

Gallais, P., Miletto, G., Corriol, J., and Bert, J.: Introduction á l' étude d'EEG physiologique du noir d'Afrique. Méd. Trop. 11:128, 1951b.

Geber, M., and Dean, R. F. A.: Gesell tests on African children. Pediatrics 20:1055, 1957.

Gwinup, G., Byron, R. C., Roush, W. H., Kruger, F. A., and Hamwi, G. J.: Effect of nibbling versus gorging on serum lipids in man. Am. J. Clin. Nutr. 13:209, 1963a.

Gwinup, G., Roush, W., Byron, R. C., Kruger, F., and Hamwi, G. J.: Effect of nibbling versus gorging on glucose tolerance. Lancet 2:165, 1963b.

Heggeness, F. W., Binoschadler, D., Chadwick, J., Conklin, P., Hulnick, S., and Oaks, M.: Weight gains of overnourished and undernourished preweaning rats. J. Nutrition 75:39, 1961.

Hejda, S., and Fábry, P.: Frequency of food intake in relation to some parameters of the nutritional status. Nutr. Dieta 6:216, 1964.

Hollifield, G., and Parson, W.: Metabolic adaptations to a "stuff and starve" feeding program. I. Studies of adipose tissue and liver glycogen in rats limited to a short daily feeding period. J. Clin. Invest. 41:245, 1962.

Jones, H. B.: The background of research in the biology of aging. Research in Gerontology: Biological and Medical. Series Number 10, Washington, D.C., Department of Health, Education, and Welfare, 1961, p. 13.

Kennedy, J. G.: The development with age of hypothalamic restraint upon the appetite of the rat. J. Endocrinol. 16:9, 1957.

Lane, P. W., and Dickie, M. M.: The effect of restricted food intake on the life span of genetically obese mice. J. Nutrition 64:549, 1958.

Lát, J., Widdowson, E. M., and McCance, R. A.: Some effects of accelerating growth. III. Behaviour and nervous activity. Proc. Roy. Soc. B. 153:347, 1961.

Lee, C. J., and Chow, B. F.: Protein metabolism in the offspring of underfed mother rats. J. Nutrition 87:439, 1965.

Marks, H. H.: Influence of obesity on morbidity and mortality. Bull. N. Y. Acad. Med. 36:296, 1960.

McCance, R. A., and Widdowson, E. M.: Nutrition and growth. Proc. Roy. Soc. B. 156: 326, 1962.

McCay, C. M., Crowell, M. F., and Maynard, L. A.: The effect of retarded growth upon the length of life span and upon the ultimate body size. J. Nutrition 10:63, 1935.

McCay, C. M., Sperling, G., and Barnes, L. L.: Growth, ageing, chronic diseases, and life span in rats. Arch. Biochem. 2:469, 1943.

Nelson, G. K., and Dean, R. F. A.: The electroencephalogram in African children: effects of kwashiorkor and a note on the newborn. Bull. World Health Organ. 21:779, 1959.

Platt, B. S., Pampiglione, G., and Stewart, R. J. C.: Experimental protein-calorie deficiency. Clinical, electroencephalographic and neuropathological changes in pigs. Develop. Med. Child. Neurol. 7:9, 1965.

Ross, M. H.: Protein, calories and life expectancy. Fed. Proc. 18:1190, 1959.

Ross, M. H.: Length of life and nutrition in the rat. J. Nutrition 75:197, 1961.

Saxton, J. A., Jr.: In Moore, R. A., (ed.): Biological Symposia, Vol. XI, Ageing and Degenerative Diseases. Lancaster, Pa., Jaques Cattell Press, 1945, p. 177.

Simms, H. S., and Berg, B. N.: Longevity and the onset of lesions in male rats. J. Gerontol. 12:244, 1957.

Simms, H. S., and Berg, B. N.: Longevity in relation to lesion onset. Geriatrics 17:235, 1962.

Stevenson, J. A. F., Feleki, V., Svlavko, A., and Beaton, J. R.: Food restriction and lipogenesis in the rat. Proc. Soc. Exp. Biol. & Med. 116:178, 1964.

Tanner, J. M.: Growth at Adolescence. 2nd ed. Oxford, Blackwell Scientific Publications, 1963.

Tepperman, H. M., and Tepperman, J.: Adaptive hyperlipogenesis. Fed. Proc. 23: 73, 1964.

Tepperman, J., and Tepperman, H. M.: Effects of antecedent food intake pattern on hepatic lipogenesis. Am. J. Physiol. 193:55, 1958.

Widdowson, E. M., Dickerson, J. W., and McCance, R. A.: Severe undernutrition in growing and adult animals. 4. The impact of severe undernutrition on the chemical composition of the soft tissues of the pig. Brit. J. Nutr. 14:457, 1960.

Widdowson, E. M., and McCance, R. A.: Some effects of accelerating growth. I. General somatic development. Proc. Roy. Soc. B. 152:188, 1960.

Winick, M., and Noble, A.: Cellular response during malnutrition at various ages. J. Nutrition 89:300, 1966.

Winick, M., and Noble, A.: Cellular response with increased feeding in neonatal rats. J. Nutrition 91:179, 1967.

Appendices

Composition of

Item No. (A)	Food and description (B)	Water (C)	Food energy (D)	Protein (E)	Fat (F)	Carbohydrate Total (G)	Carbohydrate Fiber (H)
	Baby foods: [11]	*Percent*	*Calories*	*Grams*	*Grams*	*Grams*	*Grams*
	Cereals, precooked, dry, and other cereal products:						
67	Barley, added nutrients_____	6. 6	348	13. 4	1. 2	73. 6	1. 2
68	High protein, added nutrients_____	5. 9	357	35. 2	3. 7	48. 1	2. 2
69	Mixed, added nutrients_____	6. 5	368	15. 2	2. 9	70. 6	1. 1
70	Oatmeal, added nutrients_____	7. 0	375	16. 5	5. 5	66. 0	1. 5
71	Rice, added nutrients_____	7. 2	371	6. 6	1. 6	80. 0	. 5
72	Teething biscuit_____	5. 6	378	11. 1	2. 3	78. 0	. 7
	Wheat. See Farina, instant-cooking: items 995–996.						
	Desserts, canned:						
73	Custard pudding, all flavors_____	76. 5	100	2. 3	1. 8	18. 6	. 2
74	Fruit pudding with starch base, milk and/or egg (banana, orange, or pineapple).	75. 7	96	1. 2	. 9	21. 6	. 3
	Dinners, canned:						
	Cereal, vegetable, meat mixtures (approx. 2%–4% protein):						
75	Beef noodle dinner_____	88. 2	48	2. 8	1. 1	6. 8	. 3
76	Cereal, egg yolk, and bacon_____	84. 7	82	2. 9	4. 9	6. 6	. 1
77	Chicken noodle dinner_____	88. 5	49	2. 1	1. 3	7. 2	. 1
78	Macaroni, tomatoes, meat, and cereal_____	84. 5	67	2. 6	2. 0	9. 6	. 3
79	Split peas, vegetables, and ham or bacon_____	81. 5	80	4. 0	2. 1	11. 2	. 2
80	Vegetables and bacon, with cereal_____	85. 7	68	1. 7	2. 9	8. 7	. 4
81	Vegetables and beef, with cereal_____	87. 0	56	2. 7	1. 6	7. 6	. 4
82	Vegetables and chicken, with cereal_____	87. 8	52	2. 1	1. 4	7. 7	. 2
83	Vegetables and ham, with cereal_____	85. 6	64	2. 8	2. 2	8. 3	. 3
84	Vegetables and lamb, with cereal_____	87. 0	58	2. 2	2. 0	7. 7	0. 3
85	Vegetables and liver, with cereal_____	87. 8	47	3. 1	. 4	7. 8	. 3
86	Vegetables and liver, with bacon and cereal___	87. 2	57	2. 4	1. 9	7. 5	. 3
87	Vegetables and turkey, with cereal_____	88. 9	44	2. 1	. 8	7. 2	. 2
	Meat or poultry (approx. 6%–8% protein):						
88	Beef with vegetables_____	81. 6	87	7. 4	3. 7	6. 0	. 2
89	Chicken with vegetables_____	79. 6	100	7. 4	4. 6	7. 2	. 2
90	Turkey with vegetables_____	81. 3	86	6. 7	3. 2	7. 6	. 5
91	Veal with vegetables_____	85. 0	63	7. 1	1. 6	5. 1	. 2
	Fruits and fruit products, with or without thickening, canned:						
92	Applesauce_____	80. 8	72	. 2	. 2	18. 6	. 5
93	Applesauce and apricots_____	76. 7	86	. 3	. 1	22. 6	. 5
94	Bananas (with tapioca or cornstarch, added ascorbic acid), strained.	77. 5	84	. 4	. 2	21. 6	. 1
95	Bananas and pineapple (with tapioca or cornstarch).	78. 5	80	. 4	. 1	20. 7	. 1
96	Fruit dessert with tapioca (apricot, pineapple, and/or orange).	77. 6	84	. 3	. 3	21. 5	. 2
97	Peaches_____	78. 1	81	. 6	. 2	20. 7	. 5
98	Pears_____	82. 2	66	. 3	. 1	17. 1	1. 0
99	Pears and pineapple_____	81. 5	69	. 4	. 2	17. 6	. 9
100	Plums with tapioca, strained_____	74. 8	94	. 4	. 2	24. 3	. 3
101	Prunes with tapioca_____	76. 7	86	. 3	. 2	22. 4	. 3
	Meats, poultry, and eggs; canned:						
	Beef:						
102	Strained_____	80. 3	99	14. 7	4. 0	(0)	(0)
103	Junior_____	75. 6	118	19. 3	3. 9	(0)	(0)
104	Beef heart_____	81. 1	93	13. 5	3. 8	. 4	(0)
105	Chicken_____	77. 2	127	13. 7	7. 6	(0)	(0)
106	Egg yolks, strained_____	70. 0	210	10. 0	18. 4	. 2	(0)
107	Egg yolks with ham or bacon_____	70. 3	208	10. 0	18. 1	. 3	(0)
	Lamb:						
108	Strained_____	79. 3	107	14. 6	4. 9	(0)	(0)
109	Junior_____	76. 0	121	17. 5	5. 1	(0)	(0)
110	Liver, strained_____	79. 7	97	14. 1	3. 4	1. 5	(0)
111	Liver and bacon, strained_____	77. 0	123	13. 7	6. 6	1. 3	(0)
	Pork:						
112	Strained_____	77. 7	118	15. 4	5. 8	(0)	(0)
113	Junior_____	74. 3	134	18. 6	6. 0	(0)	(0)
	Veal:						
114	Strained_____	80. 7	91	15. 5	2. 7	(0)	(0)
115	Junior_____	76. 9	107	18. 8	3. 0	(0)	(0)
	Vegetables, canned:						
116	Beans, green_____	92. 5	22	1. 4	. 1	5. 1	. 8
117	Beets, strained_____	89. 2	37	1. 4	. 1	8. 3	. 6
118	Carrots_____	91. 5	29	. 7	. 1	6. 8	. 6
119	Mixed vegetables, including vegetable soup_____	88. 5	37	1. 6	. 3	8. 5	. 5
120	Peas, strained_____	85. 5	54	4. 2	. 2	9. 3	. 8
121	Spinach, creamed_____	88. 1	43	2. 3	. 7	7. 5	. 4
122	Squash_____	92. 1	25	. 7	. 1	6. 2	. 8
123	Sweetpotatoes_____	82. 3	67	1. 0	. 2	15. 5	. 5
124	Tomato soup, strained_____	83. 4	54	1. 9	. 1	13. 5	. 2

Infant Foods ☼

Ash (I)	Calcium (J)	Phosphorus (K)	Iron (L)	Sodium (M)	Potassium (N)	Vitamin A value (O)	Thiamine (P)	Riboflavin (Q)	Niacin (R)	Ascorbic acid (S)
Grams	Milligrams	Milligrams	Milligrams	Milligrams	Milligrams	International units	Milligrams	Milligrams	Milligrams	Milligrams
5.2	736	821	53.2	452	413	(0)	3.71	1.20	32.2	(0)
7.1	815	904	63.1	653	1,078	—	3.67	1.15	24.0	(0)
4.8	820	741	56.4	470	345	—	3.15	1.35	22.3	(0)
5.0	757	734	48.2	437	374	(0)	2.58	1.05	21.3	(0)
4.6	858	646	50.2	530	208	(0)	2.56	1.24	19.7	(0)
3.0	322	347	4.6	421	250	—	.47	.57	3.0	(0)
.8	64	62	.3	150	94	100	.02	.12	.1	1
.6	27	34	.3	128	75	100	.03	.05	.1	3
1.1	12	29	.5	269	159	620	.02	.05	.5	2
.9	29	60	.8	301	36	520	.05	.06	.4	—
.9	27	30	.3	297	42	800	.03	.06	.4	1
1.3	21	35	.5	381	77	500	.14	.12	1.0	1
1.2	29	79	.7	295	112	600	.08	.05	.5	1
1.0	17	28	.6	282	130	2,200	.07	.05	.6	1
1.1	17	39	.8	307	143	2,800	.03	.04	.9	1
1.0	33	33	.4	307	55	1,000	.03	.04	.5	Trace
1.1	25	42	.3	360	90	1,000	.08	.05	.5	3
1.1	23	37	0.7	269	148	2,200	0.03	0.05	0.7	1
.9	17	57	2.7	236	162	4,700	.04	.37	1.6	3
1.0	11	42	2.6	284	131	4,600	.03	.33	1.3	2
1.0	22	26	.3	307	46	400	.01	.03	.4	1
1.3	13	84	1.2	304	113	1,100	.07	.17	1.6	2
1.2	22	85	.9	265	71	1,000	.09	.15	1.6	2
1.2	38	63	.6	348	122	1,000	.13	.13	1.8	2
1.2	11	71	.8	323	95	800	.08	.15	2.0	2
.2	4	7	.4	6	64	40	.01	.02	.1	Trace
.3	4	14	.3	(⁴)	105	600	.01	.02	.1	2
.3	13	10	.2	29	118	70	.02	.02	.2	35
.3	20	12	.2	59	72	30	.01	.01	.1	2
.3	15	9	.4	53	73	450	.02	.01	.2	4
.4	6	14	.3	(⁴)	80	500	.01	.02	.7	3
.3	7	8	.2	4	62	30	.02	.02	.2	2
.3	7	12	.2	(⁴)	72	20	.03	.02	.2	2
.3	5	12	.4	38	44	250	.01	.02	.2	2
.4	7	21	.9	33	120	400	.02	.06	.4	4
1.0	8	127	2.0	228	183	—	.01	.16	3.5	0
1.4	8	163	2.5	283	242	—	.02	.20	4.3	0
1.2	5	155	3.7	208	—	—	.06	.62	3.6	0
1.5	—	129	1.9	263	96	—	.02	.16	3.5	0
1.4	81	256	3.0	273	59	1,900	.12	.22	Trace	Trace
1.3	71	185	2.8	313	82	1,900	.10	.23	5	—
1.2	9	124	2.1	241	181	—	.02	.17	3.3	—
1.4	13	156	2.7	294	228	—	.02	.21	4.1	—
1.3	6	182	5.6	253	202	24,000	.05	2.00	7.6	10
1.4	6	157	4.2	302	192	22,000	.05	1.99	7.8	7
1.1	8	130	1.5	223	178	—	.19	.20	2.7	—
1.3	8	144	1.2	237	210	—	.23	.23	2.8	—
1.1	10	145	1.7	226	214	—	.03	.20	4.3	—
1.4	8	157	1.6	276	206	—	.03	.22	6.0	—
.9	33	25	1.1	213	93	400	.02	.06	.3	3
1.0	18	27	.7	212	228	20	.02	.03	.1	3
.9	23	21	.5	169	181	13,000	.02	.03	.4	3
1.1	22	36	.9	272	170	4,700	.05	.04	.6	2
.8	11	63	1.2	194	100	500	.08	.09	1.2	10
1.4	64	63	.6	272	142	5,000	.02	.13	.3	6
.9	24	17	.4	292	138	2,400	.02	.04	.3	8
1.0	16	34	.4	187	180	4,900	.04	.03	.4	8
1.1	24	52	.4	294	300	1,000	.05	.12	.7	3

From Composition of Foods. Agriculture Handbook No. 8. Washington, D.C., U.S. Department of Agriculture. 1963.

☼Composition per 100 gm of food.

Appendix II

Collection of Urine
and Feces and
Metabolic Balance Studies

Nutritional evaluation of infants may require quantitative collection of specimens of urine and/or feces for periods of 24 to 72 hours. Occasionally, a 72-hour metabolic balance study with accurate analysis of intake as well as urinary and fecal excretion will be helpful. It should be noted that intakes of infants receiving milk or formula as exclusive or major source of calories can be measured with much greater accuracy than can mixed diets of older children or adults. Methods previously described by the author and his associates (Fomon et al., 1958; Fomon, 1960) will therefore be reviewed in some detail. Alternate procedures for collecting urine or for carrying out metabolic balance studies with infants have been described by Newberry and Van Wyk (1955), Geist (1960) and Hepner and Lubchenco (1960).

Quantitative collections of urine from infants are necessary not only in metabolic balance studies but in determining urinary excretion of endogenous creatinine and hydroxyproline, in certain loading tests employed to detect nutritional and metabolic abnormalities, and in investigation or management of a variety of disorders unrelated to nutrition. Quantitative determination of fecal excretion of fat is often of great value even when a metabolic balance study is not performed.

282

Many reports published during the past 60 years indicate the usefulness of metabolic balance studies in at least three areas of investigation: (1) comparison of nutritional properties of foods fed to comparable groups of human subjects or experimental animals under standardized conditions, (2) comparison of performance of normal subjects or experimental animals with those having certain metabolic abnormalities, and (3) comparison of the effects of two regimens of management with a single subject.

Procedure

Metabolic Bed and Accessories

Metabolic beds of the design employed by the author and his associates (Fomon et al., 1958, 1962) are not commercially available but may be constructed from wood in almost any carpentry shop. A drawing indicating dimensions is presented in Figure A-II–1 and a photograph appears in Figure A-II–2.

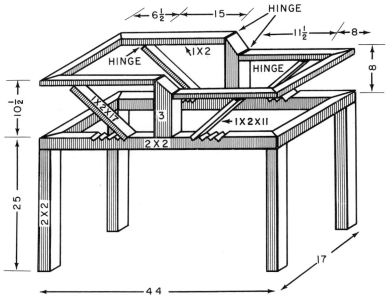

Figure A-II–1. Dimensions of frame for metabolic bed. (From Fomon, S. J., Thomas, L. N., Jensen, R. L. and Owen, G. M.: Pediatrics 29:330, 1962.)

Lacing the canvas to the frame of the metabolic bed, as shown in Figure A-II–2, requires some practice since the comfort of the infant is dependent upon having this canvas quite taut.

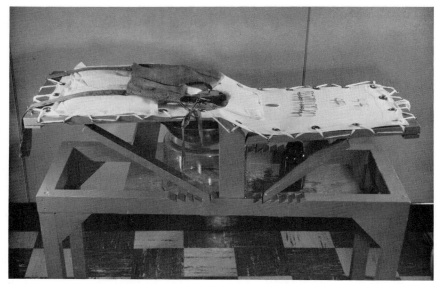

Figure A-II-2. Metabolic bed. Canvas has been laced tightly to frame and jacket is in place. Foam rubber has been placed around the larger circular hole in the canvas and covered with plastic sheeting held in place with safety pins. The metal pan for collection of feces (urine plus feces from a girl) may be seen. A smaller circular hole in the canvas permits the rubber tubing of the apparatus (for collection of urine from boys) to be led directly to the collection jar.

A piece of plastic sheeting is attached as an apron across the abdomen of a girl and pinned to the lower portion of the restraining jacket to direct urine into the metal pan. (From Fomon, S. J., Thomas, L. N., Jensen, R. L., and May, C. D.: Pediatrics 22:94, 1958.)

The restraining jacket used for maintaining the infant's position on the metabolic bed is shown in Figures A-II-3 and A-II-4.

APPARATUS FOR BOYS. Apparatus employed in urine collection from boys is prepared from a finger cot or finger of a rubber glove, adhesive tape, a glass adapter and a length of rubber tubing. A stellate perforation, large enough to accomodate the finger cot, is made toward one end of an eight-inch length of three- to four-inch-wide adhesive tape. The other end of the adhesive tape is cut down the center to make two tails that are one inch wide and at least eight inches long (Fig. A-II-5). Narrow strips of adhesive are cut diagonally to provide reinforcement pieces. The finger cot is fringed at the open end by making quarter-inch cuts into it. The cot is then pushed through the stellate perforation from the adhesive side of the tape. The fringed end of the cot is pressed to the adhesive tape and anchored with the reinforcement pieces as shown in Figure A-II-6.

The distal end of the finger cot is then cut off and the apparatus is placed on the infant so that the penis projects into the finger cot. The adhesive tails are brought around the upper posterior part of the thighs, leaving the rectum exposed; tincture of benzoin applied to

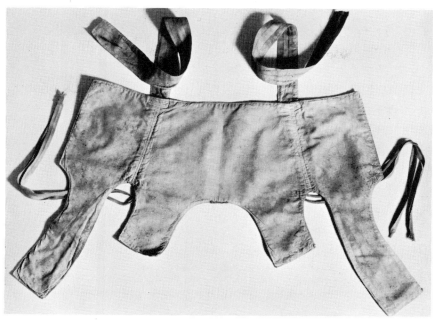

Figure A-II-3. Jacket for maintaining infant in position on the metabolic bed. The wide upper ribbons are attached to the head of the metabolic bed and the narrow lower ribbons are attached to the sides of the bed (Fig. A II-2). The central panel of the jacket is pinned to the canvas of the bed. With the infant lying supine on the jacket, the side panels are folded toward the center (Fig. A II-4) and pinned about the thighs of the infant. (From Fomon, S. J., Thomas, L. N., Jensen, R. L., and May, C. D.: Pediatrics 22:94, 1958.)

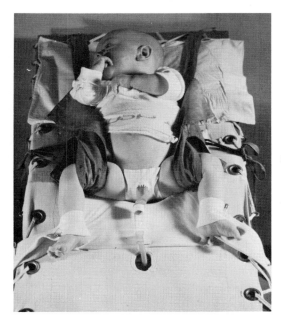

Figure A-11-4. Infant restrained on metabolic bed.

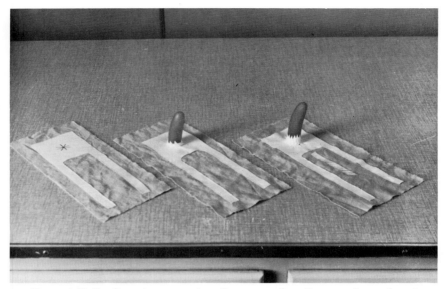

Figure A-II–5.   Steps in preparation of apparatus for collection of urine from boys. Front view. Left, Adhesive tape has been cut in the proper shape with two long strips of the tape arising from a square central portion. The adhesive tape is mounted on a piece of cloth. A stellate incision for insertion of the finger cot has been made. Center, The finger cot has been inserted from the rear. Right, Additional small strips of adhesive tape have been placed around the base of the finger cot. The end of the finger cot is then cut off and the finger cot attached to a glass adapter from which rubber tubing leads to the collection bottle.

When the adapter has been removed from the cloth and the central portion of the adhesive surface placed against the pubis with the infant's penis projecting into the finger cot, the long strips of adhesive tape are made to encircle the posterior aspect of the upper portion of the thigh. (From Fomon, S. J., Thomas, L. N., Jensen, R. L., and May, C. D.: Pediatrics 22:94, 1958.)

the appropriate area of skin affords some protection against excoriation that might otherwise arise from the tape. The free end of the finger cot is slipped over the glass adapter (made from a test tube) and secured with adhesive tape. The tapered end of the adapter is inserted into rubber tubing which leads to a urine collection bottle. Some practice is required in preparing this adapter for collection of urine. Leakage of urine will occur unless it is well-constructed.

APPARATUS FOR GIRLS.   In metabolic balance studies with girls, an adapter for separate urine collection is not employed. A piece of polyethylene sheeting attached to the abdomen of the infant is directed through the larger opening of the canvas on which the infant lies. This sheeting extends into a metal pan so constructed that the central portion is elevated 0.25 to 0.5 cm above the remaining portion. The elevated portion of this pan is placed beneath the infant in such a fashion that feces will fall onto the central elevated area while urine will flow by gravity into the shallow depression around the periphery. The method employed in obtaining an estimate of separate urinary and fecal excretion from girls will be described.

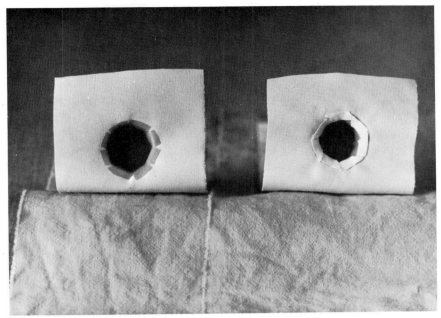

Figure A-II–6. Steps in preparation of apparatus for collection of urine from boys. Rear view. Left, The finger cot has been inserted through the stellate incision in the adhesive tape. Right, Small strips of adhesive tape have been put in place. (From Fomon, S. J., Thomas, L. N., Jensen, R. L., and May, C. D.: Pediatrics 22:94, 1958.

The infant is restrained on the metabolic bed as indicated in Figure A-II–4.

Feeding

Metabolic balance studies with infants are greatly facilitated if the sole food given during the balance study consists of formula supplied by a manufacturer in ready-to-feed disposable units. It is then probable that concentration of any one bottle of formula will be representative of that of all food consumed. However, several bottles of formula should be selected at random for analysis.

At 8 A.M. on the day the metabolic balance period is to begin, sufficient carmine is added to the milk or formula to contribute a definite pink color. The infant is placed on the metabolic bed at about 8:20 A.M., and the time of the first voiding of urine thereafter is noted. This specimen and all urine voided during the ensuing 72 hours is saved. Later in the day when the first stool containing carmine is passed, the carmine-containing portion is saved as the first aliquot of the 72-hour collection of feces. Seventy-two hours after the initial administration of carmine, another bottle of milk or formula with carmine is given. When the stool containing this second dose of carmine is passed, that portion of the stool not containing carmine is saved as the last aliquot of feces to be included in the 72-hour collection. The infant is then removed from the metabolic bed.

Collection of Urine and Feces

Urine and feces are collected separately from boys with the aid of the apparatus shown and described in Figures A-II–2 through A-II–6.

Two containers are used for storage of urine from each girl, one for "uncontaminated urine" and one for urine contaminated with feces. By close observation of the infants and by transferring urine to the storage container in the refrigerator soon after each voiding, it is usually possible to obtain the greater portion of the 72-hour specimen of urine uncontaminated with feces. The volumes of uncontaminated and contaminated urine are then measured and the contaminated specimen added to the fecal collection.

The *total excretion* of nitrogen (or mineral) is determined by multiplying the value for volume of urine with that for concentration of nitrogen in uncontaminated urine and adding to this result the volume and concentration of nitrogen in the fecal homogenate to which urine contaminated with feces was added.

The *urinary excretion* of nitrogen is estimated from the total volume of urine (contaminated with feces and uncontaminated) and the concentration of nitrogen in the uncontaminated urine. Fecal excretion of nitrogen is obtained by subtracting the estimated urinary excretion from the total.

Misuse of Metabolic Balance Studies

Successful use of metabolic balance studies in nutritional evaluation of two foods under satisfactorily controlled circumstances or in comparison of performance of normal subjects with subjects having certain metabolic abnormalities has sometimes led individuals to conclude that results of metabolic balance studies are precisely quantitative. Were this true, it would be possible on the basis of continuously or serially performed balance studies between two specified ages to make an accurate calculation of the change in one or another aspect of body composition. For example, the change in nitrogen or calcium content of the body could be calculated; from the change in nitrogen content, the change in protein content could be estimated, and from the change in calcium content, the change in skeletal mass could be estimated.

As an example, one might consider a normal infant with a birth weight of 3500 gm. If protein comprised 11 per cent of body weight at birth, content of the body at birth (assuming that nitrogen accounts for 16 per cent by weight of protein) would be 61 gm. The mean retention of nitrogen in 3-day metabolic balance studies performed biweekly from birth until six months of age, with the infant receiving a high-protein formula (3.5 gm protein in 100 ml) might be 1.25 gm/day, or 228 gm in 182 days. The total content of nitrogen in the body at six months of age would be 228 gm + 61 gm = 289 gm. With a body weight of 8.28 kg at six months of age (Table 2–6), protein would account for 21.8 per cent of the body weight.

Because a protein content of the body equal to 21.8 per cent of body weight is far more than has been found by direct chemical analysis of the human body (Chapter Two), it is clear that the calculations given above are not justified.

It seems probable that several factors must be considered jointly in explaining the falsely high body content of protein calculated on the basis of nitrogen balance studies. Of these, the most important are probably cumulative errors in balance techniques, nitrogen loss in sweat and desquamated epithelium and, especially, differences in retention of nitrogen during balance studies and in intervals between balance studies. Confirmation or refutation of the conclusion based on metabolic balance studies — that feeding of high-protein diets results in accumulation of relatively large amounts of protein in the body — must certainly come from assessments of body composition of normal infants made with techniques other than metabolic balance studies.

Similar errors are inherent in calculating body content of calcium, phosphorus, sodium, and other minerals from results of metabolic balance studies. With some substances, e.g., sodium and potassium, failure to measure losses from skin will introduce a much greater error than is the case with nitrogen or calcium.

REFERENCES

Fomon, S. J.: Comparative study of adequacy of protein from human milk and cow's milk in promoting nitrogen retention by normal full-term infants. Pediatrics 26:51, 1960.

Fomon, S. J., Thomas, L. N., Jensen, R. L., and May, C. D.: Determination of nitrogen balance of infants less than 6 months of age. Pediatrics 22:94, 1958.

Fomon, S. J., Thomas, L. N., Jensen, R. L., and Owen, G. M.: (Letters to Editor) Metabolic bed. Pediatrics 29:330, 1962.

Geist, D. I.: Round-the-clock specimens. Am. J. Nursing 60:1300, 1960.

Hepner, R., and Lubchenco, L. O.: A method for continuous urine and stool collection in young infants. Pediatrics 26:828, 1960.

Newberry, E., and Van Wyk, J. J.: A technique for quantitative urine collection in the metabolic study of infants and young children. Pediatrics 16:667, 1955.

INDEX

Page numbers set in *italics* indicate figures; those followed by a T signify a table.

Adipose tissue, significance of, 32
Advisable intake(s)
  of amino acids, 75
  of ascorbic acid, 127
  of calcium, 142T, 143
  of chloride, 140, 141T
  of copper, 187
  of fat, 85
  of fluoride, 183
  of food, 41
  of iron, 179
  of magnesium, 142T, 143
  of major minerals, 139
  of phosphorus, 142T, 143
  of potassium, 140, 141T
  of protein, 74
    estimated, 74T
  of sodium, 140, 141T
  of vitamin A, 115
  of vitamin B$_6$, 132
  of vitamin D, 119
  of vitamin E, 122
  of vitamin K, 124
  of zinc, 191
Age, influence on excretion of fat, 92T
Alacta, composition of, 205T
Albumin, serum, 71. See also *Serum, protein in.*
  concentrations of, 69
Allergy, food, definition of, 226
  milk. See *Milk allergy.*

Alpha-tocopherol, in plasma and milk, 122T
Amino acids. See also *Protein(s).*
  advisable intakes of, 75
  essential, 58–59.
  imbalance of, 58
    effects of, 59T
  requirements for, 75
  toxicity from, 58
Anemia
  hypocupremia and, 187
  iron deficiency, 166–180
    incidence among infants, 167
  megaloblastic, vitamin B$_{12}$ and, 134
  of infancy, definition of, 166
  prevention of, aims in, 169
Arginine, 58
Ascorbic acid, 126
  advisable intakes, 127
  deficiency of, 126
  in fruits and vegetables, 128T
  requirements for, 127
  scurvy and, 4
Atherosclerosis, 94–95

Barium-140, 238
Bed, metabolic, construction of, 283, 283, 284, 285

291